AF837394

Early Interaction and Developmental Psychopathology

Gisèle Apter • Emmanuel Devouche
Maya Gratier
Editors

Early Interaction and Developmental Psychopathology

Volume I: Infancy

Springer

Editors
Gisèle Apter
Groupe Hospitalier du Havre
Université de Rouen Normandie
Rouen
France

Emmanuel Devouche
Institute of Psychology
Paris Descartes University
Paris
France

Maya Gratier
University of Paris Nanterre
Nanterre Cedex
France

ISBN 978-3-030-04767-2 ISBN 978-3-030-04769-6 (eBook)
https://doi.org/10.1007/978-3-030-04769-6

© Springer Nature Switzerland AG 2019
This work is subject to copyright. All rights are reserved by the Publisher, whether the whole or part of the material is concerned, specifically the rights of translation, reprinting, reuse of illustrations, recitation, broadcasting, reproduction on microfilms or in any other physical way, and transmission or information storage and retrieval, electronic adaptation, computer software, or by similar or dissimilar methodology now known or hereafter developed.
The use of general descriptive names, registered names, trademarks, service marks, etc. in this publication does not imply, even in the absence of a specific statement, that such names are exempt from the relevant protective laws and regulations and therefore free for general use.
The publisher, the authors, and the editors are safe to assume that the advice and information in this book are believed to be true and accurate at the date of publication. Neither the publisher nor the authors or the editors give a warranty, express or implied, with respect to the material contained herein or for any errors or omissions that may have been made. The publisher remains neutral with regard to jurisdictional claims in published maps and institutional affiliations.

This Springer imprint is published by the registered company Springer Nature Switzerland AG
The registered company address is: Gewerbestrasse 11, 6330 Cham, Switzerland

Introduction

The papers in this volume all explore facets of the complex but crucially important processes by which human social interactions give rise to habitual ways of being and of experiencing the world. These can be described as more or less adaptive modes in which relationships and events are met. They tend to persist throughout life and can give rise to symptoms of illness and psychopathological conditions. Every human being grows and changes through recurrent and familiar, as well as through new social encounters. This is a remarkable fact. It urgently requires attention. Scientists and practitioners need to understand and focus on this essential dimension.

The papers gathered here bring together the accumulated scientific and clinical evidence underlining that social interactions are vital for human development.

It is not surprising that René Spitz's seminal work on relational affective deprivation in infancy was an important inspiration for Bowlby's theory of attachment and Winnicott's early emotional approach. A few decades after Spitz, Sir Michael Rutter and his colleagues showed that cognitive disorders can indeed arise as a result of severe affective and sensory deprivation. They also showed that developmental catch-up is possible at 4 years but only for children adopted into caring environments at less than 6 months of age. Social environments directly affect the neurocognitive development of young children and the first months of life are crucial for establishing solid connections between affective social experience and cognitive processes involved in learning and mastering new abilities. What has emerged from the last decades of research on the social lives of babies is that they actively get involved with other people from the get-go. Infants do this by tuning their behavior and expressions to those of the affectionate and attentive people they enlist into their everyday care. Many of the authors of this book have been directly influenced by some of the pioneers of an interactional approach to infant development, such as Beatrice Beebe, T. Berry Brazelton, Serge Lebovici, Lynne Murray, Daniel Stern, Colwyn Trevarthen, and Edward Tronick. And indeed, some chapters in this book have been written by Colwyn Trevarthen and Edward Tronick respectively.

It is now known that newborn infants are to some extent equipped for social interaction with caring partners. Throughout the first year, infants gain know-how in conducting and negotiating social interaction with a widening array of partners. This know-how is crucial for all the major developmental achievements that follow. As the chapters in this book show, when social interactions take on distorted forms during the first year of life, infants are at high risk for following deviant developmental trajectories marked by overt or latent mental illness. Epigenetic research based on animal models has shown that early interactive behavior is not only essential for offspring health but spills over to the next generation, notwithstanding initial genetic equipment of the first generation. More studies are being conducted today in order to assess how epigenetics may impact neonatal development and proceed to influence health and mental health through to adulthood.

We also know that the infant brain is well equipped to deal with adversity and that in situations where social interactions are nonoptimal, infants can develop resources and strategies that enable a variety of adaptive developmental processes. Differently organized developmental trajectories need to be studied from early infancy on. This will give professionals opportunities to guide children and parents towards more optimal ways of experiencing each other and their worlds. Gaining knowledge in the field of early developmental psychology is a precious tool for early intervention and prevention of later, more stabilized, forms of psychopathology.

The book is divided into 3 parts. The first part covers research on interactional processes in early infancy in the context of typical development. The second one focuses on identifying the pressures that parents with psychiatric disorders or premature infants come to bear on interactional relational processes. These chapters directly address the question of how psychopathology may emerge as a function of repeated maladaptive interactive patterns shaped by specific at-risk contexts. The third part of the book is concerned with assessment and therapeutic tools that are based on interactive situations and that also provide insight into which interactional patterns are most crucial for infant development.

The introductory chapter by Colwyn Trevarthen brushes in broad and vivid strokes the 20th century history of a developmental science of human relating. Trevarthen draws on his own unique experience and position as a fore-runner of the relational turn that is emerging in developmental and cognitive psychology, and in clinical and therapeutic practice. The chapter by Devouche and Gratier describes the earliest forms of social interaction between alert and calm infants and attentive parents. These authors review a number of key studies that use microanalysis to investigate the fine workings of the multimodal coordination that characterizes social engagement between healthy and happy infants and parents from birth onwards. Banella and Tronick's chapter explores the complex dynamics of regulation in social interaction between infants and parents based on decades of research using the Still Face paradigm developed by Ed Tronick in the late 1970s. They show how unique relations and relational meaning are built from repeated interactive patterns shared and shaped by infants and their close ones. The chapter includes the presentation of a study conducted on 78 mothers and their 6-month-old infants and 41 mothers and their 11-month-old infants, using the Face-to-Face Still Face paradigm and aimed at identifying behavioral patterns that reflect what they have called "unique implicit relational knowing." Their discussion of the relevance of this kind of detailed behavioral coding for clinical practice is highly insightful for practitioners. Anne Bobin-Bègue's exhaustive review of the literature on rhythmic experience in early infancy ranges from biological and genetically rooted processes to the social and cultural rhythms that organize infants' daily lives. It thus becomes obvious that various types of rhythms, circadian, physiological, behavioral, and social, are tightly interconnected and that infants' lives are held in balance by multiple and often coordinated rhythmic processes. The chapter explores how these rhythmic processes in adults and infants shape social interactions between them and goes on to describe how specific disorders or at-risk conditions in infants can be better understood in light of what we know today about rhythm in infancy.

The first chapter of Part II, by Poget, Genet, and Apter, reviews research on the impact of parental psychiatric disorder on infant and child developmental outcomes. More importantly, the authors argue, first, that parental psychopathology plays a crucial role in the mental health issues of infants and young children themselves, and second, that these issues could arise as a result of disturbed, dysfunctional or lacking social interactions. They discuss the implications of their triptych approach involving parents' mental health, parent-infant interaction, and infant mental health for peripartum care. The following chapter, by Apter and Devouche, delves deeper into the workings of various kinds of disturbance or distortion in parent-infant interaction. The authors of this chapter focus on the mother-infant dyad as a dynamically regulated system that must adapt to pressures from psychopathological conditions such as postpartum depression or borderline personality disorder. This chapter describes the budding developmental pathways of infants who must contend with their mother's psychopathological condition. The third chapter in Part II of the book is on interaction between preterm infants and their parents. Joëlle Provasi discusses how premature birth and the specific contexts of a premature infant's life in hospital condition parent-infant social interaction and relationship formation. She looks both at parents' dispositions to interact with their infants, given the biological and psychological upheavals of an untimely birth, and at preterm infants' readiness for social engagement. Provasi offers insight into the construction of attachment bonds between premature infants and parents based on their ability to interact with each other and based on the particular constraints imposed on them by various endogenous and exogenous factors. Her chapter includes a fascinating discussion on the impact of recent scientific evidence of preterm infants' social needs and abilities on the physical environments that shape their early development in Neonatal Intensive Care Units around the world, through and beyond the NIDCAP program. The next chapter, by Mueller, Beeghly, and Tronick, brings to the forefront a highly neglected issue in studies of early social interaction and emergent developmental trajectories, namely the role of parent and infant gender. Here, the authors focus on postpartum depression, not only of mothers but also of fathers, and they also identify specific vulnerabilities related to infant gender. They take into account how the infant, with its own given and acquired specificities, co-creates his/her family system. Knowledge of the specific gendered roles, vulnerabilities, and strengths of both parents appears crucial for anyone adopting a developmental approach to the early formation of psychopathology.

The first chapter of Part III, by Devouche, Dominguez, and Apter, presents a series of assessment tools used both by researchers and clinicians to identify specific behaviors and patterns in early parent-infant social interaction. These tools can be used as such or as guiding principles clinicians can use to observe the subtle, complex, and often ungraspable interactive processes that day after day orient infants' developmental trajectories towards more or less favorable outcomes. In the second chapter of Part III of the book, Drina Candilis offers a very detailed and nuanced account of T. Berry Brazelton's Neonatal Behavioral Assessment Scale. She focuses on the importance of this work in fostering and supporting adaptive and emotionally rewarding social interactions between infants and parents, from birth. The clinical case study presented in this chapter is useful not only for understanding the relevance of the assessment itself, but also because it reveals how deeply rooted it is in the clinician's observational skills. Observation is indeed presented as a tool that is difficult to master, but that no clinician working in the field of peripartum care (and beyond) can afford to ignore. The next chapter by Aude Buil describes how the French tradition of psychomotor care can provide invaluable insight to clinicians working with vulnerable infants. Psychomotor practice is an acknowledged and accredited profession in France and other francophone countries. It investigates infants' well-being through the lens of body tonus, considered a fundamental means through which infants experience the world and organize their behavior. Aude Buil proposes ways in which psychomotor therapists can provide support for parents, and thus indirectly for infants, particularly in the context of premature birth and prolonged hospitalization of infants. The last chapter of Part III, by Alecian and Medjkane, presents the 0-3R diagnostic classification and assessment tool and discusses its relevance for clinical practice. The authors borrow from their own clinical experience to illustrate how the 0-3R can be implemented in real life contexts. Finally, the last chapter by A Harrison opens new perspectives on care and treatment, focusing on "developmental formulation and scaffolding towards the goal of adaptive function."

Overall, the book aims to promote refined knowledge of very early development in its environmental context and to foster an orientation towards prevention and clinical innovation in the care given to infants, toddlers, children, and their families. The next volume will aim to disseminate further knowledge on the second year of life when the complexity of regulatory interactions is linked to new developmental skills in the growing toddler. We hope this first volume will enrich readers, widen their horizons, and encourage them to look for the second volume of this book in the near future.

Rouen, France — Gisèle Apter
Paris, France — Emmanuel Devouche
Nanterre Cedex, France — Maya Gratier

Contents

The Psychobiology of the Human Spirit 1

Colwyn Trevarthen

1.1 Discovering Kindness

This is a book about kindness in care for young children and about how we need to share the inventions of our liveliness in close relationships to help with the unhappiness of emotional disorders. When we want to help a baby or toddler who is expressing sadness, or anger, or confusion and distress and who acts as if they want to be alone, we must keep confidence in the strength and optimism of the loving human spirit of playful sympathy, which they fear they cannot show [1–3].

I have had the rewarding experience of many years as a researcher trying to record how, from birth, happy infants are ready to join in kindness with companions who accept the miracle of human being. According to the conventional, highly educated wisdom of some authorities in the science of intelligence or cognition, this way of being alive and sharing its discoveries is not only miraculous—it is impossible before we are able to talk about our experiences in conventional ways. They deny that there can be a psychology of the newborn [4]. My task, with imaginative teachers and colleagues, has been to make records of innate and developing abilities that famous experts in psychology of learning and knowing, as well as doctors caring for ill babies, have believed are not possible for the infant mind.

The biggest mystery concerns the ability of a newborn to share by imitation acts of attending, as well as delicate expressions of feelings about what is perceived together. Both Sigmund Freud [5] and Jean Piaget [6, 7] said such imitation was impossible. They believed the baby had to acquire knowing, or cognition of conscious actions, by learning with parents as teachers. Awareness of life in the human world, they said, can only become meaningful by following conventions of understanding that may be described in language.

C. Trevarthen (✉)
University of Edinburgh, Edinburgh, UK
e-mail: C.Trevarthen@ed.ac.uk

© Springer Nature Switzerland AG 2019

G. Apter et al. (eds.), *Early Interaction and Developmental Psychopathology*,
https://doi.org/10.1007/978-3-030-04769-6_1

But photographic recordings of intimate and responsive exchanges with babies in the first hours after birth proved they do wish to imitate, and with astonishing discrimination and skill. Indeed they are happy to negotiate exchanges of imitation, taking their turn and inventing new messages [8]. This attentive aiming of the baby's sense organs is imaginative and creative using the wisdom of a body feeling its movements intentionally. It is not reflexive, triggered and 'conditioned' by stimuli. Thus a blind baby can look, and a deaf baby can listen, making the required movements 'as if' they had sight or hearing, expecting new experience. Books for parents with eloquent photographs show how rich infant sociability normally is in intimate communication [9, 10].

Although it is clear that this sharing of interest opens the way to cultural learning in the human way [11–13], we still do not fully appreciate what the urges and feelings are that lead infants to imitate and to be imitated—how they 'know our minds', as Vasudevi Reddy [14] puts it. She describes the sensitive ways young babies engage expressions of interest and emotion with us. Can this be accepted as consciousness of being in company? As psychologists or neuroscientists, we do not know how our bodies and brains can do it and how they can exhibit a moral sense seeking affectionate company [15]. There are now some inspiring findings using subtle analysis of the forms of expression, and new technologies of functional brain imaging, but many features of the baby's intuitions for playful 'proto-conversation' remain mysterious. A key feature is the rhythmic coordination of movements in precise synchrony that display the dimensions of pulse and tone in melodies, a 'musicality' to which we respond to so strongly [16, 17].

One important aspect of the descriptive natural science of emotions, observing how they have evolved to build social collaboration in a community, is the evidence from ethology pioneered by Charles Darwin [18] who published pictures of how animals share emotions with shapes of expressive movement of parts of the body that are adapted to be seen or heard. Anthropological studies, since his voyage of discovery of other races in the early nineteenth century, proved for Darwin there are universal human expressions of relating in social worlds ready to support the learning of very different traditions of knowledge, art and technologies. Babies everywhere respond to loving care, imitate and enjoy play with familiar companions. That is their special human vitality prepared for joining a rich and ancient cultural life. It is the resource that psychotherapy depends on to help afraid and shamed persons of any age recover contented and optimistic vitality.

1.2 Biology Is the Science of Life. Psychobiology Is Biology of the Mind: We Are Born Sharing the Drama of Life, for Love

Every living organism, plant or animal, grows or moves with initiative and imagination, seeking with its evolved life form a healthy and rewarding existence—a self-creating and self-protecting way of being. This depends on processes that plan and evaluate actions in invented time of moving, making measured steps into the future with anticipation of rewards of well-being and avoidance of harm [19–21].

New brain science, breaking free of the idea that intelligence is built by training reflexes or 'conditioning' them, confirms that the feelings of value for human consciousness of an active and aware person arise deep in the brain with emotional power to direct knowing. 'The subcortical level would ensure basic feeling states while the cortical level would largely relate feeling states to cognitive processes such as decision-making and imagination' [22].

The Venezuelan biologist, systems theorist and language philosopher Humberto Maturana [23], Maturana and Varela [24] describes the processes of life as of two kinds with different, complementary purposes: *autopoiesis* or 'self-making' grows within the shaped vitality of a dynamic body and *consensuality*, which makes mutual support in communities of beings, appreciating and adapting to the resources of the physical environment and negotiating with other lively selves. Maturana's colleague Francisco Varela, with Evan Thompson and Eleanor Rosch, describes how the mind is 'embodied' by the animated form it grows within [25].

As human beings, we grow and prosper with mastery of the most complex and versatile animal bodies made for many new ways of moving to investigate and manipulate a rich world [26]—and we talk about it. We strive to cooperate in the great consensus of meanings we value as our culture, a history of inventive being and making by gifted individuals living through generations in artful companionship. And, as speaking creatures, we use the skill that Maturana calls 'languaging', which includes more than speaking and writing. It is ways of moving to make up stories that describe old ways of being and invent new ones [27]. We become authors of our *Self As Agent* and live as *Persons in Relation* [28, 29].

1.3 The Infant Mind Is Full of Feeling for Measures of Movement in Company

Supported by insights from new findings of anthropology and animal ethology, the veteran educational psychologist Jerome Bruner, who was always seeking new ideas about the nature of culture and its transmission, collaborated with paediatrician Berry Brazelton in the late 1960s to study infant initiatives to perceive and use objects and the intimate reciprocal imitation that develops between infants and affectionate parents and caregivers who offer playful collaboration with the child's rhythms and qualities of movement [30]. Film studies showed that young infants make complex shifts of posture and hand gestures that are regulated rhythmically in time, with measures of pulsation that match those of the same movements made by adults. In face-to-face play, a baby often takes the lead with 'narratives' of expressive acts that are imitated joyfully by the mother.

At Harvard, as a doctoral student in Bruner's group, I recorded how a baby's eyes and head move in precise synchrony to look at, or track, an object of interest, expressing the baby's sense of self. In looking, a baby's measured steps or saccades made consistent rhythms that were the same as those of an adult scanning a picture. By 6 months the infants had developed efficient binocular depth perception, and by precisely moving their eyes and head together, they could track a slowly moving object smoothly, without saccades, which is a skill that requires a mental prediction of the object's path and its velocity. Tracings I made of infants, 1 or 2 months old, reaching out to touch or grasp objects were regulated in elegant patterns with rhythms that were close to those of an adult reach and grasp [31]. There were innate rules of self-conscious vitality in human beings who were very different in body size and breadth of knowledge.

This 'motor intelligence' of the baby ready for engaging with things to be seen and grasped in the world was astonishing. But even more remarkable were the body movements of communication with attention directed to an interested mother. These were creative, prosocial and mutually regulated. They included delicate face expressions of emotion, like a smile or a scowl, deliberate eye-to-eye contact, 'pre-speech' movements of the lips and dramatic gestures of the hands [32]. These movements of a conscious self can only have a desired effect if they are sensed sympathetically by another human being. And, the baby could take the lead, in the 'dialogue'. They were not simply imitating the expressions of their mothers. They wanted a cooperative engagement of their interests and feelings to discover new ideas.

We made films at 16 frames per second, week by week, with 5 infants and their mothers from 2 to 6 months of age. We compared how each infant behaved towards the mother herself and to a suspended toy presented by her. The room was a quiet studio surrounded by heavy curtains, with subdued lighting. A camera was aimed to take a full-face view of the whole baby, and a mirror placed behind the baby gave a head-and-shoulder view of the mother. We filmed the mother and infant enjoying intimate chat, undisturbed.

A 'conversation' between 12-week-old Jody and his mother, in which the baby clearly led the engagement, was an eye-opener. This leading by the baby was confirmed by further microanalysis of the body movements of infants of the same age when they were communicating with their delighted mothers. Infants rarely imitated the mother in these 'proto-conversations'. They had their own stories to tell, and the mothers followed the plot with confirming and encouraging expressions.

When a baby is born, we, if we are ready to respond with affection, meet an active, interested and sensitive human person who senses our readiness for dialogues of expressive movement. We find ourselves measuring lifetime together and exchange expressions of love—seeking a shared gaze, a smile or puzzled look and hand gestures of enquiry, pointing with focused interest or of self-comforting—all rhythmic and immediately connected to join or alternate with our signs of affectionate companionship [33].

This partaking in sympathetic vitality is not new for the infant. It has been practised for months within the mother's body, often, in the last few months of gestation, responding to the impulses and tensions of pleasure and pain in her life as a person, sometimes aware of the lively behaviours of other people nearby, speaking, touching and moving objects. If the baby is born before term, still in the stage of a foetal apprentice in human companionship, the mother, who is now seen and heard with more immediate and complex presence, must be responsive in gently expressive ways if she is to continue giving intimate care as the baby expects she will. The sensitivity and special intimacy of her support and nurture must adapt to the strong but immature sensibilities and accommodations of the baby.

This is the intimate relationship between them which paediatrician Lou Sander described as a 'living system' [34]. The English paediatrician and psychoanalyst Donald Winnicott described the mother's care as a 'holding environment' that is essential to the child's developing self. He said, 'the foundations of health are laid down by the ordinary mother in her ordinary loving care of her own baby' [35]. This holding applies to the environment of family and society that Professor of Psychology Darcia Narvaez and her colleagues call the Evolved Developmental Niche for the human infant, a species of mammal born needing many months of support, feeding and protection of affectionate care from mother, father and a close community of neighbors of all ages [36].

The gracious and constructive emotion relating between parent and baby is what the medical caregivers call 'attunement' to the baby's expressions of need. It needs to be timed and with the right tones to complement what the baby seeks and feels and to reduce or remove any compelling and stressful intrusions in the baby's experience and sense of comfort and their enjoyment of a new and much richer awareness.

1.4 A History of Responsive Medical Care for the Newborn Person

Our post-industrial scientific culture developed a scientific medical treatment of disorders as if the receiver of care were a reflex organism, needing attention focused on anatomy and internal physiological state only. It relied on diagnosis to identify faults in development of sensory-motor or visceral functions or to detect symptoms of abnormal physiology or injuries and infections that cause harm.

Then some doctors saw this was too narrow, and they insisted on creating a new compassionate awareness of the newborn as a person with strong powers of imaginative action and human ways of signalling and responding to interests and feelings.

In 1935, René Spitz used direct observation of spontaneous mindful behaviour of children rather than tests of their reflex responses to artificial stimuli. His work revealed the serious effects of deprivation of a mother's love on her child's sense of well-being. He coined the term 'anaclitic depression' to refer to the immediate effect on a newborn baby and showed that if children are deprived of a mother's care for longer than 5 months, they will show symptoms of increasingly serious deterioration, which he called 'hospitalism'. Observing children in a foundling home in the United States, he confirmed that poor care during the children's first year results in irreparable damage to their spirit for life and learning [37]. His film *Psychogenic Disease in Infancy* changed childcare in homes and hospitals.

John Bowlby, in England, worked with maladjusted and delinquent children as a psychologist before he qualified in medicine and later as a psychoanalyst. He helped children who were evacuated from London to Cambridge during a time of war and separated from their families and nannies. One of his main findings was that children described as 'affectionless', and likely to become thieves, had experienced complete and prolonged separation before the age of 5. Bowlby's work led to his writing of the World Health Organization's report on the mental health of homeless children in post-war Europe, published as *Maternal Care and Mental Health* [38].

The attachment theory of Spitz and Bowlby confirmed the needs of the young child for affectionate protection and scare. It also encouraged growth of interest in infants' emotions for playful discovery of life in a human world, which inspired doctors responsible for care of babies at birth to treat the babies and their parents with more sympathy and humour.

In the 1960s, three doctors independently called for a revolution in the care of birth and early development and for attention to the special needs of prematurely born persons.

These three doctors, Leboyer in Paris and Sander and Brazelton in Boston (all of whom were born in 1918 at the end of a world war), perceived newborns as alert playful persons seeking love in companionship beyond attachment for comfort and feeding of weak bodies. They were led by their sensitivity and imagination to reject the prejudice of their professional training that infants have no awareness of what they are doing or sensitivity to other people's emotions or attitudes. Their attention to the powers of innate human conviviality supported a move away from Freud's psychotherapy, which, with little appreciation of the positive motives and feelings of an infant, had become preoccupied with listening to the patient's talking about memories of trauma experienced at what was understood to be a more primitive stage of the self. The three doctors urged a richer appreciation of the psychobiology of emotions and the communication of gentle love and playfulness in movement, and they promoted new ideas about the readiness of children for learning cultural skills and beliefs and how they wanted to share these with self-confidence. Their work supported a change to more intimate 'relational' psychotherapy.

Frédérick Leboyer**,** a French obstetrician who left his medical practice to become a famous author writing on the powers of the infant to stimulate loving care, is best known for his [39] book, *Pour Une Naissance Sans Violence*. He introduced the practice of immersing the newborn in a tub of warm water, known as a 'Leboyer bath', to ease the transition to the outside world. He also advocated low lighting in a quiet warm room to limit the stress of birth and that the baby be first laid on the mother's stomach and allowed to bond, instead of being taken away for tests. His own birth was traumatic with his distressed mother forcefully restrained, and Leboyer attributes his interest in birth to this experience. In *Pour Une Naissance Sans Violence*, he advises that 'sharing love is the sovereign remedy for anguish'. Other books he wrote that have been translated and become popular in English include *Loving Hands: The Traditional Art of Baby Massage* and *Inner Beauty, Inner Light*.

The paediatrician Louis Sander made two crucial contributions. With William Condon, who used microanalysis of rhythmic movements to study speech and gesture in adult conversation, Sander confirmed that a newborn baby's hand movements may synchronise with adult speech, matching, or 'attuning' to, the rhythms of two very different forms of body action [40]. This inspired careful attention to the timing and emotional intensity of infants' movements and their precise engagement with sympathetic rhythms of their mother's behaviour. Furthermore, in a project to trace the development of communication between mothers and their children from birth to age 6 years, Sander and his colleagues demonstrated that a strong and creative childhood is fostered by a collaboration of the baby's efforts to learn supported by the innate talents of the mother—her readiness to take part in an adaptive learning that responds to developments of expressions and actions in the child [41, 42]. He recognised that mother and baby form a single living system to which both are adapted [34].

Confirmation of mutual regulation of development of an imaginative mind from birth was obtained by Olga Maratos in her PhD thesis, in which she reported of the development of imitative expressions through the first 6 months of infants when they are attentive to an adult who is instinctively seeking sympathetic engagement with the baby's motives and feelings [43]. She presented her findings in 1973 to her supervisor in Geneva, Jean Piaget, who did not believe newborns are conscious enough to imitate. He remained sceptical.

The new understanding of the creative mental abilities of infants and their readiness for intimate, two-way collaborative learning, not 'instruction', was inspired by the sensitive work of the Boston paediatrician, T. Berry Brazelton. Creating his *Neonatal Behavioral Assessment Scale* for use to help early detection of developmental disorders [44, 45], Brazelton perceived that, from the very beginning of life outside the mother's body, an infant is gifted with rhythmic 'musical' sensibilities for imaginative play and ready to start cultural learning by imitating and engaging sensitively with actions and expressions of both mother and father. He said, 'The old model of thinking of the newborn infant as helpless and **ready** to be shaped by his environment prevented us from seeing his power as a communicant in the early mother-father-infant interaction. To see the neonate as chaotic or insensitive provided us with the capacity to see ourselves as acting "on" rather than "with" him'. (Brazelton [46], p. 79).

Like Sander, and Maratos, Brazelton drew attention to the developing child's initiative to pass through age-related steps, in both their own powers of activity and in readiness for collaboration, which he called 'touchpoints' [47–49]. His *Touchpoints Model of Development* has become a world famous institution to support parent's intuitive concern to accompany their children tenderly through changes in life's opportunities that come with transforming powers and feelings of human body movement [50, 51].

1.5 Affective Attunement of Vitality Dynamics, Leading to a New Psychotherapy

In 1961, Dan Stern, a young paediatrician being trained in psychoanalysis in New York, began a revolutionary career in the study of the natural origins of human compassion and understanding. He watched a film of a mother with 3-month-old twins enjoying teasing play, with precisely coordinated moves timed to fractions of a second to make collaborative patterns of the game [52]. With colleagues in Columbia University and Harvard, that work, which proved the intelligent initiative of the child to 'attune' and synchronise with an adult's intentions [53], inspired a critical reassessment of the baby's mindless, primitive and instinctive 'Id' invented by Freud, which requires a 'moralising' education to become a responsible 'ego'.

Stern was long associated with the New York City Ballet, and theatre artists, dancers and choreographers were enthralled by his microscopic investigations of how mothers and infants invent drama together in play. His subsequent clinical work led to publication in 1985 of *The Interpersonal World of the Infant*. In the Preface of the reprint in 2000 he declares 'This book attempts to create a dialogue between the infant as revealed by the experimental approach and as clinically constructed, in the sense of resolving the contradiction between theory and reality' (Stern [54], p. ix). He became committed to a psychotherapy of lived experience and 'moments of meeting' as critical for the making and remembering of 'emotional narrative envelopes' in dialogue.

In 1999 Stern took a leading part in the announcement of a group of psychotherapists who accepted that emotional foundations of self-awareness and self-confidence in relationships could be given new strength by open acceptance of momentary expressions of hope and conviction and developed in shared dynamic emotional narratives of 'implicit relational knowing' [55].

In a new Introduction to the paperback edition of *The Interpersonal World of the Infant*, he wrote:

> One consequence of the book's application of a narrative perspective to the non-verbal has been the discovery of a language useful to many psychotherapies that rely on the non-verbal. I am thinking particularly of dance, music, body, and movement therapies, as well as existential psychotherapies. This observation came as a pleasant surprise to me since I did not originally have such therapists in mind; my thinking has been enriched by coming to know them better. (Stern [56], p. xv).

Indeed, in the final decade of the twentieth century, there was an outpouring of publications on the use and beneficial effects of music therapy. A leader in this work was the musician and psychologist Mercedes Pavlicevic who developed her work at the Nordoff Robbins Music Therapy Centre in London and the Music Therapy Community Clinic, Cape Town, South Africa [57–61]. This and other 'relational therapies' give privileged attention to the non-verbal aspects of the therapeutic engagement, which are so important for any sharing of emotions of creative vitality in pairs or in groups of any size, for example, *Video Interaction Guidance* developed in the Netherlands by Harrie Biemans and colleagues in the 1980s and now practised in more than 15 countries helping professionals in social work, education and health and also in business management [62].

Throughout his highly influential career, Stern was entranced by the 'living moment' of companionship between the developing child and parent and what it can teach us about the natural foundations of psychotherapy that accepts the need for sensitive engagement of ideas and feelings between therapist and a patient of whatever age, by communication of the vitality and grace of body movements [63, 64].

1.6 Musicality of Our Body Moving Inspires Adventures of Collaboration in a Lifetime of Learning

Musician and counselor Stephen Malloch and I have used evidence of the musical abilities of young infants to develop a theory of 'communicative musicality' to describe the essential features of rhythm and attunement of vitality in body movements that put shared enjoyment of life into dance and music [17, 65]. What these expressive arts share with the ritual performances of theatre is what the anthropologist Victor Turner [66] called *The Human Seriousness of Play*. It is a serious experience of enjoyable performance because it transmits the essential powers of self-regulated body movement in any human actor, to keep alive a harmony of muscle forces and the pleasure felt as well-being in inner vital functions.

Thinking of the different media of this body-to-body communication, by sight or by sound and vibrations produced in performance of any activity, we discover that the essential messages are 'amodal' or 'transmodal' with respect to the distance senses that are adapted to explore the out-of-body world with sight, sound and touch. Music and dance communicate with or imitate proprioceptive and visceroceptive sensations inside different bodies of co-performers or between performers and audience or viewers. Like the mystery of neonatal imitation, the intrinsic forces of artful communication engage sympathetic feelings in a way that escapes the facts of external reality. The Norwegian social psychologist Stein Bråten has spent his life confronting the paradox of knowledge and reality, helping us by relating this to the communicative intuitions of infants [67–70].

Of fundamental importance is the evidence of how sensitive newborn infants, and even foetuses, are for music and for the prosody of a mother's voice. We are born transmodal communicators in the body consciousness of moving. Our ears and throats, as well as eyes, face and hands, are adapted to express tones of emotion as signals of vitality [71], as are the dynamics of locomotion by walking and running and by hand gestures. This is the language of Birdwhistell's kinesics [72] or Stern's vitality dynamics [64].

Two words grasp the principle of a transmodal sympathy in sensations of purposeful life—'attunement' and 'harmony'. Both refer to the expressive use of the voice or of actions making rhythmic patterns of the sound and sight in other individuals that evoke our inner sensations of body movement, which may be celebrated by song, instrumental performance or dance. These psychodynamic forces give vitality to any form of communication and aid the cooperative direction of interests and actions [33].

The power of music imagines into the future and recalls rich moments of our past by its natural ability to portray projects of moving in melodies that have the appealing form of narratives. They exhibit a wave of excitement and commitment with dramatic phases of *introduction*, *development*, *climax* and *resolution* (or *coda*) [65, 73]. This portrays the plan of human purposeful movement and its willingness to be shared as a drama. It appeals to the dramatic interest of a baby a few months old in a holding lullaby or a baby song accompanied by teasing hand actions.

The spiritual poetry is most evident when it is composed and enjoyed in the spontaneous playful way of an innocent young child or of a great artist. When all attention is given to abstract rules of structure and to precision of measures in repetition between performances of a given story, the beauty of living creation in the lifetime of movements with affection may be weakened or lost. Any story, conveyed by any medium, verbal or non-verbal, has forms that may become directed in the rules of syntax and grammar of language, on which the authority or 'significance' of semantics in an established vocabulary depends. Too much attention to the referential message pretending objective truth destroys the 'poetry', the subjective making of the message.

1.7 Humanistic Philosophy and Enlightened Relations

In the eighteenth century, a new philosophy of natural life in a community developed in protestant Scotland. It was led by Francis Hutcheson, a Presbyterian from Ireland educated in the University of Glasgow, who became an eloquent and very popular public speaker in that city. He became one of the founding fathers of the Scottish Enlightenment and is famous for his book *A System of Moral Philosophy* based on belief in 'natural sympathy' [74]. His followers David Hume [75], Adam Smith [76, 77] and Thomas Reid [78] developed this theory of a human nature based on compassionate common sense, which grows from the fundamental powers of non-verbal arts of expression, including music. Modern psychobiology supports this view of human well-being and effective reasoning in a life of relationships, both intimate and political, and how it depends on honest sharing of feelings of aesthetic grace and moral virtue.

1.8 Relational-Affective Psychotherapy, Recognising the Intuitive Motives of Young Children for Cultural Learning

Important developments in therapy to help children or adults who have lost confidence in their impulses to find meaning and enjoyment by sharing life experiences affectionately and playfully have gained from close attention to the way most infants happily contribute to building strong affectionate and creative relations with family and neighbours in joyful rituals of teasing play [79].

As Daniel Stern demonstrated, knowledge of how young infants participate in interpersonal life and form intimate and confident relationships with parents, siblings and friends reveals the power of shared vitality and its discoveries and values. This power grows to animate cultural creativity and symbolic communication in language, and it also leads to a more collaborative approach for therapy to aid young children who do not engage and who exhibit anxious loneliness.

Among close associates of Sigmund Freud who debated with him the theory of psychoanalysis, Sándor Ferenczi [80], in 1932, with an address entitled *Confusion of Tongues* to fellow analysts at a meeting in Germany, opened a way to mutuality in more intimate and reciprocal or relational therapy, not one in which the therapist 'stands back' and interprets the patient's recollections of trauma. Forty years later the psychobiology of infancy confirmed that, indeed, it is our nature to find shared meaning for the actions we can perform with our agile and expressive bodies. From birth we seek collective urges and ambitions. This view of self-creative and cooperative development encouraged therapists working with children who had lost confidence in their social desires and who could not share joyful feelings with trusted friends, to try to find revitalization of their spirit. It was clear they needed help to recall and trust the experience of love in kindness, not just courage to overcome memories of trauma.

As we have noted, Donald Winnicott, like Louis Sander, drew attention to the natural support of a mother's intimate, affectionate care for her baby [81]. In *The Maturational Process and the Facilitating Environment* [82], he observed that mental health of a child is developed by 'the continuation of reliable holding in terms of the ever-widening circle of family and school and social life'. Renouncing the primary aim of his psychoanalytic training, he sought positive ways to restore the deep sympathetic spirit of companionship, and he wrote, 'A correct and well-timed interpretation in an analytic treatment gives a sense of being held physically that is more real … than if a real holding or nursing had taken place. Understanding goes deeper'. His trust in the infant's experience of loving maternal care also led him to give special importance to play in the development of a rich and real experience of the meaning of life [83]. He was thus, with René Spitz [84], a pathfinder to kinds of psychotherapy that require gentle invitation to negotiate joy in moving with playful invention. This approach was developed by Ann Jernberg as Theraplay [79, 85, 86].

Other clinicians, seeking to give effective help to children with weakened social responsiveness, or who had suffered from loss of kind maternal care and were taken into adoption, followed Winnicott's lead. Peter Hobson, a professor of developmental psychopathology at University College London, became known for his work on autism and experimental child psychology, which lead him to question the prevailing cognitive psychology of thinking [87] and to adopt a theory of the growth of human intelligence in intimate, affectionate communication, summarised in *The Cradle of Thought* [88]. He considered the main weakness of children diagnosed as autistic was not lack of a 'theory of mind' but an inability to use emotions for reaching out to others [89–92]. They do not feel intimate engagement with the playful and caring impulses of parents and other companions. He, with Jessica Hobson, came to appreciate how this casts light on the role of feelings in normal development and their changes as the infant and young child gain new powers of moving to use the world and to communicate experiences in shared learning [93].

Peter Hobson's inviting or encouraging method of therapy for autistic children, helping them to appreciate and identify with the attitudes of other people, became a highly influential 'conversational model'. He has also studied the relations of a mother with her infant when she displays the abnormal, insensitive behaviour of borderline personality disorder and how she transmits her pathology to her child [94].

Hobson's conversational model has been taken up by Emeritus Professor of Psychiatry Russell Meares of the University of Sydney [95]. The use of Hobson's method led him to develop effective methods of treatment for borderline personality disorder [96], proving the value of assistance for more intimate engagement of purposes and feelings with people who experience a fragile sense of self. Meares has written two thought-provoking books on the importance of artful play with engagements for freeing psychiatric patients from anxieties and shame in relationships—*The Metaphor of Play: Origin and Breakdown of Personal Being* [97] and *The Poet's Voice in the Making of Mind* [98]. Both books acknowledge the insights gained from research on the development of intimate communication and shared imagination in infancy.

In the past 30 years, a clinical psychologist Dan Hughes has tested a treatment to support families with adopted or fostered children, giving them guidance to build strong affectionate relationships with boys and girls who had experienced neglect and abuse in their birth families and were suffering from developmental trauma [99, 100]. He was inspired by the attachment theory of Spitz and Bowlby and new understanding of how normal development of a healthy childhood depends on the active and creative life from birth in affectionate and playful companionship with parents and children [101].

Hughes draws on the 'relational neuroscience' of Dan Siegel [102] and Alan Schore [103, 104] who report remarkable developments in understanding of how the developing human brain actively seeks to share motives for discovery of meaning in the world and how the body and brain are designed to build memories of life's meanings in affectionate relationships, with loved ones. Within a relationship, the brain can function in a more integrative and restorative manner in spontaneous communication of impulses and feelings with a trusted other to help to make sense of highly stressful events in order to reduce the fear or shame they inspire. Stephen Porges [71] describes regions of the brain that make up the social engagement system, in which individuals learn about themselves and others with a sense of safety.

When the therapist and caregiver using the insights of DDP are able to establish safety and acceptance, the adopted child is less likely to be defensive and withdrawn and more ready to enjoy sharing habits with pride, in attunement.

'In healthy families, a baby forms a secure attachment with her parents as naturally as she breathes, eats, smiles and cries. This occurs easily because of her parents' attuned interactions with her. Her parents notice her physiological/affective states and they respond to her sensitively and fully. Beyond simply meeting her unique needs, however, her parents "dance" with her. Hundreds of times, day after day, they dance with her. There are other families where the baby neither dances nor even hears the sound of any music. In these families she does not form such secure attachments. Rather, her task—her continuous ordeal—is to learn to live with parents who are little more than strangers. Babies who live with strangers do not live well or grow well'. (Hughes [100], p. ix).

Hughes' experience with neglected and abused children led him to change his communication with them by adopting a more hopeful and cooperative invitation to share life with pride.

'Many, many years ago I reflected on my frequent inability to help children who had been abused and neglected ... My initial goals were to help them to be less terrified by the traumatic events of their past. When I found I wasn't successful with this I developed other goals, which focused on helping them to reduce the deep sense of shame they felt and which underpinned their conviction that they deserved the maltreatment that they had received'.

He developed his practice for 'dyadic developmental psychotherapy' now used in many countries. The DDPI (Dyadic Developmental Psychotherapy Institute) provides training, certification and supervision for dyadic developmental psychotherapy and practice in Portland Maine, USA [101].

1.9 Reaching to the Source of Values to Be Shared and Remembered in Lively Movement

The human spirit is motivated for sharing the meaning and pleasure of life with excitement and rituals that confirm rewarding conventions of practice. These are based on the vitality of a mammal with special powers of cooperation in large creative and adventurous societies. Sometimes these powers are betrayed or misguided in ways that harm relations and confuse meanings they should live by with actions that are destructive and cruel [105]. Then we must seek to recover contact in harmony with the basic values of the first stages of innocent life with other persons.

I would like to end by confirming that we find both aesthetic and moral values expressed in joyful play with children too young to appreciate talk about how to behave. The source of the emotions of grace and kindness appears to be in the way movements of a very complex body are harmonised through self-generated time of vitality, as Goodrich explains, and how they seek to cooperate in the graceful rhythms of their energy with other actors who wish to share and contribute to their invention with beauty [106, 107].

From the meticulous science of motor control developed by Bernstein and the analysis of vitality dynamics by Stern, we appreciate the importance of a sense of the future in this moving that makes stories that need no words. This supports a psychotherapy which the Harvard-trained medical doctor Mark Epstein in *Thoughts Without a Thinker* describes as 'from a Buddhist perspective' [108]. In that book the Foreword by the Dalai Lama begins with this confession: 'The purpose of life is to be happy. As a Buddhist I have found that one's own mental attitude is the most influential factor in working toward that goal. In order to change conditions outside themselves, whether they concern the environment or relations with others, we must first change within ourselves'. Epstein's therapy values inner grace and harmony and moral responsibility in relationships. Stephen Malloch ([73], p. 69), with his life as a violinist, conductor and therapist, and as someone who holds to the Buddhist faith, declares that 'the therapeutic relationship is a piece of music, experienced in the unfolding present', in which the participants seek to improvise a balance of responsibility.

A turn in relational neuroscience accepts the primacy of feelings in the inspiration of practical and rational awareness, in the graceful economy of actions and in the moral concessions of kind relations. Recognising these as the fundamental processes of all our endeavours is what characterises relational therapies, especially to assist young children who need to retrieve happiness in friendship in rhythms of relating [106].

References

1. Trevarthen C (2001) Intrinsic motives for companionship in understanding: Their origin, development, and significance for infant mental health. Infant Ment Health J 22:95–131
2. Trevarthen C (2016) Sharing joyful friendship and imagination for meaning with infants, and their application in early intervention. In: Acquarone S (ed) Surviving the early years: the importance of early intervention with babies at risk. Karnak, London, pp 19–55
3. Trevarthen C (2017) The affectionate intersubjective intelligence of the infant, and its innate motives for relational mental health. Int J Cognit Anal Therap Relat Mental Health 1(1):11–53
4. Nagy E (2011) The newborn infant: a missing stage in developmental psychology. Infant Child Dev 20:3–19
5. Freud S (1923) Das Ich und das Es (The Ego and the Id). Internationaler Psycho-Analytischer Verlag/W.W. Norton & Company, Vienna/New York
6. Piaget J (1958) The child's construction of reality. Routledge and Kegan Paul, London
7. Piaget J (1966) The psychology of intelligence. Littlefield Adams, Totawa, NJ
8. Nagy E, Molnár P (2004) Homo imitans or homo provocans? Human imprinting model of neonatal imitation. Infant Behav Dev 27:54–63
9. Murray L, Andrews L (2000) The social baby: understanding babies' communication from birth. CP Publishing, Richmond, Surrey
10. Nugent K, Morell A (2011) Your baby is speaking to you: a visual guide to the amazing behaviours of your newborn and growing baby. Haughton Mifflin, New York
11. Trevarthen C (1988) Universal cooperative motives: how infants begin to know language and skills of culture. In: Jahoda G, Lewis IM (eds) Acquiring culture: ethnographic perspectives on cognitive development. Croom Helm, London, pp 37–90
12. Trevarthen C (1989) Motives for culture in young children—Their natural development through communication. In: Koch W (ed) The nature of culture. Bochum, Brockmeyer, pp 80–119
13. Trevarthen C (2011) The generation of human meaning: how shared experience grows in infancy. In: Seemann A (ed) Joint attention: new developments in philosophy, psychology, and neuroscience. MIT Press, Cambridge, MA, pp 73–113
14. Reddy V (2008) How infants know minds. Harvard University Press, Cambridge, MA
15. Narvaez D (2014) Neurobiology and the development of human morality. W.W. Norton & Company, New York
16. Altenmüller E, Finger S, Boller F (2015) Music, neurology, neuroscience evolution, the musical brain, medical conditions, and therapies, Progress in Brain Research, vol 217. Elsevier, Amsterdam
17. Malloch S, Trevarthen C (eds) (2009) Communicative musicality: exploring the basis of human companionship. Oxford University Press, Oxford
18. Darwin C (1872) The expression of emotion in man and animals. Methuen, London
19. Bernstein N (1966) The active search for information: from reflexes to the model of the future. (In Russian) Republished in English by Feigenberg, I. M., & Meijer, O. G. (1999). The active search for information: from reflexes to the model of the future. Mot Control 3:225–236
20. Bernstein N (1967) The coordination and regulation of movements. Pergamon, Oxford

21. Goodrich BG (2010) We do, therefore we think: time, motility, and consciousness. Rev Neurosci 21:331–361
22. Damasio A, Damasio H, Tranel D (2013) Persistence of feelings and sentience after bilateral damage of the insula. Cerebral Cortex 23:833–846. https://doi.org/10.1093/cercor/bhs077
23. Maturana HR (1978) Biology of language: the epistemology of reality. In: Miller GA, Lenneberg E (eds) Psychology and biology of language and thought: essays in honor of eric lenneberg. Academic Press, New York, pp 27–63
24. Maturana HR, Varela FJ (1980) Autopoiesis and cognition. D. Reidel, Dordrecht
25. Varela FJ, Thompson E, Rosch E (1991) The embodied mind. MIT Press, Cambridge, MA
26. Bernstein N (1996) Dexterity and its development. In: Latash ML, Turvey MT (eds) Dexterity and its development. Lawrence Erlbaum, New Jersey, pp 1–235
27. Bruner JS (2003) Making stories: law, literature, life. Harvard University Press, Cambridge, MA
28. Macmurray J (1959) The self as agent (Volume I of The form of the personal). Faber and Faber, London. (Paperback, 1969)
29. Macmurray J (1961) Persons in relation (Volume II of The form of the personal). Faber and Faber, London. (Paperback, 1970; New edition, with introduction by F. G. Fitzpatrick, Humanities Press International, 1991; reissued by Faber and Faber, 1995)
30. Bruner JS (1968) Processes of cognitive growth: infancy. (Heinz Werner Lectures, 1968). Clark University Press with Barri Publishers, Worcester, MA
31. Trevarthen C (1974) Conversations with a two-month-old. New Scientist, 2 May, pp 230–235.
32. Trevarthen C (1979) Communication and cooperation in early infancy. A description of primary intersubjectivity. In: Bullowa M (ed) Before speech: the beginning of human communication. Cambridge University Press, London, pp 321–347
33. Osborne N (2017) Love, rhythm and chronobiology. In: Daniel S, Trevarthen C (eds) Rhythms of relating in children's therapies: connecting creatively with vulnerable children. Jessica Kingsley, London, pp 14–27
34. Sander LW (2008) In: Amadei G, Bianchi I (eds) Living systems, evolving consciousness, and the emerging person: a selection of papers from the life work of Louis Sander. Taylor & Francis, Abingdon
35. Winnicott DW (1964) The child, the family and the outside World. Penguin Books, London
36. Narvaez D, Braungart-Rieker JM, Miller-Graff LE, Gettler LT, Hastings PD (eds) (2016) Contexts for young child flourishing: evolution, family, and society. Oxford University Press, New York
37. Spitz RA (1945) Hospitalism—An inquiry into the genesis of psychiatric conditions in early childhood. Psychoanal Study Child 1:53–74
38. Bowlby J, World Health Organization (1952) Maternal care and mental health: a report prepared on behalf of the World Health Organization as a contribution to the United Nations programme for the welfare of homeless children/John Bowlby, 2nd edn. World Health Organization, Geneva. http://www.who.int/iris/handle/10665/40724
39. Leboyer F (1974) Pour une naissance sans violence. Éditions du Seuil, Paris
40. Condon WS, Sander LS (1974) Neonate movement is synchronized with adult speech. Interactional participation and language acquisition. Science 183:99–101
41. Sander LW (1962) Issues in mother-child interaction. J Am Acad Child Psych 1(1):141–166
42. Sander LW (1964) Adaptive relationships in early mother-child interaction. J Am Acad Child Psych 3:231–264
43. Maratos O (1982) Trends in development of imitation in early infancy. In: Bever TG (ed) Regressions in mental development: basic phenomena and theories. Hillsdale, NJ, Erlbaum, pp 81–101
44. Brazelton TB (1973) Neonatal behavioural assessment scale (Clinics in developmental medicine, 50. Spastics International Medical Publications). Heinemann Medical Books, London
45. Brazelton TB, Nugent JK (1995) The neonatal behavioural assessment scale, 3rd edn. MacKeith Press, London

46. Brazelton TB (1979) Evidence of communication during neonatal behavioural assessment. In: Bullowa M (ed) Before speech: the beginning of human communication. Cambridge University Press, London, pp 79–88
47. Brazelton TB (1982) Joint regulation of neonate-parent behavior. In: Tronick EZ (ed) Social interchange in infancy: affect, cognition and communication. University Park Press, Baltimore
48. Brazelton TB (1993) Touchpoints: your child's emotional and behavioral development. Viking, New York
49. Brazelton TB (2002) Strengths and stresses in today's families: looking toward the future. In: Gomes-Pedro J, Nugent JK, Young JG, Brazelton TB (eds) The infant and family in the twenty-first century. Brunner-Routledge, New York/Hove, UK, pp 23–30
50. Brazelton TB, Sparrow JD (2006) Touchpoints 0-3: your child's emotional and behavioral development, 2nd edn. Da Capo Press, Cambridge, MA
51. Lester B, Sparrow JD (eds) (2012) Nurturing young children and their families: building on the legacy of T. B. Brazelton. Wiley-Blackwell Scientific, Oxford
52. Stern DN (1971) A micro-analysis of mother-infant interaction: behaviors regulating social contact between a mother and her three-and-a-half-month-old twins. J Am Acad Child Psych 10:501–517
53. Stern DN, Beebe B, Jaffe J, Bennett SL (1977) The infant's stimulus world during social interaction: a study of caregiver behaviors with particular reference to repetition and timing. In: Schaffer HR (ed) Studies in mother-infant interaction. Academic Press, New York, pp 177–202
54. Stern DN (1985) The interpersonal World of the infant: a view from psychoanalysis and development psychology. Basic Books, New York
55. Stern DN, Bruschweiler-Stern N, Harrison AM, Lyons-Ruth K, Morgan AC, Nahum JP, Sander L, Tronick EZ (1999) The process of therapeutic change involving implicit knowledge: some implications of developmental observations for adult psychotherapy. Infant Ment Health J 19(3):300–308
56. Stern DN (2000) The interpersonal World of the infant: a view from psychoanalysis and development psychology, 2nd edn. Basic Books, New York
57. Pavlicevic M (1997) Music therapy in context: music meaning and relationship. Jessica Kingsley, London. ISBN: 1-85302-434-1
58. Pavlicevic M (1999) Music therapy: intimate notes. Jessica Kingsley, London
59. Pavlicevic M, Ansdell G (2009) Between communicative musicality and collaborative musicing: a perspective from community music therapy. In: Malloch S, Trevarthen C (eds) Communicative musicality: exploring the basis of human companionship. Oxford University Press, Oxford, pp 357–376
60. Pavlicevic M, Trevarthen C (1989) A musical assessment of psychiatric states in adults. Psychopathology 22:325–334
61. Pavlicevic M, Trevarthen C, Duncan J (1994) Improvisational music therapy and the rehabilitation of persons suffering from chronic schizophrenia. J Music Ther 31(2):86–104
62. Kennedy H, Landor M, Todd L (eds) (2011) Video interaction guidance: a relationship-based intervention to promote attunement, empathy and wellbeing. Jessica Kingsley Publishers, London
63. Stern DN (2007) Applying developmental and neuroscience findings on other-centred participation to the process of change in psychotherapy. In: Bråten S (ed) On being moved: from mirror neurons to empathy. John Benjamins Publishing Company, Amsterdam/Philadelphia, pp 35–47
64. Stern DN (2010) Forms of vitality: exploring dynamic experience in psychology, the arts, psychotherapy and development. Oxford University Press, Oxford
65. Malloch S (1999) Mother and infants and communicative musicality. In: Deliège I (ed) Rhythms, musical narrative, and the origins of human communication. Musicae Scientiae, Special Issue, 1999–2000. European Society for the Cognitive Sciences of Music, Liège, Belgium, pp 29–57

66. Turner VW (1982) From ritual to theatre: the human seriousness of play. PAJ Publications, New York
67. Bråten S (1988) Between dialogical mind and monological reason: postulating the virtual other. In: Campanella M (ed) Between rationality and cognition. Albert Meynier, Turin, pp 205–235
68. Bråten S (1998) Intersubjective communion and understanding: development and perturbation. In: Bråten S (ed) Intersubjective communication and emotion in early ontogeny. Cambridge University Press, Cambridge, pp 372–382
69. Bråten S (2007) On being moved: from mirror neurons to empathy. John Benjamins Publishing Company, Amsterdam/Philadelphia
70. Bråten S (2009) The intersubjective mirror in infant learning and evolution of speech. John Benjamins Publishing Company, Amsterdam/Philadelphia
71. Porges SW (2011) The polyvagal theory: neurophysiological foundations of emotions, attachment, communication, and self-regulation. W.W. Norton & Company, New York
72. Birdwhistell R (1970) Kinesics and context. University of Pennsylvania Press, Philadelphia
73. Malloch S (2017) Establishing a therapy of musicality: the embodied narratives of myself with others. In: Daniel S, Trevarthen C (eds) Rhythms of relating: stories from children's therapies. Jessica Kingsley Publishers, London, pp 63–81
74. Hutcheson F (1755/2013) A system of moral philosophy 2 volume set: a system of moral philosophy: in three books: volume 1 (Cambridge Library Collection-Philosophy) Reprint Edition, 2013. Cambridge University Press, New York
75. Hume D (1739) A treatise on human nature: an attempt to introduce the experimental method of reasoning into moral subjects. John Noon, London
76. Smith A (1759) Theory of moral sentiments. Edinburgh (Modern Edition: D. D. Raphael and A. L. Macfie, General Editors, Glasgow Edition. Oxford: Clarendon, 1976). Reprint, Liberty Fund, Indianapolis, p 1984
77. Smith A (1777/1982) Of the nature of that imitation which takes place in what are called the imitative arts. In W. P. D. Wightman and J. C. Bryce (eds.) with Dugald Stewart's account of Adam Smith (ed. I. S. Ross), D. D. Raphael and A. S. Skinner (General eds.), Essays on philosophical subjects. Liberty Fund, Indianapolis, 1982, pp 176–213
78. Reid T (1764) An inquiry into the human mind on the principles of common sense. A. Millar, A. Kincaid and J. Bell, London/Edinburgh
79. Jernberg AM (1979) Theraplay: new therapy using structured play for problem children and their families. Jossey-Bass, San Francisco, CA
80. Ferenczi S (1933) Confusion de langue entre les adultes et l'enfant. In: Psychanalyse 4. Payot, Paris, p 1982
81. Winnicott DW (1987) In: Winnicott C, Sheperd R, Davis M (eds) Babies and their mothers. Addison Wesley, Reading, MA
82. Winnicott DW (1965) The maturational process and the facilitating environment. Hogarth, London
83. Winnicott DW (1958) Playing and reality. Tavistock, London
84. Spitz RA (1957) No and yes: on the genesis of human communication. International Universities Press, New York
85. Booth P, Jernberg AM (2010) Theraplay: helping parents and children build better relationships through attachment-based play. John Wiley and Sons. Jossey-Bass, San Francisco, CA
86. Jernberg AM, Booth PB (2001) Theraplay: helping parents and children build better relationships through attachment-based play, 2nd edn. Jossey-Bass, San Francisco, CA
87. Hobson RP (1989) Beyond cognition: a theory of autism. In: Dawson G (ed) Autism: nature, diagnosis, and treatment. Guilford Press, New York, NY, pp 22–48
88. Hobson P (2002) The cradle of thought: exploring the origins of thinking. Macmillan, London
89. Hobson RP (1984) Early childhood autism and the question of egocentrism. J Autism Dev Disord 14:85–104
90. Hobson RP (1991) Against the theory of 'theory of mind'. Br J Dev Psychol 9:33–51. On the affective basis of interpersonal understanding

91. Hobson RP (1993) Autism and the development of mind. Lawrence Erlbaum, Hove
92. Hobson RP, Ouston J, Lee A (1988) Emotion recognition in autism; coordinating faces and voices. Psychol Med 18:911–923
93. Hobson RP, Hobson JA (2011) Joint attention or joint engagement? Insights from autism. In: Seemann A (ed) Joint attention: new developments in philosophy, psychology, and neuroscience. MIT Press, Cambridge, MA, pp 115–135
94. Hobson RP, Patrick M, Crandell L, García-Pérez R, Lee A (2005) Personal relatedness and attachment in infants of mothers with borderline personality disorder. Dev Psychobiol 17(2):329–347
95. Meares R (2004) The conversational model: an outline. Am J Psychother 58(1):51–66
96. Meares R, with Bendit N, Haliburn J, Korner A, Mears D, Butt D (2012) Borderline personality disorder and the conversational model: a clinician's manual. W.W. Norton & Company, New York
97. Meares R (2005) The metaphor of play: origin and breakdown of personal being. Routledge, London/New York
98. Meares R (2016) The poet's voice in the making of mind. Routledge, London/New York
99. Hughes D (1997) Facilitating developmental attachment: the road to emotional recovery and behavioral change in foster and adopted children. Jason Aronson, New York
100. Hughes D (2006) Building the bonds of attachment: awakening love in deeply traumatized children, 2nd edn. Rowman and Littlefield, Lanham, MD
101. Hughes D (2011) Attachment-focused family therapy workbook. W.W. Norton & Company, New York
102. Siegel DJ (2012) The developing mind, 2nd edn. Guilford, New York
103. Schore AN (2001) Effects of a secure attachment on right brain development, affect regulation, and infant mental health. Infant Ment Health J 22:7–67
104. Schore AN (2003) Affect regulation and the repair of the self. W.W. Norton & Company, New York
105. Bråten S (2013) Roots and collapse of empathy: human nature at its best and at its worst. John Benjamins Publishing Company, Amsterdam/Philadelphia
106. Daniel S, Trevarthen C (eds) (2017) Rhythms of relating in children's therapies: connecting creatively with vulnerable children. Jessica Kingsley, London
107. Trevarthen C, Malloch S (2017) Chapter 8: Grace in moving and joy in sharing: the intrinsic beauty of communicative musicality from birth. In: Bunn S (ed) Anthropology and beauty: from aesthetics to creativity. Taylor & Francis/Routledge, London, pp 115–130
108. Epstein M (1995) Thoughts without a thinker: psychotherapy from a Buddhist perspective. Basic Books, New York

Part I

Early Interactive Development

The Beginning of Parent-Infant Communication

2

Emmanuel Devouche and Maya Gratier

For several decades, the way mothers and infants communicate, through forms of dynamic relating, has constituted a privileged field of research for understanding human development. Communication, which etymologically refers to the idea of "making common" or sharing, is indeed a central aspect of the life of every baby, right from birth [1]. Many theorists interested in early forms of communication, including specialists of parent-child attachment [2], of language development [3, 4], or of developmental psychopathology [5], have highlighted that early face-to-face communication is the cradle of all subsequent social abilities such as joint engagement, coordinated attention and joint attention, and processes of intentional communication leading to language use [6–9]. Yet, caregiving and caring adults are in an asymmetrical position with regard to developing infants, and it is not obvious that adults' and infants' communicative abilities can or do match each other. One theoretical model that can account for this asymmetry and the potential mismatch it entails is system's theory. According to this approach, adults and infants strive to maintain a state of balance by continuous co-regulation of each other's behavior [10–13]. This approach entails that not only adults adapt to changes in the infant's behavior but also that infants are active in adjusting to their physical and social surroundings.

One crucial point that continues to divide the scientific community is the question of whether or not socio-cognitive skills underlie early communication, and if so which ones. Some authors argue that it is not until the end of the first year or even the second year that the baby becomes truly aware of the mental state of others and thus able to communicate [14–16]. According to this perspective, inherited from Piagetian constructivism, the baby would be devoid of the cognitive structures and

E. Devouche (✉)
Laboratoire de Psychopathologie et Processus de Santé, Paris Descartes University, Paris, France

M. Gratier
Paris Nanterre University, Nanterre Cedex, France

© Springer Nature Switzerland AG 2019

G. Apter et al. (eds.), *Early Interaction and Developmental Psychopathology*,
https://doi.org/10.1007/978-3-030-04769-6_2

mental representations on which knowledge of the world is based. Thus, the kinds of early discriminations researchers may observe in young infants would be merely sensory, and behaviors like imitation of expressions and gestures would be mere reflex responses to stimulation, at least at the very beginning. For other researchers, the baby has an innate capacity for communication and is born with the means to achieve intimate, perhaps prenoetic, understanding of an attentive partner's state [6–8, 17–19]. According to this approach, the infant is born with an interest in the emotions and motives of his partner and, by engaging from the beginning into immediate sympathetic contact with others, acquires both new communicative skills and knowledge and people and objects. Trevarthen [9] describes this innate capacity for sympathetic sharing as "primary intersubjectivity." It is brought about through coordinated expressive behavior enabling a direct sharing of subjective states and experiences.

Legerstee [17] suggests this controversy is based on an opposition between defenders of developmental continuity and defenders of stage-based approaches. Continuity theorists conceive of the baby as predisposed to an early form of communication that is a rudimentary form of the one that takes shape over the following months [9, 19]. Other researchers see "true" communication, that is one that implies an intention to communication, as an emergent process and one that emerges only late in the first year of life [20]. Understanding intentions to communicate is, in this view, rooted in an understanding of others' mental states. According to Trevarthen [9], however, the newborn is predisposed to grasp many higher-order invariants in the expressive behavior of social partners (sensitivity to the human voice, to the human face, to facial expressions, etc., see previous section), which orient its perceptions and actions. In this perspective, the kind of communication that characterizes the first weeks of life, which is essentially dyadic (or person-person), gradually gives way to a more elaborate form of social engagement, described as triadic because it involves referential processes in person-person-person and then person-person-object configurations [21–24].

2.1 Co-construction of the Dyadic Space

Feldman and Eidelman [25] demonstrated that a 2-day-old newborn sporadically manifests gaze toward social partners and that mothers adapt their own behavior to the state of alertness that they consider appropriate for communication. This maternal adjustment may thus enable the newborn to experience continuity between his/her own internal state and his mother's behavior toward her/him. Feldman and Eidelman [25] observe that the baby spends more time in an alert state (i.e., "calm and attentive," state 4 on the Brazelton scale) when the mother behaves contingently, that is, responds in a timely manner. These findings are in line with Stern's [18] earlier observations that mothers were adjusted to their babies from the start, closely monitoring and interpreting their signals, states of alertness, and expressive behavior. Maternal adjustment seems crucial in facilitating and promoting the engagement of the baby in social interaction from the first days of postnatal life [26].

Stern [27] describes the intermodal reciprocity of behaviors and affective expressions as "affect attunement" and suggests it creates for the infant the feeling of being accompanied in his movements and emotions. Most mothers and fathers spontaneously "tune in" to even very young infants' affective states, and they match and mirror them dynamically so as to support positive states and dampen negative states. Interestingly though, some mothers, even those with no known psychopathology, are less affectively attuned to their infants, and their infants in turn are less responsive than infants of mothers who display high affect attunement [28].

In recent years, much debate has centered on parental behavior toward infants. Indeed, parents acquire a great deal of practical knowledge about their infants' needs and abilities and about risks encountered while caring for them. But they also appear to have in-built knowledge of how to hold or soothe or talk to a baby. Much research has been conducted on the seemingly universal characteristics of baby talk or infant-directed speech, which all infants prefer to the faster-paced and less melodious adult-directed version [29, 30]. This form of speech, which is highly redundant and associated with expressive gesture and facial expression, has been described as "intuitive parenting" [31, 32] and points to biological determinants of a species-specific human parenting. Thus, infants' predispositions for adjusted, sensitive communication is matched to parental predispositions to support and scaffold communicative behavior.

The bidirectional process of communicating motivation and affect in face-to-face interaction and the active role played by the baby in this first partnership is now widely recognized [33]. Co-construction [34], synchrony and turn-taking [35, 36], co-regulation [12, 37], shared rhythmic sensibility [38, 39], and sharing of a common time base [40] are all dynamic processes based on reciprocity and complementarity within the dyadic interaction between parent and infant.

Video-based microanalysis of parent-infant interaction has enabled many researchers to establish the behavioral patterns characteristic of a contingent adjustment between a mother and her baby [38, 41–43]. Stern [44] apprehended early interaction by focusing on its structure and temporal organization. He described face-to-face exchange as composed of well delimitated phases in which the behaviors of each partner are interpreted according to their position in time. Interactional engagement is thus initiated by an introductory phase characterized by the mother's intention to capture and maintain the infant's attention. A shared rhythm, to which both adults and infants are sensitive, enables the coordination of each partner's expressions during the exchange [38].

2.2 Rhythm and Protoconversation

Both partners establish a common beat [45], and "this shared rhythm enables them to meet at the intersection of their vocal and bodily expressions" ([38], p. 55). The infant seems particularly attracted by the natural rhythm of the mother's speech. It is a rhythm that is neither random nor completely predictable and offers both partners a range of expressive possibilities [46]. Expressive timing refers to small temporal shifts in the onset of expected events, as in peekaboo play [47]. Mothers use expressive timing when they talk, play, and sing to young infants [18, 48], and infants are more socially engaged when mothers use expressive timing compared with more predictable or incoherent timing [46, 49]. Several studies have shown that the baby comes into the world with a remarkable capacity for rhythm (for a review, see [50]). Before birth, the fetus manifests an attraction to rhythmic events [51], and preterm infants born up to 2 months before term are able to synchronize their vocal expressions with those of an adult, thus participating in protoconversations [52].

Several researchers have demonstrated the early coordination between the behaviors of mothers and infants, as well as the precise regularity of interactive timing from 2 months of age which is associated with shared biological and behavioral rhythms [40, 53–56].

Condon and Sander [36] were perhaps the first researchers to suggest that rhythmic sense is what enables newborns to synchronize their own behavior with their mother's speech. Synchrony can indeed be considered a crucial foundation for any communicative process [57]. According to Trevarthen [45], early mother-infant communication is much like a dialogue, or what he calls protoconversation, emphasizing its reciprocal nature and flexible coordination, which is surprising given young infants' limited motor and cognitive skills. According to this view, social skills precede and drive the development of abilities in other domains.

By 2 months infants display a triad of expressive behaviors that index their social orientation and motivation for dyadic engagement [58]. The combination of knit-brow gaze concentration, directed smile, and coo vocalization powerfully elicits contingent positive reactions from all social partners and is interpreted as an intention to communicate. Cooing, which appears between 6 and 8 weeks after birth, is in fact described by specialists of vocal development as "speech-like" vocalization [59, 60]. Adults respond more often to coo vocalizations than to other sorts of vocalizations [59], and they do so in a timely manner. They also tend to embed them in meaningful talk, that is, talk that is referential and often narrative.

Thus mother-infant interaction must be thought of as more than just a two-way transfer of feelings or representations. Dual interaction involves meaningful shared and remembered contexts that can be summoned to reenact and improvise new encounters. Mother-infant interaction, from the very beginning and well before referential processes become explicit, is embedded in implicit semiotic processes, which involve styles of reciprocity and unique signatures of expressive movement [46, 61, 62]. Mother-infant interaction must be understood as a dynamic process fostering historic time, bridging the experienced past and the anticipated future. Researchers must focus on the dyad as a unit of analysis, taking into account its immediate context and its intimate history in order to describe how the behaviors of the two partners coordinate over time. The behaviors of each partner may be seen to constitute an extension of those of the other, generating forms of shared intentionality that are made possible not by shared mental representations but by the temporal and rhythmic dimensions intrinsic to social interaction.

2.3 Interactive Timing and Social Contingency

Through reciprocal engagement, the baby gradually develops his or her sense of experience sharing (intersubjectivity) enabling better anticipation of the mother's behavior and the formation of generalized social expectations. Separately from each other, mother and baby do not experience the same social and biological time, that is, their temporal worlds are quite distinct. By interacting with each other, they build a shared temporality. Being in time together fosters the experience of a mental or imaginative space within which emotions and motivations or common projects can be lived through together. Interactive timing requires a mutual adaptation to each other's spontaneous tempo [50]. This shared rhythm and sense of time thus supports the integration of behavioral schemes that have a certain temporal organization and the integration of interactive routines specific to the dyad. Indeed, over the first weeks of life infants come to identify regularities in their environment and form clear expectations about recurrent events and routines [63–65].

The repetition of temporal sequences facilitates the detection of contingent relations between behaviors and contributes to make the world less unpredictable for the baby. The dyad's own intersubjective space constitutes the cradle of these acquisitions by offering the baby an accessible and predictable temporal world. By internalizing interactive routines, the baby carries a piece of interactive time into his own temporal world. This progressive integration of expressive behavioral associations allows the baby to anticipate the development of an expressive action, to project the future behavior, and to play a more and more active role in shaping social exchanges. Security and confidence are constructed in and through time.

Several authors have sought to define the time window that enables infants to appreciate the contingency of expressive behaviors during a social interaction. Van Egeren et al. [43] reviewed a large number of studies using the habituation paradigm and showed that a latency period greater than 3 s between stimuli tends to cause discouragement or withdrawal in young infants. These authors thus confirm the finding from microanalytic observations of naturalistic social interactions according to which pauses lasting more than 3 s in infant-directed behavior cause infants to disengage from social interaction [44, 45] Van Egeren et al. [43] also highlight the fact that research that has focused on response times in the dyad mostly uses time windows with a short duration (less than 2 s). It is possible that the temporal window for contingent responsiveness varies between adults and infants, that it changes as infants develop, and that it varies according to which expressive modalities are involved. For example, contingent responsiveness between maternal utterances and infant non-cry vocalization is centered around 1 s, regardless of the language and culture of the mother [66]. Recent evidence suggests that mothers respond to infants within a shorter temporal window than infants respond to mothers [67]. However, it is highly probable that 3 s represents an important psychological boundary for marking the contours of a meaningful event. This is supported by the finding that mothers package their speech into units lasting on average 3 s [67–69]. This duration roughly corresponds to the perceived present and to the span of working memory as well as to units such as phrases in speech and music or lines of poetry [70, 71].

According the Hains and Muir [72], infants learn to form expectations based on their experiences of contingency between their own actions and their consequences. Other researchers consider that infants are born with a "contingency detection module" that predisposes them to prefer perfect contingency or co-occurrence between events in the first months of life and, progressively after the age of 3 months, to integrate imperfectly contingent events [73]. Stern [44], however, sees the repetition and variation of rhythmic maternal behavior as the basis on which infants form expectations and perceive contingency. Repetition would enable infants to predict the partner's behavior based on strict contingency, and variation would enable infants to adjust to ongoing change within a flexible temporal window. Contingency detection is, according to this view, flexible from the beginning and is based on appropriate timing (not too regular and not too variable) from social partners. From a theoretical standpoint, the concept of timing formulated by researchers like Trevarthen, Beebe, or Brazelton implies that each partner actively takes into account the predictability of the other in the course of interaction within a shared temporal framework. Each partner thus builds a memory of the other and of their shared temporality, upon which their capacity to anticipate each other is founded [9, 40].

The appreciation of social contingency through the idea of a time window is not evident, and few studies have explored this question. However, quantifying the time lapse that defines the causality that imparts combinatorial meaning to consecutive behaviors is of great interest for understanding the dynamics of early interactions. The stake is all the more important because it is inseparable from the question of intentionality in the behavior of the baby, a question that was evoked at the beginning of this chapter. Recent research on early vocal exchange presented below sheds some light on these critical issues for early communication.

Another important characteristic of expressive behavior that is known to foster an experience of unity, continuity, and coherence is imitation. Papoušek and Papoušek [31, 32] emphasize the primacy of parental imitation as an integral part of the intuitive didactic support that parents provide for their baby. And infants imitate adults' gestures, facial expressions, and vocal sounds from the very start of life [74–76]. In naturalistic social interaction, imitation is largely contingent, that is, it occurs within temporal windows that do not exceed 3 s. But the reproduction by one partner of some aspect of the other partner's behavior certainly serves to reinforce the experience of interpersonal connectedness that contingency in itself enables. For example, in spontaneous vocal interaction between mothers and 3-month-olds, infants imitate the intonation contours of the mother's preceding utterance far more often than they imitate the sound itself [7], suggesting that young infants are much more active in driving and shaping social interaction than most researchers acknowledge. Furthermore, multiple forms of imitation are at play from birth in naturalistic social interaction. Forms of imitation and their various functions deserve more attention.

2.4 The Roots of Turn-Taking

From the first weeks of life, the baby produces vocalizations that lead to responses from the social environment [59]. The emergence of these vocalizations rapidly primes the first exchanges with the entourage turning them into protoconversations characterized by the alternating vocalizations of both partners with contingency-relevant pauses [7, 35, 55, 69, 77, 78]. Research on vocal interaction shows that around 2 months, the turn-taking exchange is characterized by vocalizations of the mother and the baby separated by pauses ranging from 500 ms to 1 s [66, 79]. It also appears that pauses rarely exceed 3 s and, when they do, mark the end of an episode of engagement between mother and baby [49, 69, 80].

Ginsburg and Kilbourne [81] observed that the interaction between a mother and her 7–18-week-old infant presented more overlap in vocalizations than with younger infants. In a recent longitudinal study of vocal interaction with infants aged 3–18 months, Hilbrink et al. [82] also found a reduction in overlap after the age of 5 months. In the same study, the pauses separating the vocalizations of the two partners were found to lengthen after infants reached the age of 9 months. However, Gratier et al. [78] showed an increase in pause duration between partners in the vocal interactions of 2–3-month-old infants and 4–5-month-olds. The fact that older babies take longer to respond may paradoxically be a reflection of their increasing communicative skills. Indeed, by 4 months of age, infants' attention is less focused on their partner's facial expressions because it alternates between environmental stimuli and the partner. Gratier et al. [78] also observed very precisely timed vocalizations already with 2-month-olds, where infants vocalize less than 100 ms after the end of a maternal utterance. This finding suggests that infants are highly skilled in anticipating and initiating vocal turns.

In line with this work, Dominguez et al. [83] studied the turn-taking of newborn infants and their mothers in the hospital environment. Indeed, considering what we know today about very early socio-cognitive abilities and newborns' sensitivity to social partners [84], it is not inconsistent to assume newborns are expert at turn-taking interaction. Indeed, some recent research shows that turn-taking interaction is common even in other animal species [85]. Dominguez et al.'s [83] study showed that the vocalizations of newborn infants are rarely isolated, that is, maternal utterances are highly concentrated after the vocalizations made by the newborn, occurring for the vast majority within the second following the end of the newborn vocalization. Another interesting finding was that two thirds of the infant vocalizations that follow a maternal vocalization also occur within the second that follows. These results suggest that at birth already a 1-s window is appropriate for understanding social contingency [26, 86–88] and that newborns are already responsive to their mother's behavior.

2.5 How Does Research on Early Parent-Infant Communication Inform Our Understanding of Interactive Disturbance?

A number of early interaction specialists have focused on developing paradigms designed to highlight aspects of interactive functioning, many of which have proved useful tools for studying interactive dysfunction. We propose to conclude this chapter by highlighting two such research paradigms, one of which has been widely used in clinical contexts. The closed-circuit double-television setup and the still-face paradigm procedure have both shed light on young infants' social expectations and initiatives.

Murray and Trevarthen [89] developed the double-TV setup to study the role of interactional synchrony during dyadic exchange. They developed a system in which the dyad interacts through two television screens with sound and vision transmitted electronically in real time. Thus, a 2-month-old baby could be presented either with a live television broadcast of her mother eliciting and responding in her usual manner or with a delayed retransmission of the mother. During deferred transmission, the behavior of the mother is no longer synchronized with the behavior of the baby. Studies conducted with this setup and procedure have shown that infants are extremely sensitive to the contingent aspect of adult behavior [90]. Indeed, even when maternal behavior is well adapted to the infant's state and age and reflects a positive, affectionate disposition, infants become upset and disengage from interaction when it is not well timed. This research shows that timing, and not just appropriate emotions, is crucial for communication in the first months of life. Interestingly, mothers are as sensitive as infants to a lack of contingency between their own behavior and the infant's responses. Murray and Trevarthen [91] report a breakdown in the narrative flow of the infant-directed speech of a mother presented with the non-contingent video of her happy, expressive baby.

With the still-face paradigm, Cohn and Tronick [92] have shown that young infants are able to detect the quality of the mother's emotional engagement and respond accordingly. Infants react strongly to a breakdown in communication by displaying distress behaviors. Hundreds of studies to date, using the still-face procedure, have shown that infants have clear expectations about a social partner's communicative behavior. When the mother displays an expressionless face, the baby shows signs of agitation or even distress, as evidenced by gaze avoidance, increase in number of short glances, reduction of smiling, and self-comforting behavior [93–96]. The sequence of infant behavior during the still-face episode is perhaps the most relevant aspect for clinical work. Infants manifest surprise at a discontinuation of communicative behavior when no other environmental distractor is present. They then display strong motives to re-engage the partner and finally become overtly distressed as a last straw strategy to repair the loss of social engagement. In line with Weinberg and Tronick's [97] previous work on the effects of postnatal depression on mother-infant interaction, Diego et al. [98] compared dyads with depressed mothers and non-depressed mothers who were asked to "look depressed" during part of the interaction with their 3-month-old babies. They observed that infants interacting with their non-depressed mothers vocalized more frequently and had more positive and less negative expressions than infants with their depressed mothers. Moreover, as soon as non-depressed mothers interrupted the interaction, their infants, who were not accustomed to this type of attitude, expressed more distress than the infants of depressed mothers whose reactions were far less manifest.

As we have seen, from the get-go, social interaction implies a sophisticated exchange, with both partners seeking to capture the attention of the other and trying to respond appropriately, thus contributing to mutual regulation and emerging habitual styles of interaction. Early interaction is made possible by the development of a coordination of action and expression based on the sharing of interactive goals, a lexicon of communicative acts, interactive rules, and rhythm. It can be seen thus to constitute "true" communication well before babies have access to referential and symbolic meaning or have some explicit "thing" they want to communicate to another person.

However, the quality of exchange can be hindered most notably by individual characteristics stemming from either parents or infants. It is important to understand, however, that when parents are not disposed to communicate expressively and effectively with their baby or when babies are not responsive or lack motivation to communicate, the whole dyadic system misses the beat. Communication, as a fundamentally two-way process, is both hindered by individual particularities and impacts personal characteristics of each individual involved in it. An important issue that merits attention for better understanding dysfunctions and disturbances of communication with preverbal infants is whether communication itself is either efficient or flawed or admits of degrees of success. In other words, failures in establishing and maintaining communication may be less damaging than flawed or inconsistent patterns of communication where a rewarding interaction can disintegrate inexplicably.

References

1. Reddy V, Legerstee M (2007) What does it mean to communicate? Infant Behav Dev 30(2):177–179
2. Bowlby J (1969) Attachment and loss, vol 1. Basic Books, New York
3. Bruner JS (1978) The role of dialogue in language acquisition. In: Sinclair A, Jarvelle RJ, Levelt WJM (eds) The child's concept of language. Springer-Verlag, New York
4. Vygotsky L (1962) Thought and language. The MIT Press, Cambridge, MA
5. Sroufe LA, Rutter M (1984) The domain of developmental psychopathology. Child Dev:17–29
6. Bruner JS (1990) Acts of meaning. Harvard University Press, Cambridge, MA
7. Gratier M, Devouche E (2011) Imitation and repetition of prosodic contour in vocal interaction at 3 months. Dev Psychol 47(1):67–76
8. Reddy V (2008) How infants know minds. Harvard University Press, Cambridge MA
9. Trevarthen C (1998) The concept of foundations of infant intersubjectivity. In: Bråten S (ed) Intersubjective communication and emotion in early ontogeny. Cambridge University Press, Cambridge, pp 15–46
10. Beebe B, Jaffe J, Markese S, Buck K, Chen H, Cohen P et al (2010) The origins of 12-month attachment: A microanalysis of 4-month mother–infant interaction. Attach Hum Dev 12(1-2):3–141

11. Fogel A (1992) Movement and communication in human infancy: the social dynamics of development. Hum Mov Sci 11(4):387–423
12. Tronick EZ (1989) Emotions and emotional communication in infants. Am Psychol 44:112–119
13. Tronick EZ, Cohn JF (1989) Infant-mother face-to-face interaction: age and gender differences in coordination and the occurrence of miscoordination. Child Dev:85–92
14. Barresi J, Moore C (1996) Intentional relations and social understanding. Behav Brain Sci 19(1):107–154
15. Carpenter M, Nagell K, Tomasello M (1998) Social cognition, joint attention, and communicative competence from 9 to 15 months of age. Monogr Soc Res Child Dev 63(4):i–vi. 1-143
16. Perner J, Davies G (1991) Understanding the mind as an active information processor: do young children have a 'copy theory of mind?'. Cognition 39(1):51–69
17. Legerstee M (2009) Infants' sense of people: precursors to theory of mind. Cambridge University Press, Cambridge
18. Stern DN (1985) The interpersonal world of the infant: a view from psychoanalysis and developmental psychology. Basic Books, New York
19. Trevarthen C (1993) The self born in intersubjectivity: an infant communicating. In: Neisser U (ed) The perceived self: ecological and interpersonal sources of self-knowledge. Cambridge University Press, New York, pp 121–173
20. Tomasello M (2009) The cultural origins of human cognition. Harvard university press, Cambridge, MA
21. Bakeman R, Adamson LB (1984) Coordinating attention to people and objects in mother-infant and peer-infant interaction. Child Dev 55:1278–1289
22. Hubley P, Trevarthen C (1979) Sharing a task in infancy. New Dir Child Adolesc Dev 1979(4):57–80
23. McHale J, Fivaz-Depeursinge F, Dickstein S, Robertson J, Daley M (2008) New evidence for the social embeddedness of infants' early triangular capacities. Fam Process 47(4):445–463
24. Trevarthen C, Hubley P (1978) Secondary intersubjectivity: confidence, confiding and acts of meaning in the first year. In: Lock A (ed) Action, gesture and symbol: the emergence of language. Academic Press, London, pp 183–229
25. Feldman R, Eidelman AI (2007) Maternal postpartum behavior and the emergence of infant–mother and infant–father synchrony in preterm and full-term infants: the role of neonatal vagal tone. Dev Psychobiol 49(3):290–302
26. Papoušek H, Papoušek M, Bornstein MH (1985) The naturalistic environment of young infants: on the significance of homogeneity and variability in parental speech. In: Field T, Fox N (eds) Social perception in infants. Ablex, Norwood, NJ, pp 269–297
27. Stern DN (1993) The role of feelings for an interpersonal self. In: Neisser U (ed) The perceived self. Cambridge University Press, New-York, pp 205–215
28. Markova G, Legerstee M (2006) Contingency, imitation, and affect sharing: foundations of infants' social awareness. Dev Psychol 42(1):132
29. Cooper RP, Aslin RN (1990) Preference for infant-directed speech in the first month after birth. Child Dev 61:1584–1595
30. Fernald A (1985) Four-month-old infants prefer to listen to motherese. Infant Behav Dev 8(2):181–195
31. Papoušek M, Papoušek H (1989) Forms and functions of vocal matching in interactions between mothers and their pre-canonical infants. First Lang 9:137–158
32. Papoušek H, Papoušek M (1989) Intuitive parenting: aspects related to educational psychology. Eur J Psychol Educ 4(2):201–210
33. Reddy V, Hay D, Murray L, Trevarthen C (1997) Communication in infancy: mutual regulation of affect and attention. In: Bremner G, Slater A, Butterworth G (eds) Infant development. Psychology Press, Hove, pp 247–274
34. Bruner JS, Hickman M (1983) La conscience, la parole et la « zone proximale » : Réflexions sur la théorie de Vygostky. In: Bruner JS (ed) Le développement de l'enfant: savoir faire, savoir dire. Presses Universitaires de France, Paris, pp 281–292

35. Bateson MC (1979) The epigenesis of conversational interaction: a personal account of research development. In: Bullowa M (ed) Before speech: the beginning of human communication. Cambridge University Press, Cambridge, pp 63–77
36. Condon WS, Sander LW (1974) Synchrony demonstrated between movements of the neonates and adult speech. Child Dev 45:456–462
37. Fogel A (1993) Two principles of communication: co-regulation and framing. In: Nadel J, Camaïoni L (eds) New perspectives in early communicative development. Routledge, London/New York, pp 9–21
38. Devouche E, Gratier M (2001) Microanalyse du rythme dans les échanges vocaux et gestuels entre la mère et son bébé de 10 semaines. Dev Dent 13(2):55–82
39. Trevarthen C (2001) Intrinsic motives for companionship in understanding: their origin, development, and significance for infant mental health. Infant Ment Health J 22(1-2):95–131
40. Brazelton TB, Koslowski B, Main M (1974) The origins of reciprocity: The early mother-infant interaction. In: Lewis M, Rosenblum L (eds) The effect of infants on its caregiver. Wiley, New York, NY, pp 49–77
41. Cohn JF, Tronick EZ (1987) Mother–infant face-to-face interaction: the sequence of dyadic states at 3, 6, and 9 months. Dev Psychol 23(1):68–77
42. Symons DK, Moran G (1987) The behavioral dynamics of mutual responsiveness in early face-to-face mother-infant interactions. Child Dev 58(6):1488–1495
43. Van Egeren LA, Barratt MS, Roach MA (2001) Mother-infant responsiveness: timing, mutual regulation, and interactional context. Dev Psychol 37(5):684–697
44. Stern DN (1977) Structure et réglage temporel. In: Stern D (ed) Mère Enfant, les premières relations. P. Mardaga, Bruxelles, pp 111–134
45. Trevarthen C (1999) Musicality and the intrinsic motive pulse. Musicae Scientiae, Special Issue 1999–2000:155–215
46. Gratier M, Apter G (2009) The improvised musicality of belonging: repetition and variation in mother-infant vocal interaction. In: Malloch S, Trevarthen C (eds) Communicative musicality: exploring the basis of human companionship. Oxford University Press, Oxford, pp 301–327
47. Gratier M (2003) Expressive timing and interactional synchrony between mothers and infants: cultural similarities, cultural differences, and the immigration experience. Cogn Dev 18(4):533–554
48. Delavenne A, Gratier M, Devouche E (2013) Expressive timing in infant-directed singing between 3 and 6 months. Infant Behav Dev 36(1):1–13
49. Delavenne A, Gratier M, Devouche E, Apter G (2008) Phrasing and fragmented time in "pathological" mother-infant vocal interaction. Music Sci 12(1 Suppl):47–70
50. Provasi J, Anderson DI, Barbu-Roth M (2014) Rhythm perception, production, and synchronization during the perinatal period. Front Psychol 5:1048
51. Lecanuet JP, Granier-Deferre C, Busnel MC (1995) Human fetal auditory perception. In: Lecanuet JP, Fifer WP, Krasnegor NA, Smotherman WP (eds) Fetal development: a psychobiological perspective. Lawrence Erlbaum Associates, Hillsdale, NJ/England, pp 239–262
52. Trevarthen C, Kokkinaki T, Fiamenghi GA (1999) What infants' imitations communicate: with mothers, with fathers and with peers. In: Nadel J, Butterworth G (eds) Imitation in infancy. Cambridge University Press, Cambridge, pp 127–185
53. Brazelton TB, Tronick EZ, Adamson L, Als H, Wise S (1975) Early mother-infant reciprocity. In: Hofer M (ed) Parent-infant interaction. Elsevier, Amsterdam
54. Feldman R (2003) Infant–mother and infant–father synchrony: the coregulation of positive arousal. Infant Ment Health J 24(1):1–23
55. Trevarthen C (1977) Descriptive analysis of infant communicative behavior. In: Schaffer H (ed) Studies in mother-infant interaction. Academic Press, New York, pp 227–270
56. Van Puyvelde M, Loots G, Vanfleteren P, Meys J, Simcock D, Pattyn N (2014) Do you hear the same? Cardiorespiratory responses between mothers and infants during tonal and atonal music. PLoS One 9(9):e106920
57. Condon WS (1976) An analysis of behavioral organization. Sign Lang Stud (13):285–318

58. Lavelli M, Fogel A (2013) Interdyad differences in early mother–infant face-to-face communication: real-time dynamics and developmental pathways. Dev Psychol 49(12):2257
59. Bloom K, Russell A, Wassenberg K (1987) Turn taking affects the quality of infant vocalizations. J Child Lang 14(2):211–227
60. Oller DK (1980) The emergence of the sounds of speech in infancy. In: Yeni-Komshian G, Kavanagh J, Ferguson C (eds) Child phonology, Production, vol 1. Academic Press, New York, pp 93–112
61. Gratier M (2007) Musicalité, style et appartenance dans l'interaction mère-bébé. In: Imberty M, Gratier M (eds) Temps, geste et musicalité. L'Harmattan, Paris, pp 69–99
62. Trevarthen C (1990) Signs before speech. In: Sebeok TA, Umiker-Sebeok J (eds) The semiotic web. Mouton de Gruyter, Berlin, pp 689–755
63. Reddy V, Markova G, Wallot S (2013) Anticipatory adjustments to being picked up in infancy. PLoS One 8(6):e65289
64. Rochat P, Querido JG, Striano T (1999) Emerging sensitivity to the timing and structure of protoconversation in early infancy. Dev Psychol 35(4):950
65. Rovee-Collier C (1997) Dissociations in infant memory: rethinking the development of implicit and explicit memory. Psychol Rev 104(3):467
66. Keller H, Lohaus A, Völker S, Cappenberg M, Chasiotis A (1999) Temporal contingency as an independent component of parenting behavior. Child Dev 70(2):474–485
67. Infanti, R, Guellai, B, Parlato-Oliveira, E, Devouche, E, & Gratier, M (2019).Timing patterns of mother-infant turn-taking in France and Brazil
68. Beebe B, Gerstman LJ (1980) The "packaging" of maternal stimulation in relation to infant facial-visual engagement: a case study at four months. Merrill-Palmer Q Behav Dev 26(4):321–339
69. Stern DN, Beebe B, Jaffe J, Bennett SL (1977) The infant's stimulus world during social interaction: a study of caregiver behaviors with particular reference to repetition and timing. In: Schaffer H (ed) Studies in mother-infant interaction. Academic Press, New York, pp 177–202
70. Stern DN (1999) Vitality contours: the temporal contour of feelings as a basic unit for constructing the infant's social experience. In: Rochat P (ed) Early social cognition: understanding others in the first months of life. Lawrence Erlbaum, Mahwah, NJ, pp 67–80
71. Wittmann M, Pöppel E (1999) Temporal mechanisms of the brain as fundamentals of communication-with special reference to music perception and performance. Music Sci 3(1 suppl):13–28
72. Hains SMJ, Muir DW (1996) Effects of stimulus contingency in infant–adult interactions. Infant Behav Dev 19(1):49–61
73. Gergely G, Watson JS (1996) The social biofeedback model of parental affect-mirroring. Int J Psychoanal 77(6):1181
74. Kugiumutzakis G (1993) Intersubjective vocal imitation in early mother- infant interaction. In: Nadel J, Camaioni L (eds) New perspectives in early communicative development. Routledge, London, pp 23–47
75. Meltzoff AN, Moore MK (1977) Imitation of facial and manual gestures. Science 198:75–80
76. Nagy E, Molnar P (2004) Homo imitans or homo provocans? Human imprinting model of neonatal imitation. Infant Behav Dev 27:54–63
77. Bloom K (1988) Quality of adult vocalizations affects the quality of infant vocalizations. J Child Lang 15(3):469–480
78. Gratier M, Devouche E, Guellai B, Infanti R, Yilmaz E, Parlato-Oliveira E (2015) Early development of turn-taking in vocal interaction between mothers and infants. Front Psychol 6:1167
79. Jaffe J, Beebe B, Feldstein S, Crown CL, Jasnow MD, Rochat P et al (2001) Rhythms of dialogue in infancy: coordinated timing in development. Monogr Soc Res Child Dev 66:1–8
80. Stern DN, Gibbon J (1979) Temporal expectancies of social behaviours in mother-infant play. In: Thoman EB (ed) Origins of the Infant's Social Responsiveness. Lawrence Erlbaum Associates, Hillsdale, NJ, pp 409–429
81. Ginsburg GP, Kilbourne BK (1988) Emergence of vocal alternation in mother-infant interchanges. J Child Lang 15:221–235

82. Hilbrink EE, Gattis M, Levinson SC (2015) Early developmental changes in the timing of turn-taking: a longitudinal study of mother-infant interaction. Front Psychol 6:1492
83. Dominguez S, Devouche E, Apter G, Gratier G (2016) The roots of turn-taking in the neonatal period. Infant Child Dev
84. Nagy E (2008) Innate intersubjectivity: Newborns' sensitivity to communication disturbance. Dev Psychol 44(6):1779
85. Takahashi DY, Fenley AR, Ghazanfar AA (2016) Early development of turn-taking with parents shapes vocal acoustics in infant marmoset monkeys. Phil Trans R Soc B 371(1693):20150370
86. Bigelow AE, Rochat P (2006) Two-months-old Infants' sensitivity to social contingency in mother-infant and stranger-infant interaction. Infancy 9(3):313–325
87. Mayer NK, Tronick EZ (1985) Mothers' turn-giving signals and infant turn-taking in mother-infant interaction. In: Field T, Fox NA (eds) Social perception in infants. Ablex, Norwood, NJ, pp 199–216
88. Watson JS (1985) Contingency perception in early social development. In: Field TM, Fox NA (eds) Social perception in infants. Ablex, Norwood, NJ, pp 157–176
89. Murray L, Trevarthen C (1985) Emotional regulation of interaction between two-month-olds and their mothers. In: Field M, Fox N (eds) Social perception in infancy. Ablex, Norwood, NJ, pp 177–198
90. Nadel J, Carchon I, Kervella C, Marcelli D, Réserbat-Plantey D (1999) Expectancies for social contingency in 2-month-olds. Dev Sci 2(2):164–173
91. Murray L, Trevarthen C (1986) The infant's role in mother–infant communications. J Child Lang 13(1):15–29
92. Cohn JF, Tronick EZ (1983) Three-month-old infants' reaction to simulated maternal depression. Child Dev 54:185–193
93. D'Entremont B, Muir DW (1997) 5-month-olds' attention and affective responses to still-face emotional expressions. Infant Behav Dev 20:563–568
94. Ellsworth C, Muir DW, Hains SMJ (1993) Social competence and person-object differentiation: an analysis of the still-face effect. Dev Psychol 29:63–73
95. Kisilevsky BS, Hains SMJ, Lee K, Muir DW, Xu F, Fu G, Zhao ZY, Yang RL (1998) The still-face effect in Chinese and Canadian 3- to 6-month-old infants. Dev Psychol 34(4):629–639
96. Tronick EZ, Als H, Adamson L, Wise S, Brazelton TB (1978) The infant's response to entrapment between contradictory messages in face-to-face interaction. J Am Acad Child Psychiatry 17(1):1–13
97. Weinberg MK, Tronick EZ (1994) Beyond the face: an empirical study of infant affective configurations of facial, vocal, gestural, and regulatory behaviors. Child Dev 65(5):1503–1515
98. Diego MA, Field T, Hart S, Hernandez-Reif M, Jones N, Cullen C, Schanberg S, Kuhn C (2002) Facial expressions and EEG in infants of intrusive and withdrawn mothers with depressive symptoms. Depress Anxiety 15(1):10–17

3 Mutual Regulation and Unique Forms of Implicit Relational Knowing

Fabia Eleonora Banella and Ed Tronick

In this chapter, we focus on the mutual regulation model (MRM, [1]). The MRM conceptualizes infant and caretaker as components of a larger dyadic regulatory system, in which each person—infant and adult—influences and is being influenced by the communications of the other, in a circular, moment-by-moment, continuous manner. Since the organization of the system is inherently messy, a co-created relationship emerges out of the ongoing process of mutual exchange of expressive actions and affects relational intentions. The mutual regulatory process is seen as the formative process for attachment and the varied forms taken by relationships [2, 3]. These co-creative processes lead to changes in the infant's and child's moods and state of knowing about themselves in relation to the world and generates *implicit relational knowing* and implicit ways of being together [4–8].

We develop the concepts of the co-creative process, the process of mutual regulation, and recent research on the development of implicit relational knowing in infants and mother-infant dyads and then draw some implications for psychopathology and therapy.

3.1 The Mutual Regulation Model

The central concept of the MRM is that infants and caregivers, even in their earliest interpersonal exchanges, have a specific interactive goal of achieving reciprocity of shared intentions and meanings [9–13]. To achieve this goal, both infant and caregiver actively (intentionally) employ their psychobiological affective communicative capacities to make possible mutually coordinated and bidirectional interactions

F. E. Banella
Sapienza University, Rome, Italy

E. Tronick (✉)
University of Massachusetts Boston and Harvard Medical School, Boston, MA, USA
e-mail: ed.tronick@umb.edu

© Springer Nature Switzerland AG 2019

G. Apter et al. (eds.), *Early Interaction and Developmental Psychopathology*,
https://doi.org/10.1007/978-3-030-04769-6_3

[1, 11, 14–16]. The concept is based on evidence that from the beginning of their life, infants intentionally seek and engage in interpersonal and affectionate relationships, demonstrating what Trevarthen and Tronick referred to as innate intersubjectivity or what could be thought of as an interpersonal intelligence [1, 17–20]. Specifically, infants are receptive to subjective states in other persons and are capable of appreciating the meaning behind or embedded in the affective displays of others [1]. Furthermore, infants have the capacity to display communicative intentions, primarily but not only, through affective displays that express a variety of neurosomatic meanings, meanings created by the operation of systems such as the autonomic nervous system (ANS), or even the immune system [11]. Cytokines, for example, affect individual's moods and feelings of fatigue. These displays are organized into coherent multimodal configurations of the face, voice, gesture (i.e., reaching gestures), posture, gaze, and less well understood or still unknown forms of neurosomatic displays (i.e., hormones level) [21, 22].

To illustrate this conceptualization, we can imagine a typical spontaneous interaction between a mother and her 9-month-old baby playing a peek-a-boo game. While the mother is gesturing and modulating the game with her tone of voice and facial expressions of surprise and happiness, her baby is participating with smiling and vocalizing positively, showing joyfulness. Imagine now that at a certain moment of the game, the baby turns his head away and makes an unhappy, gloomy facial expression. The mother stops playing and leans back, watching the baby. In this specific interaction with a responsive caregiver, infants' positive, as well as negative, affective configurations express an underling internal subjective state that conveys meaning, perhaps his intention to keep playing the game or to stop it. Thus, infants' affective responses serve interpersonal functions of expressing infants' intentions and at the same time regulating the interaction [11, 22]. To put it simply or perhaps to overstate it, one partner reads the other partner's subjective intention and expresses their own subjective intention. These intentions convey meanings using behavioral displays. Brazelton [23] referred to the behaviors in these displays as substitutable or what Freud saw as redundancy; that is, the same intention could be expressed by different particular behaviors.

An important implication of this conceptualization of mutual interactive regulation is that infants are also capable of regulating their own affective and psychobiological states and reactivity [23–28], an implication which dismantles the old model of the infant as a blank slate shaped by his environment. Specifically, self-organizing neurobehavioral capacities enable the infant to organize behavioral states, such as sleep, alertness, and distress, and other biopsychological processes, such as arousal, attention, temperature regulation, moods, hunger, and social engagement [11, 29, 30]. Clearly, these self-regulatory capacities are limited and immature at the beginning of the infants' life, and the parent plays a crucial role in scaffolding and sustaining the infants' appropriate development of self- and interactive regulatory capacities [14].

In the dyadic interactive process between adult and infant, self- and interactive regulatory patterns are integrated, since each person must both regulate their inner state and coordinate with their partner's state [31]. According to the results of studies examining early mother-infant face-to-face interactions using time series analysis [11, 32, 33], self- and interactive regulation have been demonstrated to be simultaneous and reciprocal processes, each affecting the outcome of the other. This view was influenced by Louis Sander's work on the organization of infant sleep in the first days of life. Sander proposed that "the organization of the interpersonal exchanges between infant and caregiver is based on the idea that these behaviors are first and foremost in the service of regulation of behavior, and of the interaction. In other words, the behavior of each, which we can observe in their interaction, serves to regulate both the behavior of the other and of their own complement of component functions" ([34], p. 14). Therefore, the same interactive repertoire that allows the infant to initiate, maintain, modify, or avoid and terminate interactions simultaneously enables him to perform self-regulatory functions.

3.2 The Still-Face Paradigm

Major contributions to our understanding of parent-infant interactive regulatory processes and infants' affective communication come from studies on face-to-face interaction employing the Face-to-Face Still-Face (FFSF) experimental paradigm [12, 13]. It was initially developed to study infants' response to a social stressor—an unresponsive Still-Faced mother. The FFSF procedure is composed of three episodes, each one typically lasting 2 min. In the first episode, the caregiver is instructed to play with her infant in a face-to-face interaction as she would do at home. In the second episode, she is asked to stop talking or touching the baby and to display a flat unresponsive face. Finally, the caregiver is asked to resume interacting with her baby. What has been observed in the large number of studies that employed the FFSF is that infants are able to detect the disruption in the communication and are able to employ clear signals to elicit responses from the caregiver in attempts to get the interaction back into its usual patterns. Specifically, studies conducted in a typically developing population highlight a typical infant response to the Still-Faced mother: the infant attempts to solicit mother's attention, showing an array of typical signaling behaviors, such as smiling, vocalizations, pick-me-up gestures, or other gestural signals. As long as the Still-Faced episode persists and infants' attempts to elicit maternal response fail, infants will also engage in self-regulatory behaviors, such as looking away to avoid the stressful stimulus, withdrawal, self-soothing behaviors, and protest, with sad and angry affects [35, 36].

Research using the FFSF with its experimental break in the interaction also emphasizes the more typical and frequent lack of coordination in interactions, or mismatches between infant and caregiver, as well as the key process of reparation of mismatches back to matches. This matching to mismatching to reparation occurs in all kind of human interactions. As the MRM postulates, mother-infant interactions are jointly regulated to achieve a state of reciprocity, characterized by a state of matching (attunement, synchrony). However, states of reciprocity don't happen all the time. Normal states of mismatches occur frequently in typical successful social exchanges, approximately two thirds of the time, and they may occur for different reasons, such as misreading of the other partner's signal, mistimed behaviors, a changing of intention, and so forth [37]. Nevertheless, in most cases (70% on average), when a state of mismatch is entered, the two persons return to matched states within two seconds and experience a reparation of the communicative and affective disruption. In essence, the typical interaction is a messy and dynamic process that moves back and forth between matching states, characterized by coordination and synchronicity, and mismatching states followed by jointly and actively accomplished reparatory states [38–40].

Although reciprocity is important, perhaps the experience of reparation of mismatches has an even more central role, serving a multiplicity of functions essential for the infant's development. First and foremost, successful interactive reparations provide opportunities to develop self- and interactive regulatory skills useful for coping with stress [1, 12, 13]. In interactions characterized by typical rates of reparation, the infant learns how to use effectively coping and communicative strategies that facilitate the reparation and in turn reinforce his coping and interactive skills. Microanalytic data reveal that the mean duration of reparation during the reunion episode of the FFSF is significantly correlated with infant cortisol reactivity [41], suggesting that quicker interactive repair provides better physiological stress regulation in infants [29].

The repeated successful transformation of mismatches with their associated negative affect into matches with positive affect establishes a positive affective core [42] and promotes the development of a sense of efficacy, as well as a representation of interactions as reparable, and of the caregiver as reliable and trustworthy. By contrast, repeated failures in reparations cause problematic effects and negative developmental outcomes. In that case, self-regulation becomes the predominant goal of the infants, at the expense of interactive regulation. A self-directed style of regulatory behavior aims to control negative affects and hampers the infant's engagement in interactions with the world of people, things, and themselves. Moreover, repeated failure of reparation leads infants to establish a negative affective core primarily characterized by sadness and anger. As demonstrated in the interactions of depressed mothers and their infants, the process of reparatory failure disrupts the dyad's capacity to mutually regulate the interaction [21], and the infant develops a representation of her- or himself as less effective and helpless and simultaneously a representation of their caregiver as untrustworthy and unresponsive.

3.3 Implication for Psychopathology

Dyadic regulatory processes have important implication for the development of psychopathology. As hypothesized by DiCorcia and Tronick [43], everyday stressors, especially micro stressors such as mismatches, sculpt the regulatory systems and lead to resilience or vulnerability depending on the quality of their resolution. Ham and Tronick [44] found that effective behavioral regulation promotes better infant regulation at other, physiologic regulatory levels, such as the HPA axis (hypothalamic–pituitary–adrenal axis).

Even apparently minor maladaptive interactive patterns (e.g., lack of typical levels of reparatory contingency) can have long-term effects on child development because of their chronic reiteration and self-amplification. When self- and interactive regulation are not balanced and self-regulation in the service of maintaining self-organization becomes the predominant goal, the infant's vulnerability to psychopathology is heightened. Such disruptions of mutually regulated patterns are often associated with problematic or derailed outcomes in the infants [14, 45].

Potential maladaptive regulatory processes have been studied in the presence of infant, parental, and familial risk factors. For example, interactive reparatory processes of miscoordinated dyadic states that characterize typical infant-parent interactions are disturbed in dyads where the mother is anxious and/or depressed [1, 46–50]. Specifically, research on postpartum depression has shown that infants of depressed mothers were more likely to show more self-comforting and self-directed regulatory behaviors, as well as less interactive regulatory behaviors. Similarly, Cohn and Tronick [51] described a specific pattern of disengagement and sad effect in the infants of withdrawn-depressed mothers. Furthermore, dyads with depressed mothers showed less coordination of positive matched states and longer latencies when repairing interactive mismatching states into positive matched states [52].

Deviations from typical interactive patterns were also observed in dyads with high-risk infants, drug-exposed infants, high levels of parental stress, and high levels of parental risk factors [53–55]. Patterns of negative affective exchanges have also been observed in dyads with cocaine-exposed infants, who show higher levels of mismatched engagement states compared to nonexposed dyads, including more negative engagement when the infants were in states of neutral engagement. Infants exposed to heavier levels of cocaine also showed more passive/withdrawn negative engagement and were more likely to engage in negative affective matching with their mothers, highlighting the critical role of prenatal cocaine exposure for infants' social and emotional development [56].

3.4 Meaning Making and States of Consciousness

A broader understanding of possible developmental pathways is supported by an open system dynamic perspective and the meaning-making processes of human beings. Bruner [57] initially argued that humans are meaning makers. Humans can be viewed as complex open psychobiological system that continuously work to gain a sense of their self in relation to the world of people and things. The meaning they make may be known, conscious, and symbolizable but also unknown and out of awareness (e.g., reactivity thresholds). These meanings are held in the individual's state of consciousness [38, 39, 58] that involves a multilevel cascade of meaning, both in and out of awareness—including emotions, purposes, intentions, thoughts, perceptions and actions, as well as biological goals, operating in every moment and on every component and process in the human system.

The meaning-making processes are complex: meaning is self-organized, private and regulated internally, and dyadically organized, shared, and regulated with others. When self-organized, meaning making is successful, new meanings are made, and the individual's state of consciousness changes and expands, increasing complexity and coherence. When meanings are dyadically organized, a dyadic state of consciousness emerges between individuals, which contains new co-created meanings that are incorporated by each individual into their own private state of consciousness [29]. Clearly, these dyadic states are more complex and more coherent than either partner's single state and have the potential to expand each partner's complexity and coherence.

The growth of states of consciousness is governed by principles from dynamic systems theory [57, 59–63]. All living systems require energy and information (meaning) from the world in order to maintain and increase a dynamic state of organization (a state of consciousness). The open systems (humans) become more coherent, complex, and integrated when they are successful in acquiring resources; thus, they remain as distant as possible from entropy and dissipation.

Especially infants and children have limited energy for self-organized meaning making, and when it is drained, they lose coherence of their state of consciousness. To overcome this limitation, the dyadic forms of meaning making and the dyadic state of consciousness are crucial. Each person uses behaviors and other cues to exchange intentions, affects, states of mind, cognitive meaning, and the like with another individual to maintain and increase their coherence. This, in turn, leads to an emotional experience of expansion, wholeness, and growth. As Tronick stated [38, 39] the creation of new meaning with another person is the constitutive process for forming and growing relationships: "individuals create something new together and consequentially feel connected to each other, and this connection is unique because each relationship makes new meaning in different ways" ([39], p. 7).

In infancy, meaning-making processes are determined by the qualities of infants' environment as well as their unique internal characteristics. Disruption or distortion of meaning making can lead to developmental difficulties. A simple analogy is to think of meaning as the food provisioned by the caretaker feeding the infant. Though the infant has a capacity for self-feeding, feeding is a dyadic process in which the caretaker scaffolds the infants' resources. The nutrients are required by the body to grow and for physical activity, for the infant to become a more complex system. If the dyadic system fails to access needed nutrients, the system decomposes.

When infants interact with a responsive and reliable caregiver, they exchange meanings and (both) gain in complexity and coherence, which in turn shapes their ongoing engagement with the world of people, things, and themselves and influences their meaning-making process. As a consequence, they have gained resources to allow them to become more flexible and capable of reorganizing to cope with perturbations. In contrast, infants who continuously interact with unresponsive caregivers experience states of disorganization that undermine their meaning-making ability. As a consequence, they lose complexity and flexibility and may be more vulnerable to the effects of later perturbations [40]. Effectively, the infant who typically experiences failed reparation develops a sense of failure and wariness in their sense of self in the world.

3.5 Co-creation, Uniqueness of Relationship, and Implicit Relational Knowing

A dynamic systems framework for the MRM helps us to understand early parent-infant interactions, the complexity of infant's development, and the formation of individuals' ways of being in relation to the world of people and things and in relation to his or her self. The term "co-creation" implies that the dyadic regulation—not only between mother and infant but in every relationship—of a communicative exchange is an unpredictable and variable or messy process which creates continuous changes in the relationship that sculpt its uniqueness and specificity.

Sander [34] observed evidence of early specificity (uniqueness) in the interctions between infant and the caregiver by the end of the first week of life. He hypothesized that the regulation of the mother-infant pair becomes more and more specific for every dyad and leads to the distinctive and idiosyncratic characteristics of exchange. Sander added that "This specificity can be thought of as a complex gestalt involving timing, sequence, cue, etc., a complex in which the familiar sequence of caretaking activities over the awake span is carried out" ([34], p. 22). Hinde [64] also emphasized the uniqueness of relationships when he described, in contrast to the limited categories of attachment theory, different dimensions of relationships, such as their intensity, their rhythm, their intimacy, their attunement, the quality of what the infant and mother actually do together, and how they use particular gestures and facial expressions [65].

To use an analogy, parent-infant pairs can be seen as couples dancing. We could think about the different kinds of dance that couples perform together—like tango, two-step, waltz—as well as how differently they perform even the same dances—i.e., with different degrees of intensity, coordination, and rhythm. These features make the dancing couples different from one another. In an analogous way, infant-parent relationships are as uniquely different from one another as are couples dancing together. They show unique and specific ways of "being together" which arise from a dynamic process of co-creation. In this way, relationships are unique and have unique effects on each of the individuals within them, and over time, their way of being together becomes highly specific and increasingly differentiated from others.

Unique ways of being together are procedurally and implicitly generated. Infant research has highlighted how infants make sense of the world and of their relationship with others through implicit messages related to nonverbal cues, body movements, sensation, affect, and expectations (e.g., [1, 66–68]). Therefore, the interactional experiences are organized and held by the infant in an implicit representation that is nonsymbolic, nonverbal, procedural, and primarily out of awareness [69].

These representations, referred to as implicit relational knowing (IRK), emerge from the daily reiteration of co-created moment-by-moment interactions [5, 6, 65, 70]. IRK refers to "representations of the ways individuals relate to one another that are outside both focal attention and conscious verbal experience" ([70], p. 905). In other words, it is the implicit knowledge that two interactants—infant and adult—have about their ways of being together, how to proceed, and *do* things with the other that gradually arises in the interactional processes that take place between baby and caretakers [1, 4].

The IRK is an important domain of implicit psychobiological memory processes. It is different from other forms of procedural knowledge, such as how to ride a bicycle or drive a car, because it emerges and grows in the dynamic and mutual exchange of affect and relational intentions between infant/child and others. The implicit memory has a special regulatory function, which acts in an automatic and unconscious way. It is not only cognitive, in the way that neuroscientists think of cognitive/brain processes, but also affective and interactive. The BCPSG emphasized that IRK does not contain semantic knowledge and is thought to continue to operate implicitly throughout life and, over time, though it can be expanded into more conscious, articulated, coherent, and complex states in collaboration with another person, especially during therapeutic relationships.

Implicit procedures and knowing are specific and unique to each relationship the child experiences. An example of how uniqueness in relationship is generated can be seen in the course of all the repetitive activities related to specific time and context of an infant's and parent's daily life together (sleep, waking up, feeding, diapering, playing, changing, etc.). These "time activity contexts" ([65], p. 479) are co-experienced and mutually regulated by the infant and the caregivers and over time develop a specificity of temporal organization and sequential relations that also differs from other time activity contexts regulated by another dyad. The extent to which different relationships have different numbers of different time-activity contexts is referred to by Tronick [65] as "thickness." Thickness refers to the ways of being together that are generated in the many time activity-contexts that are experienced repeatedly often on a daily basis. Importantly, the thickness of different relations varies from one relationship to the next.

3.6 Forms of Implicit Relational Knowing

The co-creative communicative process leads to unique characteristics of the interaction both at a micro-temporal level through micro-affective mutual regulation and at a macro-level through the generation of IRK about how to be together [4, 5, 65]. IRK has various forms. One form of IRK is micro-interactive and constitutes an integration of the repeated relational micro-interactive moves of the dyad [69]. This micro-interactive knowing comprises the features and details of different exchanges, such as unique games played by the infant with someone (i.e., mother, father, or others). Clearly behavioral routines such as games can manifest themselves in several dyads but will have different meaning and form in each relationship and specific context. For example, the infant wrinkling his nose with the father could be part of a face-to-face game and means "let's start to play!" whereas with the mother may carry the meaning "I don't like what we are doing, let's stop!" Tronick [3] has hypothesized that much of the IRK generated at this level may not be transferable to other relationships, because the meaning of specific behaviors between two persons may remain exclusive to a particular relationship, that is cryptic to other individuals.

The second kind of IRK is meta-procedural, and it is related with how two persons are able to "work out" things together (e.g., how we repair mismatches).

Compared to the micro-interactive form, it has to do with a more general way of "working together," no matter what the content of the mismatch is. For example, the infant and the caretaker could share the IRK that "we can move from a mutual negative state to a positive state." The variety of meta-procedural knowing generates ways of feeling about one's self in relationship, such as "I feel my efficacy," "I feel trustful," or "I feel helpless" and "I feel hopeless." Although they are specific to a particular relationship, contrary to micro-interactive knowing, these feelings can be transferable and affect other kind of relationships.

3.7 Unique Interactive Patterns: How IRK Procedures Are Used to Overcome a Social Stress

Despite the uniqueness of relationships being generally acknowledged [3], there is a lack of research that pays attention to the individual differences of the interactive regulatory patterns which lead to stable and unique dyadic characteristics. Research studies on mother-infant exchanges in typically developing populations have primarily focused on mutual regulatory processes, their variation, and development, in order to understand the organization of the interaction and to explore potential maladaptive regulatory patterns in the presence of infant, parental, and familial risk factors. However, this search for generalities regarding the organization or structure of relationships needs to be balanced with the recognition of the specificity, uniqueness, differentiation, and complexity of the features of human relationships [71].

It is now well established that uniqueness in relationships emerges out of mutual regulated co-creative interactive processes that generate unique implicit and procedural knowing of "how we are together." Starting from this basic finding, the study of the ways in which unique mother-infant relationships are generated needs to focus on dyadic regulatory processes including IRK.

Consistent with this premise, we explored and described what we think of as unique implicit relational knowing (UIRK) and examined if these unique behaviors had effects on the infant regulation of the interaction. UIRKs were hypothesized to be an expression of the infant's IRK of how to interact with his/her mother in unique ways.

To examine the occurrence and function of UIRKs, we used the FFSF [12, 13]. Infant behavior was observed and coded at two different ages, 6 and 11 months, in two different episodes, Play and Still-Face.

Infants' reaction to the Still-Faced mother has been widely explored, and an abundant literature on FFSF paradigm [35, 36] reveals that infants react to the Still-Face with behaviors aimed at eliciting mothers' return to playful interaction. Most infants might use what can be thought of as typical eliciting behaviors (TEBs), such as smiles, pick-me-up gestures, "fake" cries, or other gestural signals. However, we sought to explore whether infants might also use UIRKs as communicative and coping strategies, to elicit the mother's response. That is, do they utilize unique interactive behaviors (e.g., finger games, arms gestures, etc.) seen during their play with the mother to elicit her attention during the Still-Face? Thus, we looked at the Play episodes to identify UIRKs, as well as TEBs and then at the Still-Face episode to see if the infant used UIRKs and/or TEBs to elicit the mother in a different context and with a different goal.

The differentiation between TEBs and UIRKs is not as easy to determine as it might appear. What we categorize as a TEB, an action seen in many infants which seems to be part of the neurotypical developmental repertoire of eliciting behaviors (e.g., pick-me-up gestures, pointing), nonetheless might be a unique behavior specific to a particular dyad. For example, an UIRK during the Still-Face episode might be one in which the infant reproduces part of an interactive game—such as mutual clapping—played with the mother in the Play episode, by holding up and clapping her hands while looking at the mother. The clapping is something they did together in the Play episode, and it is part of their own interactive repertoire and easy to see during the SF episode. However, a pointing gesture might be seen as a TEB because many infants use it, even though it might actually also be a UIRKs in a particular dyad (i.e., the pointing gesture could express a mother-infant unique way of playing together when the infant may use it in the interactions with his mother but may not use it when he is playing with other people). Our approach to this categorization dilemma was conservative. We determined a set of behaviors we categorized as TEBs for 6- and 11-month-old babies (see Table 3.1). These behaviors occur

Table 3.1 Description of the typical eliciting behavior of 6- and 11-month-old babies occurring in the Still-Face episode

Typical eliciting behavior	Description
Positive vocalization	The infant vocalizes in a positive manner (laughing, babbling, squealing, etc.)
Negative vocalization	The infant vocalizes in a negative manner (fret, whimper, growl, protest, fussy, shrill, etc.)
Neutral vocalization	The infant vocalizes in a neutral manner
Cry	The infant cries, his/her eyes are scrunched up, the mouth must be open, and there is an increase in pitch of the voice
Smile	The infant displays a smile face with upturned mouth, crinkly eyes, and raised cheeks
Raspberry	The infant sticks out his/her tongue and makes a jeering sound made by vibrating lips
Grimace	The infant displays a grimace face
Reaching	The infant moves his/her arms or legs in an organized manner in the direction of the mother
Pointing	The infant indicates with his index finger a point
Leaning	The infant leans his/her trunk and head toward the mother
Oscillate head	The infant swing his/her head repeatedly from one side to the other
Oscillate trunk	The infant swing his/her head and trunk back and forth in the infant seat
Shake arms	The infant flails his/her arms
Kick feet	The infant kicks his/her feet repeatedly
Wave hand	The infant waves one or both hands in the air

Note: All these behaviors were coded with a gaze criterion: the infant's eyes must be oriented toward the adult's face. Each of these categories can co-occur (they are not mutually exclusive)

frequently and are noted in the literature as eliciting behavior [22]. We disregarded the possibility that they might actually be unique in a particular dyad (e.g., "we point together").

Thus, to be a UIRK, a behavior had to be seen in the Play episode as distinct and dyadic, and then the infant had to display components of it during the Still-Face episode. Furthermore, if the infants displayed a particular behavior to elicit mother's attention during the Still-Face (e.g., clapping) that didn't occur in the play interactions, this behavior too was not counted as a UIRK. Effectively, this approach results in an under-accounting of UIRKs.

The aims of the study were (1) to observe if infants used components of their interactive play behaviors as UIRKs during the Still-Face episode to elicit the mother's return to interactive play and (2) to examine, in two different age groups (6-and 11 month), if UIRKs were displayed. Our hypothesis was that both groups of infants, during the Still-Face, would utilize an UIRK with the intention of reinstating their way of being and playing together, as an expression of the infants' IRK of what we do together.

Two different groups of mother and their infants were observed during the FFSF paradigm. The first group was composed of 78 mothers and their 6-month-old infants. The second group was composed of 41 mothers and their 11-month-old infants. After being videotaped in FFSF, independent coders coded the Play and the Still-Face episodes of the paradigm for the presence of UIRKs. In the Still-Face, the frequency of UIRKS and TEBS was coded. The infants' UIRKs coded during the Still-Face are described in Table 3.2.

All of the infants at both ages displayed UIRKs in the Play episode. Only 12 11-month-old babies displayed UIRKs (29.3% of the infants) during the Still-Face episode, whereas no UIRKs were observed in the 6-month-old infants (see Fig. 3.1). When comparing UIRKs in the Still-Face across age groups, as would be expected, Chi-square revealed a significant difference between the two groups, χ^2 [72, 73] ($N = 119$) = 25.390, $p < 0.001$.

These findings have several implications for infants' development and meaning-making processes and how forms of IRK are co-created and give shape to uniqueness in the relationships.

Table 3.2 Description of the unique dyadic interactive behaviors (UIRKs) of 11 month olds and count of infants who display UIRKs

Unique IRK	Description	Number
Clapping hands	The infant strikes the palms of the hands together	6
Tapping hands	The infant taps his/her palms of the hands on the middle bar of the infant's seat	1
Peek-a-boo	The infant places the palms of the hands peripheral to both eyes	1
Total		**8**

Note: All these behaviors were coded with a gaze criterion: the infant's eyes must be oriented toward the adult's face. Each of these categories can co-occur (they are not mutually exclusive)

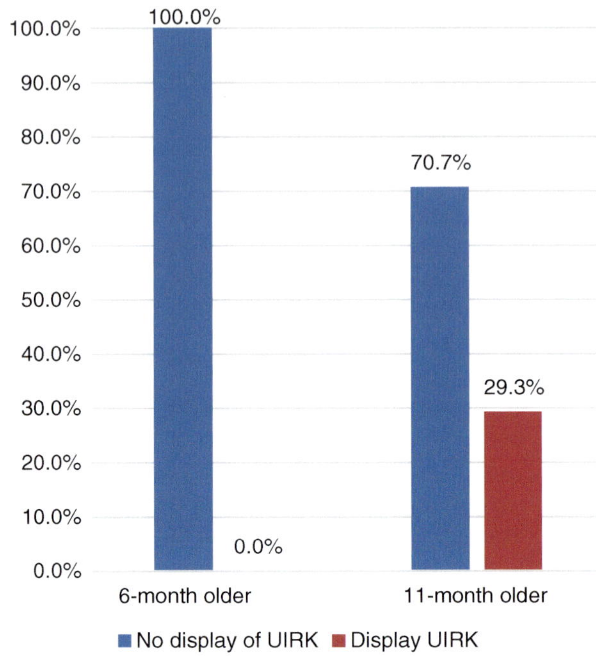

Fig. 3.1 Frequency of the occurrence of UIRKs among 6- and 11-month older

A primary consideration concerns the evidence that both 6- and 11-month-olds engage in UIRKs during the Play episode; that is, there are established dyadic interactions between the infant and the parent at both ages. The finding of this type of interaction is not surprising but confirms findings from longitudinal studies that reveal a clear age-related transformation of the infant's motives through the middle of the first year [74–82]. These studies show that infants gradually develop an intricate, precise, and selective coordination with the mother's expressions of communication and dramatized actions of play, which become more repetitive and increasingly richly modulated and rhythmically patterned [20].

The finding that UIRKs were not observed in any of the 6-month-old babies in the Still-Face episode, while 11-month-old do use UIRKS in it, points to an important early developmental change between 6 and 11 months of age. By the first year of life, infants develop more coherent socio-emotional, cognitive, and motor capacities. The capacity of older infants to utilize UIRKs purposefully to elicit a response from an unresponsive Still-Faced mother demonstrates a form of mutually adjusted intentionality that is not yet developed at 6 months of age. That is, 6-month-olds have interactive routines with their mothers, but in a new and unfamiliar situation, the Still-Face, they are unable to use them with a different intent, which the older infants can do. This developmental change is consistent with the evidence of secondary intersubjectivity of older infants [83] compared to the primary intersubjectivity of younger infants (1980; [84]). Trevarthen's secondary intersubjectivity develops around 9 months. It is a new form of cooperative intersubjectivity, a mutually adjusted intentionality of joint attention and a fluent person-person-object triangular awareness.

Further consideration needs to be given regarding the presence of UIRKs among the group of older infants, who also show evidence of IRK which are generated through repetition of an activity in their play interactions. Infants' UIRKs are exemplars of IRK, both at micro-interactive and meta-procedural levels. At a micro-interactive level, mother-infant UIRKs are found in the Play episode, in the details of their unique and intimate play with its specific timing and degree of rhythm and intensity, qualities that may reflect intimacy. At a meta-procedural level, infants' use of UIRKs during the Still-Face shows infants' implicit knowledge that "If I play this way, you will react and engage in playing with me in a positive way" that is also an expression of infants' sense of mastery and efficacy.

Another key aspect of these processes is the emergence of meaning for the infant and the formation of dyadic state of consciousness [2]. We observed that infants at 11 months of age use the behavior developed with an intention such as "let's play this way together" and then utilize it in another context with a different intent—"stop being unresponsive and play with me!". This shows infant's capacity to use a dyadic behavior learned in one context (Play) in another different context (Still-Faced mother) but with a different meaning and purpose (i.e., to capture mother's attention). It is also noteworthy that the older infants engage in the UIRK even without the mother engaging in her role.

From the perspective of the dyadic expansion of consciousness model [2, 70], an implication of UIRKs is that when mother and infant play together, a new dyadic intersubjective state of shared consciousness is generated, with the potential to expand each partner's state of consciousness. Each partner expands its state incorporating elements of the other's state of consciousness in a new form of meaning, which increases each partner's socio-affective complexity and coherence. According to this model, mother-infant UIRKs during Play Game can be seen as a shared consciousness, what Sander [34] called a moment of meeting that leads to the expansion of each partner's state of consciousness. Put another way, we might see UIRK as a result of an early presymbolic neurosomatic internalization process of making meaning that shows that the infant has interiorized the regulatory interaction [67]. This view of the origins of internalization in the first year is developed from an interactive model that view internalization as based on what "both the organism and the environment construct" ([67], p. 155). As suggested by Beebe and Lachmann [67], "both partners bring to the interaction organized behavior and mutually construct modes of regulating their joint activity. These dyadic modes include mutual as well as self-regulation. The expectation and representation of the dyadic modes of regulation constitute the internal organization" (p. 156).

Given these developmental observations, inferences about the clinical situation can be drawn. What happens if the mutually regulation processes are chronically disrupted and self-regulation becomes the predominant goal for the infants? When dyadic intersubjective states of shared consciousness fail to be generated, the way infants make meaning of themselves and of the world is undermined. As a consequence, they lose complexity and flexibility and do not develop a sense of mastery and efficacy. In these cases, it is possible to hypothesize that through the micro-interactive process, infants learn the meta-message that "It is useless to try engaging with you when you are unresponsive!" and do not develop complex strategy such as UIRKs.

This research contributes to the understanding of IRK as a form of procedural knowledge that arises in the interactional processes between infants and caregivers. Further studies could clarify the process of the formation of IRK in the interaction and also the concept of transferability and non-transferability of unique features of the interaction to other relationships. Other questions could be examined, such as: Would infants utilize the same UIRKs learned with one familiar person as a strategy to repair a prolonged mismatched state with another person? Furthermore, what could be observed in high-risk mother-infant interaction and how does IRK develop in that situation?

There are implications for clinical work with adults. One is that in the transference, UIRK may play a critical role. The patient may be using a behavior or way of being from their early experience that has an intent that is far from obvious. In a way, it is an implicit enactment, but it is obscure to the therapist and may further disrupt their therapeutic work. It is of course possible that the therapist engages in UIRKs in a similar fashion with equally disruptive effects. UIRKs may also be characteristic ways individuals with personality disorders engage others. They engage in an UIRK but, as in the Still-Face, in failing to get back what they expected, they respond with fury, disengagement, and a demeaning attitude toward the other. Of course, it generates a feeling of nonexistence in the other. One cannot avoid the implication that adults who were children of depressed parents developed and now utilize UIRKs that function to generate past depressed ways of being together. Aside from the impacts and problems they create in everyday living and being with others, the therapeutic problem is that they can be hard to identify and detect. We expect that one way they can become known in therapy is not unlike the reaction of the infant to the Still-Face; that is, they generate confusion, then frustration and anger, and finally helplessness and a state of consciousness that feels senseless.

The last implication of the findings on the differences between the 6 months old and the 11 months old warrants fuller consideration. In general terms, in most therapies and developmental, especially psychodynamic theories, the earliest aspects of past experience are thought to still affect the present, in some implicit form or another. One way to think about the past being brought into the present is in terms of transference and/or in some ways in terms of enactments by the neurosomatic meaning-making processes that create IRK. However, the finding suggests another possibility. Early dyadic experience prior to 6 months or so, which lead to the development IRK may in fact not be "bringable" into the present. The findings suggest that IRK formed in the first 6 months is limited to occurring only in the actual early interaction with a particular person. The earliest IRK is not functional in other contexts; it does not generalize to other relationships. Where this constrains the case, we would need to revise our views of the effects of early experience, including trauma. We also would have to revise the idea from attachment and psychodynamic theories that the mother (primary caretaker) relationship is prototypical for later relationships because the earliest prototypical IRK may not be in a transferable form. Moreover, in therapy, we would have to change our stance in relation to patients claiming to know or to be able to experience these earliest of relational experiences. Most importantly we need to change how we think about the role of a patient's history.

3.8 Conclusion

Interactive regulation is a key concept to understand relational processes between humans. In this chapter, we described the mutual ongoing regulation of child-parent relationship in the early years, focusing on implicit relational knowing that arises in the interactional processes.

While the interaction unfolds, the infant comes to recognize, remember, and expect specific patterns of regulation that shape the uniqueness of his or her relationship. The infant-parent dyadic system creates new forms of meaning for each partner, which are incorporated into memory, with or without consciousness, increasing each partner's socio-affective complexity. The memories that young children have of the parent are neurosomatic body based and interactive so that the earliest mental representations consist of the ways the parent did things with the child.

But why we have felt the need to study and explore how IRK are generated? Why IRK seems to be so important for the infant's organization? IRK as well as UIRKs permeate infants and likely adults' ways of being in the world, and this suggests that interventions cannot refrain from taking into account aspects of dyadic organization as well as IRK shaped in the past but operating in the present.

More research on IRK and UIRKS would add to our understanding of how to identify ones that arrive from the past and distort the present. Importantly, greater understanding of these processes would aid in the development of techniques for changing them in effective and security enhancing ways for moving forward in the therapy given how deeply rooted in the past and in our neurosomatic meaning-making systems the IRK may be.

It would be interesting to verify the hypothesis that, as it happens between the mother and child, also the analyst and the patient develop increasingly unique implicit relational knowing about one another and about their relationship. This happens in time and over the course of their being together. Future research study on implicit relational knowing in the context of therapy could also evaluate if repeated patient-therapist interactions generate changes in the patient's (and in the therapist) implicit relational knowing, with the possibility for new and more coherent ways of being with the therapist and, in turn, with other.

To conclude, it is clear that the study of mutual regulatory processes and the meanings made out of it during development have great importance for our understanding of infants and children, their earliest relationships, and for our understanding and practice of therapy.

Acknowledgment A version of this paper was presented by E. Tronick and made possible by support from the *Reiss-Greenberg Chair, an endowed chair of the Reiss-Davis Child Study Center & Institute, Los Angeles, January 2017.* Additional support came from the Bial Foundation, National Institute of Child Development, and the National Science Foundation, E.Tronick PI.

References

1. Tronick E (1989) Emotions and emotional communication in infants. Am Psychol 44(2):112–119
2. Tronick E (2001) Emotional connections and dyadic consciousness in infant-mother and patient-therapist interactions: commentary on paper by Frank M. Lachmann. Psychoanal Dialogues 11(2):187–194
3. Tronick E (2003) "Of course all relationships are unique": how co-creative processes generate unique mother–infant and patient–therapist relationships and change other relationships. Psychoanal Inq 23(3):473–491
4. Stern DN, Sander LW, Nahum JP, Harrison AM, Lyons-Ruth K, Morgan AC et al. (The Boston Change Process Study Group)(1998) Non-interpretive mechanisms in psychoanalytic therapy: the 'something more' than interpretation. Int J Psychoanal 79(5):903–921
5. The Boston Change Process Study Group (2002) Explicating the implicit: the local level and the microprocess of change in the analytic situation. Int J Psychoanal 83(5):1051–1062
6. The Boston Change Process Study Group (2005) The "something more" than interpretation revisited: sloppiness and co-creativity in the psychoanalytic encounter. J Am Psychoanal Assoc 53(3):693–729
7. Tronick E (2002) A model of infant mood states and Sandarian affective waves. Psyechoanal Dialogues 12(1):73–99
8. Tronick E, Als H, Adamson L (1979) Structure of early face-to-face communicative interactions. In: Bullowa M (ed) Before speech. Cambridge University Press, Cambridge, pp 349–371
9. Beebe B, Stern DN (1977) Engagement-disengagement and early object experiences. In: Freedman N, Grand S (eds) Communicative structures and psychic structures. Springer, New York, pp 35–55
10. Brazelton TB, Koslowski B, Main M (1974) The origins of reciprocity: the early mother-infant interaction. In: Lewis M, Rosenblum L (eds) The effect of the infant on its caregiver. Wiley, New York, pp 49–76
11. Gianino A, Tronick EZ (1988) The mutual regulation model: the infant's self and interactive regulation and coping and defensive capacities. In: Field T, McCabe P, Schneiderman N (eds) Stress and coping. Erlbaum, Hillsdale, NJ, pp 47–68
12. Tronick E, Als H, Adamson L, Wise S, Brazelton TB (1978) The infant's response to entrapment between contradictory messages in face-to-face interaction. J Am Acad Child Psychiatry 17(1):1–13
13. Tronick E, Brazelton TB, Als H (1978) The structure of face-to-face interaction and its developmental functions. Sign Lang Stud 18(1):1–16
14. Beeghly M, Tronick E (2011) Early resilience in the context of parent–infant relationships: a social developmental perspective. Curr Probl Pediatr Adolesc Health Care 41(7):197–201
15. Cohn JF, Tronick EZ (1983) Three-month-old infants' reaction to simulated maternal depression. Child Dev 54(1):185–193
16. Tronick E (1980) On the primacy of social skills. Exceptional Infant 4:144–158
17. Trevarthen C (1974) The psychobiology of speech development. In: Lenneberg EH (ed) Language and brain: developmental aspects: neurosciences research program bulletin, vol 12. Neuroscience Research Program, Boston, MA, pp 570–585
18. Trevarthen C (1979) Communication and cooperation in early infancy. A description of primary intersubjectivity. In: Bullowa M (ed) Before speech: the beginning of human communication. Cambridge University Press, London, pp 321–347
19. Trevarthen C (1998) The concept and foundations of infant intersubjectivity. In: Bräten S (ed) Intersubjective communication and emotion in early ontogeny. Cambridge University Press, Cambridge, pp 15–46
20. Trevarthen C, Aitken KJ (2001) Infant intersubjectivity: research, theory, and clinical applications. J Child Psychol Psychiatry 42(1):3–48

21. Tronick E (2009) Social interaction. In: Haith M, Benson J (eds) Social and emotional development in infancy and early childhood. Elsevier, San Diego, CA, pp 429–436
22. Weinberg MK, Tronick EZ (1994) Beyond the face: an empirical study of infant affective configurations of facial, vocal, gestural, and regulatory behaviors. Child Dev 65(5):1503–1515
23. Brazelton TB (1974) Does the neonate shape his environment? Birth Defects Orig Artic Ser 10(2):131–140
24. Field TM (1977) Effects of early separation, interactive deficits, and experimental manipulations on infant-mother face-to-face interaction. Child Dev 48(3):763–771
25. McCall RB, McGhee PE (1977) The discrepancy hypothesis of attention and affect in infants. In: Užgiris I, Weizmann F (eds) The structuring of experience. Springer, New York, pp 179–210
26. Spitz RA (1965) The first year of life: a psychoanalytic study of normal and deviant development of object relations. International University Press, New York
27. Stern DN (1974) The goal and structure of mother-infant play. J Am Acad Child Psychiatry 13(3):402–421
28. Stern DN (1977) The first relationship. Harvard University Press, Cambridge, MA
29. Tronick E (2007) The neurobehavioral and social-emotional development of infants and children. Norton, New York, NY
30. Tronick EZ, Olson K, Rosenberg R, Bohne L, Lu J, Lester BM (2004) Normative neurobehavioral performance of healthy infants on the neonatal intensive care unit network neurobehavioral scale. Pediatrics 113(3):676–678
31. Beebe B, Lachmann FM (2015) The expanding world of Edward Tronick. Psychoanal Inq 35(4):328–336
32. Beebe B, Jaffe J, Markese S, Buck K, Chen H, Cohen P, Feldstein S (2010) The origins of 12-month attachment: a microanalysis of 4-month mother–infant interaction. Attach Hum Dev 12(1–2):3–141
33. Jaffe J, Beebe B, Feldstein S, Crown CL, Jasnow MD, Rochat P, Stern DN (2001) Rhythms of dialogue in infancy: coordinated timing in development. Monogr Soc Res Child Dev 66(2):i–149
34. Sander L (1977) The regulation of exchange in the infant-caretaker system and some aspects of the context-content relationship. Interact Convers Dev Lang 5(40):579–593
35. Adamson LB, Frick JE (2003) The still face: a history of a shared experimental paradigm. Infancy 4(4):451–473
36. Mesman J, van IJzendoorn MH, Bakermans-Kranenburg MJ (2009) The many faces of the still-face paradigm: a review and meta-analysis. Dev Rev 29(2):120–162
37. Cohn JF, Tronick EZ (1988) Mother-infant face-to-face interaction: influence is bidirectional and unrelated to periodic cycles in either partner's behavior. Dev Psychol 24(3):386
38. Tronick E (2008) Multilevel meaning making and dyadic expansion of consciousness theory: the emotional and the polymorphic polysemic flow of meaning. In: Fosha D, Siegel DJ, Solomon M (eds) The healing power of emotion: affective neuroscience, development, and clinical practice. Norton, New York, NY, pp 86–110
39. Tronick E (2008) Meaning making and the dyadic expansion of consciousness model. Festschrift in honor of Arnold Modell, Boston Psychoanalytic Society, March, 28
40. Tronick E, Beeghly M (2011) Infants' meaning-making and the development of mental health problems. Am Psychol 66(2):107
41. Müller M, Zietlow AL, Tronick E, Reck C (2015) What dyadic reparation is meant to do: an association with infant cortisol reactivity. Psychopathology 48(6):386–399
42. Emde RN (1983) The prerepresentational self and its affective core. Psychoanal Study Child 38(1):165–192
43. DiCorcia JA, Tronick E (2011) Quotidian resilience: exploring mechanisms that drive resilience from a perspective of everyday stress and coping. Neurosci Biobehav Rev 35(7):1593–1602
44. Ham J, Tronick E (2009) Relational psychophysiology: lessons from mother–infant physiology research on dyadically expanded states of consciousness. Psychother Res 19(6):619–632

45. Deater-Deckard K, Petrill SA (2004) Parent–child dyadic mutuality and child behavior problems: an investigation of gene–environment processes. J Child Psychol Psychiatry 45(6):1171–1179
46. Beebe B, Lachmann FM, Markese S, Buck KA, Bahrick LE, Chen H et al (2012) On the origins of disorganized attachment and internal working models: paper II. An empirical microanalysis of 4-month mother–infant interaction. Psychoanal Dialogues 22(3):352–374
47. Beebe B, Steele M, Jaffe J, Buck KA, Chen H, Cohen P et al (2011) Maternal anxiety symptoms and mother–infant self-and interactive contingency. Infant Ment Health J 32(2):174–206
48. Goodman SH, Brand SR (2009) Infants of depressed mothers. In: Zeanah CH Jr (ed) Handbook of infant mental health. Guildford Press, New York, pp 153–170
49. Tronick E, Field TM (1986) Maternal depression and infant disturbance. Jossey-Bass, San Francisco, CA
50. Tronick E, Reck C (2009) Infants of depressed mothers. Harv Rev Psychiatry 17(2):147–156
51. Cohn JF, Tronick E (1989) Specificity of infants' response to mothers' affective behavior. J Am Acad Child Adolesc Psychiatry 28(2):242–248
52. Reck C, Noe D, Stefenelli U, Fuchs T, Cenciotti F, Stehle E et al (2011) Interactive coordination of currently depressed inpatient mothers and their infants during the postpartum period. Infant Ment Health J 32(5):542–562
53. Beeghly M, Tronick EZ (1994) Effects of prenatal exposure to cocaine in early infancy: toxic effects on the process of mutual regulation. Infant Ment Health J 15(2):158–175
54. Lester BM, Boukydis CF, Twomey JE (2000) Maternal substance abuse and child outcome. In: Zeanah CH Jr (ed) Handbook of infant mental health. Guildford Press, New York, pp 161–175
55. Strathearn L, Mayes LC (2010) Cocaine addiction in mothers. Ann N Y Acad Sci 1187(1):172–183
56. Tronick EZ, Messinger DS, Weinberg MK, Lester BM, LaGasse L, Seifer R et al (2005) Cocaine exposure is associated with subtle compromises of infants' and mothers' social emotional behavior and dyadic features of their interaction in the face-to-face still-face paradigm. Dev Psychol 41(5):711–722
57. Bruner JS (1990) Acts of meaning. Harvard University Press, Cambridge, MA
58. Tronick E (2005) Why is connection with others so critical? The formation of dyadic states of consciousness and the expansion of individuals' states of consciousness: coherence governed selection and the co-creation of meaning out of messy meaning making. In: Nadel J, Muir D (eds) Emotional development: recent research advances. Oxford University Press, New York, NY, pp 293–315
59. Fogel A (2006) Dynamic systems research on interindividual communication: the transformation of meaning-making. J Dev Processes 1(1):7–30
60. Greenspan SI (2008) A dynamic developmental model of mental health and mental illness. In: Fogel A, King B, Shanker S (eds) Human development in the twenty-first century: visionary ideas from systems scientists. Cambridge University Press, New York, pp 157–175
61. Prigogine I, Stengers I (1984) Order out of chaos: man's new dialogue with nature. Bantam Books, New York
62. Seligman S (2005) Dynamic systems theories as a metaframework for psychoanalysis. Psychoanal Dialogues 15(2):285–319
63. Smith LB, Thelen E (2003) Development as a dynamic system. Trends Cogn Sci 7(8):343–348
64. Hinde RA (1979) Towards understanding relationships. Academic Press, London
65. Tronick E (2002) The increasing differentiation and non-transferabilty ways of being together. The primary attachment is specific, not prototypical. J Infant Child Adolesc Psychother 2(4):47–60
66. Ainsworth MD, Blehar MC, Waters E, Wall S (1978) Patterns of attachment: a psychological study of the strange situation. Erlbaum, Hillsdale, NY

67. Beebe B, Lachmann FM (1994) Representation and internalization in infancy: three principles of salience. Psychoanal Psychol 11(2):127
68. Montirosso R, Tronick E, Morandi F, Ciceri F, Borgatti R (2013) Four-month-old infants' long-term memory for a stressful social event. PLoS One 8(12):e82277
69. Tronick EZ, Bruschweiler-Stern N, Harrison AM, Lyons-Ruth K, Morgan AC, Nahum JP et al (1998) Dyadically expanded states of consciousness and the process of therapeutic change. Infant Ment Health J 19(3):290–299
70. Tronick E (1998) Interventions that effect change in psychotherapy: a model based on infant research. Infant Ment Health J 19(3):277–279
71. Hinde RA (1995) A suggested structure for a science of relationships. Personal Relationships 2(1):1–15
72. Fisher RA (1922) On the interpretation of χ 2 from contingency tables, and the calculation of P. J R Statist Soc 85(1):87–94
73. Pearson K (1900) X. On the criterion that a given system of deviations from the probable in the case of a correlated system of variables is such that it can be reasonably supposed to have arisen from random sampling. London Edinburgh Dublin Philosophical Magaz J Sci 50(302):157–175
74. Beebe B, Jaffe J, Feldstein S, Mays K, Alson D (1985) Interpersonal timing: the application of an adult dialogue model to mother-infant vocal and kinesic interactions. In: Field TM, Fox NA (eds) Social perception in infants. Ablex, Norwood, NJ, pp 217–247
75. Beebe B, Stern D, Jaffe J (1979) The kinesic rhythm of mother-infant interactions. In: Sieqman AW, Feldstein S (eds) Of speech and time: temporal speech patterns in interpersonal contexts. Laurence Erlbaum Associates, Mahwah, NJ, pp 23–34
76. Bruner JS, Sherwood V (1975) Peekaboo and the learning of rule structures. In: Bruner JS, Jolly A, Sylva K (eds) Play: its role in development and evolution. Penguin, Middlesex, pp 277–285
77. Fogel A (1977) Temporal organization in mother-infant face-to-face interaction. In: Schaffer HR (ed) Studies in mother-infant interaction. Academic Press, London, pp 119–152
78. Jasnow M, Feldstein S (1986) Adult-like temporal characteristics of mother-infant vocal interactions. Child Dev 57(3):754–761
79. Mayer NK, Tronick EZ (1985) Mothers' turn-giving signals and infant turn-taking in mother-infant interaction. In: Field TM, Fox NA (eds) Social perception in infants. Ablex, Norwood, NJ, pp 199–216
80. Ratner N, Bruner J (1978) Games, social exchange and the acquisition of language. J Child Lang 5(03):391–401
81. Stern DN (1971) A micro-analysis of mother-infant interaction: behavior regulating social contact between a mother and her 3 1/2-month-old twins. J Am Acad Child Psychiatry 10(3):501–517
82. Stern DN, Beebe B, Jaffe J, Bennett SL (1977) The infant's stimulus world during social interaction: a study of caregiver behaviors with particular reference to repetition and timing. In: Schaffer HR (ed) Studies in mother-infant interaction. Academic Press, London, pp 177–202
83. Trevarthen C, Hubley P (1978) Secondary intersubjectivity: confidence, confiding and acts of meaning in the first year. In: Lock A (ed) Action, gesture and symbol: the emergence of language. Academic Press, London, pp 183–229
84. Tronick E, Als H, Brazelton TB (1980) The infant's communicative competencies and the achievement of intersubjectivity. In: Key MR (ed) The relationship of verbal and nonverbal communication. Mouton Publishers, New York, pp 261–274

Rhythms in Early Development

4

Anne Bobin-Bègue

4.1 State of the Art: A Literature Review

Rhythm, in its everyday usage, is often thought to be close in meaning to several similar words, such as tempo, duration, and frequency. For instance, we talk of rhythm when an event, such as a physiological modification or a motor behavior, is repeated with an identical interval separating the successive events. This gives rise to a periodicity associated with a tempo. The most striking feature of a periodic rhythmic event is that it is predictable. Thus in this case, an event's rhythmic property affords the anticipation of the next identical event.

In the context of social interactions between a caregiver and an infant, rhythms are based on the temporal organization of behavior. During the peripartum, there are many physiological temporal regularities in the fetus' and newborn's functioning. Notwithstanding, the environment provides regularly repeated sensory, motor, and emotional experiences. In this chapter, physiological and behavioral rhythms will first be described in order to underline their centrality. In the second part, I will describe how these rhythms are involved in early interactions in typical development. In the final section, I will discuss how disruptions in early rhythms may be involved in various clinical and pathological conditions.

4.1.1 Circadian Rhythms

A very important source of rhythmicity is imposed by the rotation of the Earth and the latitude at which the individual lives: the alternation of day and night is a very powerful indicator for daily biological rhythms that exist in all organisms [1]. These endogenous

A. Bobin-Bègue (✉)
Laboratory Ethology, Cognition, Development, Paris Nanterre University,
200 avenue de la République, Nanterre, 92000, France
e-mail: anne.bobin_begue@parisnanterre.fr

© Springer Nature Switzerland AG 2019

G. Apter et al. (eds.), *Early Interaction and Developmental Psychopathology*,
https://doi.org/10.1007/978-3-030-04769-6_4

rhythms of approximately 24 h are called circadian rhythms. Those physiological and behavioral circadian rhythms occur even in the absence of the main external synchronizer, the alternation of day and night. Other external synchronizers, with lower impacts, such as external temperature, availability of resources, and social factors, allow the individual to adapt to this fundamental external rhythm. Humans, like all mammals, have a brain structure called the suprachiasmatic nuclei (SCN) that generates the circadian biological rhythms and modulates them to match the 24 h cycle due to the information provided from the external environmental changes. Thus, circadian rhythms are an adaptative process allowing the individual to coordinate physiological and behavioral needs according to external environmental constraints. However, there is some variability from one individual to another, partly explained by genetic factors, which results in a different circadian functioning. Thus, individuals may vary in their so-called chronotype [1]. These chronotypes are consistent with circadian physiology and sleep patterns, including in the toddler [2], and thus should be considered when individuals show difficulties in sleeping, for example.

Since quality of life is highly determined by circadian rhythmicity, how and when does it appear? It is essential that the newborn and its mother (or more generally its caregivers) be synchronized to the same circadian rhythms, in order that infant's needs and activities such as sleep-wake rhythms, meals, etc. be coordinated with that of the caregivers. Data obtained in nonhuman mammalian species suggest that the circadian system is immature before birth [3]. In humans, the SCN appears during the 18th week of gestation ([4], cited in [5]), and some circadian rhythms have been detected in the fetus [3]. Nevertheless, it is impossible to separate the fetal circadian rhythm, generated independently by its endogenous circadian system, from the influence the mother's own circadian system exerts on it. Moreover, as some rhythmicities are not found after birth, it is possible that there is a form of circadian rhythm driven by the mother's own system. The study of rhythmicities observed in preterm infants has provided elements to understand how autonomous circadian rhythms are established during the perinatal period. In these studies, premature infants were in specific conditions that theoretically excluded maternal social and behavioral influence. Their results show that although the circadian system may produce some rhythms starting at 29 weeks of gestation, maternal timing factors are required for optimum functioning [6]. Therefore, prenatal circadian rhythms prepare for autonomy of the human system after birth [6] in order for it to synchronize with its environment. It could be noticed that the mode of delivery may induce changes in a newborn's rhythms. Infants born vaginally have their own distinct circadian activity compared to infants born by cesarean (planned or unplanned). The mode of delivery affects the circadian rhythms of sleep, although the amount of sleep time does not differ significantly [7]. One explanation is that the postnatal environment, in terms of the rhythm of brightness and of social interaction with parents, is different for children born vaginally, who quickly integrate a rhythmic lifestyle, and for children born by cesarean who stay longer in the hospital with a mother who is probably more tired.

After birth, some of rhythms experienced by the fetus could be experienced by the newborn, such as maternal heart rate when the infant is held close to the mother, the mother's walking pace when the infant is carried (involving proprioceptive and vestibular rhythmic stimulations), and circadian rhythms of activity (noise, movements, and activities). As the suprachiasmatic nuclei mature, the newborn experiences new situations in its environment that will contribute to the synchronization of its physiological and behavioral rhythms. One study looked at the influence of photic and non-photic factors in the implementation of the training of circadian rhythms in the newborn [8]. The researchers recorded the awake and sleep phases, temperature, melatonin levels, and food intake from birth to 6 months as indicators of circadian synchronization. Their results show that temperature is the first indicator that describes a circadian rhythm, and it becomes significant in the first week after birth. The circadian sleep/wake and melatonin rhythmicities then appear later almost concurrently, from the 45th day after birth. The circadian rhythm of sleep is based on regularly paced 90–120 min sustained awake periods during the second month. The results also showed that the infant's night sleep period begins with the sunset and subsequently with the slowing of the family's social activity. These observations suggest that the development of circadian rhythms in infants is guided first by photic cues and then by social cues.

Furthermore, fetal life seems to prepare the newborn for adaptation to circadian rhythms. The fetus appears to have an endogenous biological clock that can, to some extent, generate circadian rhythms that are synchronized with or entrained to maternal signals [6]. Thus, through the influence of maternal synchronization signals (such as daily activities, sleep/awake rhythms), fetal circadian rhythms are indirectly driven by the light/dark cycle. At birth, the circadian rhythms of the newborn result from a combination of the influence of pre- and postnatal environmental signals [9].

4.1.2 Circadian Physiological Rhythms

With the establishment of the circadian system (maturation of the suprachiasmatic nuclei), physiological circadian rhythmicities are set up. We now turn to a description of how the infant establishes physiological rhythms during the perinatal period. We begin with a brief description of how maternal physiological rhythms lead the fetus' rhythms and their mutual coordination.

4.1.2.1 Maternal Rhythms as Driving Factors of Circadian Rhythms in Fetuses

Pregnant women possess a set of circadian rhythms, generated by their own physiological system, which sets up the fetus's circadian rhythms [6]. These are:

- Circadian rhythms of maternal melatonin, which pass through the placenta. They could synchronize the activity of the fetal and maternal suprachiasmatic nuclei.
- Circadian rhythms of a corticosterone-releasing factor (CRF) and cortisol. Some studies suggest that the cycle of maternal cortisol influences fetal rhythms.
- Body temperature.

- Glucose level in blood is directly related to maternal diet and its rhythmic regulation (regulation of glucose concentration and glucose availability to the fetus).
- Uterine contractions during the last trimester of pregnancy are a source of tactile stimulation. By the end of pregnancy, the fetus has been rocked by the circadian rhythm of uterine contractions ([10], cited in [3]).

In addition, one of the main physiological rhythms during the peripartum stems from oxytocin[1] whose secretion is pulsatile. Oxytocin has been shown to impact the quality of the relationship between the caregiver and infant. Oxytocin is involved in the maturation of circadian rhythms and plays an essential role in attachment and breastfeeding. For the mother, this hormone is a key factor of attachment behavior to infants (oxytocin is also present in infants [11]). Oxytocin is also involved in the bond with the partner/father, participating in the emotional link between the two parents. In fathers, oxytocin acts as a relationship facilitator, making them more emotionally available and involved in interactions with their family members (child and spouse). However, oxytocin is only effective for fathers who show a good level of synchrony in their social interactions (Weisman et al. 2014, quoted in [11]). The quality of triadic interactions (including the father) is predicted by the levels of maternal and paternal oxytocin as well as a low daytime maternal cortisol level [11], suggesting a link between oxytocin levels and the hypothalamic-pituitary-adrenal (HPA) system in the development of attachment.

In addition to these maternal physiological rhythmicities, other factors of circadian synchronization are indirectly transmitted to the fetus through maternal behaviors and social activities, such as alternations between movement and rest phases and such as alternations between phases when the fetus is exposed to environmental sound such as social conversation or music and quieter and silent phases. All these driving factors overlap and interact with the infant's own circadian activity.

4.1.2.2 Melatonin

Melatonin is produced by the pineal gland. This hormone is involved in the organization of circadian rhythms in mammals [4, 12] and particularly that of sleep/wake rhythms. Data on infant melatonin rhythmicity are rare because melatonin levels are too low and difficult to measure. However, melatonin levels increase during development [8, 13, 14]. Burnham [13] showed that the rhythmicity of melatonin evolves toward that observed in adults between 1 and 3 months of age. In fact, their results highlight that the peak of melatonin production is around noon for 1-month-olds and shifts to 5 am for 3-month-olds. This peak in melatonin level occurs in the same time slot (between 2 am and 6 am) as for adults.

---

[1] Oxytocin is a hormone produced in the hypothalamus that regulates homeostasis, thermoregulation, etc.

4.1.2.3 Cortisol

While melatonin prepares the body for sleep, cortisol prepares it for alertness with a circadian rhythm acrophase[2] in the morning upon awakening, which mobilizes the energy reserves of the body after overnight fasting. Cortisol passes through the placenta, and maternal cortisol has been shown to be involved in the regulation of fetal circadian rhythms [6]. A more recent study has shown that cortisol rhythms set in as early as 1 month postpartum [15]. However, these researchers also found high individual variability in a large sample of healthy full-term infants during the first year of life.

4.1.2.4 Body Temperature

The circadian rhythmicity of body temperature has been observed before the infant manifests stable and long periods of wakefulness [16]. In term infants with normal development (neurological, behavioral, and somatic), clear rhythmicity appears as early as 6 weeks postpartum for some children and is well organized in all by the age of 10 weeks [16]. Nevertheless, there is no obvious circadian rhythmicity at 3 weeks of age. Like melatonin and cortisol rhythms, the circadian rhythm of body temperature does not settle before the end of the first month after birth.

4.1.3 Heart Rate and Respiration Rhythms

The first heartbeats appear as early as 3–4 weeks gestational age [17], and a regular heartbeat is detectable from 22 weeks of gestation [18]. Breathing movement patterns appear later, at 10 weeks gestational age, and are generated spontaneously [17]. Heart and breathing rhythms can be modified by environmental factors (such as external stimuli perceived by the fetus) and are therefore good indicators of the individual's state. Thus, variations in heart and respiration rhythms can be considered a response of the fetus and then newborn to changes in their environment [19]. In addition, these two rhythms show interrelated modifications through the mobilization of the autonomic parasympathetic system [20, 21]. Heart rate increases during inhalation and then decreases during exhalation. This interrelationship is measured by the RSA (respiratory sinus arrhythmia) and reflects the activity of the vagal tone. The RSA is immature at birth but adjusts to the maternal RSA during the first 2 months after birth, on a seeming continuum with fetal life. Interestingly, from 3 months postpartum, the physiological synchrony of heart and respiratory rhythms between mother and infant is no longer observed [21], suggesting a progressive physiological decoupling of the mother and infant.

---

[2] The acrophase is the position on the time axis of the maximum variation in a temporal biological rhythm.

4.1.4 Motor Rhythms

During the first year, the infant has a wide repertoire of rhythmic and stereotypic movements, which evolve according to age and maturity of the nervous system [22]. This repertoire includes kicking, arm waving, banging, bouncing, rocking, twirling, scratching, and swaying. Stereotypic movements of the legs and torso, for example, are associated with states of high or low arousal and with contextual events, such as interactions with the caregiver or body positioning [23]. Although stereotypic behavioral features greatly depend on age, their frequent manifestation during infancy suggests they are inherent to the maturation of the neuromuscular system. However, since some of these behaviors also appear in social interactive contexts, it is possible that they play an active role in communication [23]. Recent studies have considered contexts in which the infant is exposed to different sound stimuli and found that at 5 months, infants produce more rhythmic movements during exposure to music than to other sounds [24]. However, the pace of their body movements does not correspond precisely to the beat of the music [25] although when the tempo of the music accelerates, the pace of movement is faster too [24]. The infant can adapt its spontaneous motor rhythms to auditory rhythms in the environment.

4.1.4.1 Hiccups and Respiratory Movements

Hiccups could be considered rhythmic manifestations. During gestation, two successive hiccups have been shown to occur with a time interval ranging from 1 to 3 s. For breathing movements, their range is between 2 and 3 s at 12 weeks gestational age, from 0 to 1 s at 19 weeks gestational age and from 1 to 1.3 s after 30 weeks gestational age [26].

4.1.4.2 Sucking

One of the most pervasive infant behaviors is sucking. There are two sucking modes, nutritive and non-nutritive sucking. The first involves a regular rhythm of one suck per second in full-term 4-month-old infants [27]. This rhythm changes between the beginning and the end of feeding [28]. Non-nutritive sucking is a spontaneous rhythmic activity that appears around 10 weeks gestational age [17]. It consists of a regular alternation of sucking bursts with pauses. The rhythm of nutritive sucking (inter-suck interval) is influenced by the quality of the food, including its sweetness [29]. Non-nutritive sucking remains steady for several dozens of minutes. However, the pause length may be influenced by external events [30]. Two-month-old infants can accelerate their sucking rhythm when they perceive an auditorily presented tempo that is 15% faster than their initial sucking rhythm (measured in the absence of any auditory stimulations), while newborns do not significantly change their sucking rhythm [31]. When the auditory tempo is identical to the initial sucking rhythm or 15% slower, modification of the sucking rhythm is not significant, although a slight acceleration can be observed in newborns as well as in 2-month-old infants [31]. This tendency suggests that infants perceive the tempo of external stimuli.

4.1.4.3 Spontaneous Motor Tempo and Internal Tempo

The spontaneous motor tempo is the tempo of a motor activity repeated at regular intervals and in the absence of any external temporal cue. It can be detected very early in development through rhythmic activities (such as sucking). With the maturation of the neuromuscular system, spontaneous motor tempo can be observed with other effectors (rhythmic and stereotypic movements). The spontaneous motor tempo task has been used by many researchers to assess the internal tempo of an individual. It involves producing a comfortable and steady tempo in the absence of any external time cue. Most often, a "tapping task" is used, in which the effector is the hand or a finger. Studies converge in showing that internal tempo is a personal and individual characteristic which evolves with age, slowing down and becoming more stable in adulthood [32–35]. Moreover, this internal tempo is subject to circadian variations, at least in adults [36]. It is dependent on the functioning of the suprachiasmatic nuclei [37] and is influenced by many environmental factors [32, 34]. The internal tempo could be used to support other higher-level skills, such as social interactions or musical skills, by facilitating adaptions to environmental situations.

4.1.4.4 Vocalizations

Vocal production also involves rhythm. At birth, the infant produces vocalization, cries, and vegetative sounds. Vocalizations will gradually become organized into structured forms of communication contributing to the appearance of language. Vocal development which involves gain in motor control is supported by more general processes of neuromuscular development and crucially by scaffolding in social interactions. Infant crying, right from birth, is organized around a rhythm that requires coordination between breathing and contraction of skeletal muscles: expiratory sound (0.6–1.3 s)/pause (0.2 s)/inspiratory sound (0.1–0.2 s)/pause (0.2 s) ([38], cited in [39]), which corresponds to a rhythm ranging between 1100 and 2400 ms [40]. Non-cry vocalization, involving variation in rhythm, intensity, and melody, is the precursors of the first canonical vocalizations of language that is babbling sounds [41]. The temporal (and acoustic) organization of crying has been shown to be shaped from birth by the native language the newborn has been exposed to in utero [42]. This adaptation of newborn productions could be due to the infant's ability to synchronize cries with external rhythmic stimuli [43].

4.1.5 Sleep-Wake Rhythms and Activity Rhythms

After 10 weeks postpartum, most infants adjust to the circadian sleep-wake rhythm [44]. From fetal life, it is possible to detect circadian rhythms in alternating rest and activity movements [6]. Along with the maturation of the nervous system, various behavioral sleep states appear. At 32 weeks gestational age, the quiet sleep state is distinguishable from the active sleep state. However, fetuses spend a significant amount of time in an indeterminate sleep state [45]. These indeterminate sleep phases decrease until the 40th week of gestation in favor of quiet sleep phases.

Then, along with the maturation of the nervous system, sleep organization[3] gradually evolves during the first 2 years in terms of quality, quantity, and distribution between day and night [44]. After birth, sleep represents 15 h per day, with 20–25% devoted to daytime naps [48]. Up until 2 years of age, the proportion of daytime sleep gradually decreases until only nighttime sleep becomes the norm.

These changes in sleep patterns are associated not only with physiological and neurological maturation but also with the daytime organization of social life and cultural practices [48]. Even before birth, there are rhythms that are shared between the fetus and its family, which they continue to share after birth. While the circadian rhythm of the mother in the third week after birth is influenced by nighttime awakenings to care for her infant, an important synchronizing factor of the sleep/wake rhythms of the infant is the activity/interaction between mother and infant [49]. In a longitudinal study recording the activities of several families from the 37th week of pregnancy until the first 4 months of the infant, research showed that there is a match in the patterns of the ultradian activity of the mother and her infant at 1, 2, and 4 months after birth [50]. Synchronization of activities between the mother and her infant is always better than between the father and infant. The circadian rhythm of the mother-infant dyad's daily activities changes over the first 12 weeks. In general, at 3 months postpartum, the rhythm of the infant anticipates by 60 min the acrophase of the mother's activities [51]. Thus, social factors and daily routines support the implementation of the sleep-wake rhythm during the day. In preterm infants, the amount of daytime sleep has a positive impact on maternal affect and involvement [48].

4.1.6 Feeding Rhythms

Rhythms do not clearly appear in perinatal nutrition, yet, they do exist either before or after birth. During fetal life, nutrient needs are met continuously, but the amniotic fluid composition varies with maternal food intake and fetal urination. The fetus becomes sensitive to its chemical environment (including through smell[4]) during the last 2 months of gestation. By swallowing amniotic fluid, the fetus responds to a number of flavors, such as garlic, cumin, fennel, carrot, cheese, alcohol, and tobacco. These findings suggest that, depending on maternal dietary habits, the fetus is exposed to stimuli that it perceives not directly through the food per se but through the taste of the amniotic fluid. These stimulations follow the swallowing and maternal food intake rhythms. At birth, the newborn shows preferences for substances experienced in utero, demonstrating that it has already been oriented by cultural choices and maternal food preferences.

[3] For details on the assessment of sleep states in infants, see Grigg-Damberger and Gozal [46]; for a recent review on the quality and quantity of sleep from 0 to 12 years, see Galland et al. [47].

[4] It has been shown in animals that the fetal olfactory system works better in the aquatic environment than in air [52].

After birth, nutrient inputs become discontinuous following the temporal organization of food intake. The newborn is fed by the caregiver either at its request, following its physiological rhythms, or at an imposed rhythm. During the first 2 months, the amount of milk ingested via bottle feeding remains constant during the day, while in the breastfeeding mode, the quantities of milk ingested decrease during the day (a daily pattern appears during the first month) [28]. These authors think that this difference could be explained by the infant keeping a form of control on food intake and learning to adjust to the feeling of satiety. The nature of the milk, breastfed or formula, also impacts the rhythmic nutritive sucking (itself dependent on breathing and sucking/swallowing rhythms).

Indeed, in the same meal/food intake, the temporal organization of sucking bursts and pauses is not the same between the two feeding modes, breast or bottle, and depends on the nature of the milk: newborns that are bottle-fed with cow's milk all have the same temporal pattern of sucking, while there are large individual differences in the sucking patterns of infants that are bottle-fed with breast milk (Johnson and Salisbury 1975, cited in [28]). The assumption is that the composition of breast milk may explain these differences in temporal pattern. In fact, breast milk composition changes over time (with the development of the child), under the influence of substances ingested by the mother and even during a feeding. In addition, breast milk contains endogenous substances that vary depending on the circadian rhythm (melatonin) or the sucking rhythm (oxytocin, which is involved in the ejection of milk from the nipple). Melatonin is a circadian synchronizer, and the breast milk melatonin concentration follows this circadian variation [9]. However, the link between melatonin levels found in breast milk and circulating melatonin levels in infants has not been demonstrated. The extrapolation of data from adults taking melatonin and the corresponding dose of melatonin circulating in the blood suggests, given the melatonin concentrations in breast milk, almost no effect in breastfed infants [14]. Concerning oxytocin in breast milk, the pattern of burst discharge in the maternal hypothalamus is linked to the sucking rhythm of the infant. Various rhythms can be found during infant feeding, which are dependent on the frequency of meals, the feeding method, the nature of the milk, and other habits (i.e., extracting breast milk to give at another time, breaking the rhythms in the milk composition). These are all parameters that influence the infant's rhythmic experience. Consequently, infants experience satiety and different flavors (the taste of breast milk after breakfast may differ from that after lunch) with different rhythms, various sucking rhythms, and even arousal rhythms.

4.1.7 Attentional/Arousal Rhythms

Attention or, more precisely, attentional processes are fundamental during development because they help to process information from the environment efficiently and selectively. During ontogeny, attentional capacity (quantitative) and states of awareness (qualitative) gradually evolve from the different sleep-wake states (see Sect. 4.1.5) toward more passive awake or quiet alert states. Gradually, attentional abilities become increasingly efficient [53]. The infant learns to disengage from a "sticky fixation" which parallels its ability to inhibit behavior. Indeed, it has been showed that between 1 and 3 months, the infant starts to inhibit movement when the direction of gaze changes, i.e., when the infant attention disengages [54].

The time spent in a non-attentive state significantly decreases from about 5.42 min/h between 4 and 10 weeks to less than 1 min/h from 44 to 50 weeks. Meanwhile, attention paid to objects increases from 0.92 min/h after birth to 13.33 min at 1 year. Lastly, the time devoted to social interaction (6.5 min/h) remains almost constant from 20 weeks to 1 year (maximum age of children in the study) [23].

In one-month-old infants, stimuli, whether auditory, audiovisual, proprioceptive/touch, or thermic, if administered continuously, lead to a rapid decrease in the level of arousal assessed by physiological (cardiac and respiratory) and behavioral (motor activity, wakefulness) indices [55]. Later, infants show a cyclical pattern in the organization of their attention, especially at 3 months when their inhibition capacity is still very limited. This cyclic organization of attentional level allows them to be more efficient in terms of processing speed and memory: in a habituation/novelty task, infants with a cyclic attentional organization reach the criterion of habituation faster [56]. These results are coherent with the dynamic attending theory, initially proposed by Jones [57], which states that attention spontaneously focuses on events that occur at a tempo close to the individual's internal tempo. This also means that the closer the internal tempo is to the external stimulus, the better the attention paid to the event [58]. This dynamic allocation of attention occurs in individuals over the age of 4 years [33] although the spontaneous motor tempo can be ascertained before this age [31, 32]. The importance of spontaneous rhythms in infants and the fact that infants focus attention better on rhythmical events in their environment suggest that this model is valid from the beginning of life; the development of attentional abilities in infants is conditioned by the fact that their environmental stimuli are rhythmic. The social environment is also concerned; the dynamic features of social interactions should present rhythmical features.

Through an interaction whose rhythm is adapted to the attentional rhythms of the infant, the partner will support the development of attentional control processes. These include both the attentional engagement process[5] and the disengagement process, which allows the infant to control voluntarily where to focus and maintain attention, thus enabling the infant to explore other parts of the environment. From 3 months of age, the infant can track the attention of a social partner and alternate between paying attention to the same object as its social partner and the partner (passive joint engagement) [59]. According to the researchers we just cited, the transition from passive joint engagement to the attention directed at an object (situation in which the infant is actively exploring a subject) emphasizes the role of social

[5] There are six types of attentional commitment: uncommitted, look, commitment to the person, commitment to the object, passive joint commitment, and coordinated joint commitment [53, 59].

context. The role of parents is thus to orient the attention of the infant to the environment before they can actively explore it on their own. Caregivers frequently interact with infants through rhythmical games like peekaboo [60], songs, and action songs. These highly rhythmic interactions support the development of the infant's attentional abilities. These games and songs are very well structured and, in time, create attentional expectations in infants; the fun of these routines comes from the interruption of the rhythmical patterns [61] (see Sect. 4.2.3).

In contrast, rhythmical activities (such as regular rocking) allow parents to regulate the attention of their infants. Typically, rhythmic rocking (vestibular stimulation) is used by the caregiver to calm or lull an infant to sleep. The infant has experienced this since fetal life through maternal movements (walking) and studies have shown that vertical rocking, about 10 cm in amplitude with a frequency of 1 cycle every 850 ms (rhythm timescale), is most effective for calming infants [62, 63]. These results were obtained not with rocking by parents but using a mechanical rocking device to compare the effectiveness of different rocking settings on the wakefulness of the infant. Currently, no clear data are available to explain how body rhythms modulate attention and states of awareness, although this effect seems to persist in adults.[6]

While social interactions with the infant initiated by the caregiver use the rhythmicity of attention to stimulate the development of the infant's attention, another field of research suggests that social interactions, through the modulation of attention, in turn affect circadian rhythms and consequently influence sleep-wake rhythms, temperature, and melatonin secretion [8, 13, 65]. Social events could be considered to act as synchronizers of the circadian clock. The complexity of these data and the lack of their precision highlight the many interrelationships between physiological and behavioral rhythms, in which social rhythms play a supporting/facilitating role in the development of different skills in infants.

4.2 Impact on Early Interactions

Numerous biological and physiological rhythms are essential for harmonious development, especially during the perinatal period. One of the key issues of rhythmicities is that they allow the individual to adapt to their physical environment and, more importantly, to their immediate social environment. The previous section demonstrated that the infant possesses a strong ability to process rhythms from the immediate environment and that parents use rhythms to support and stimulate interactions with their infants. The next section explores the impact of social rhythms on early interactions.

[6] Note that in adults, rhythmic movements are sometimes still present at the time of falling asleep [64].

4.2.1 Perception of Environmental Rhythms

The environment of the fetus and then the newborn and the infant offers a wide variety of rhythmic sources, many of which are likely perceived and differentiated before birth. Thus, during gestation, the mother, when walking or rocking, generates rhythmic stimuli to which the fetus is sensitive [66, 67]. If the rhythmic stimuli are multimodal, then the responses of the fetus are greater than when they are presented in one modality [68]. Similarly, music, songs, and language are rhythmic auditory sources to which the fetus is sensitive. Shortly before birth, the fetus can discriminate the voice of the mother [69]: it can identify, memorize, and recognize the acoustic characteristics of her voice [70]. The fetus is sensitive to a variation of plus or minus 10% of a tempo of 600 ms (i.e., it can discriminate a tempo of 540 ms vs. 600 ms and 600 ms vs. 660 ms) [71]. After birth, the infant is sensitive to different auditory tempi. Nevertheless, it is only from 2 months of age that the infant can adapt its sucking rhythm to an external auditory tempo [31]. Intersensory[7] and intrasensory redundancy allow the 2-month-old infant to detect a change in tempo more easily [73]. At 7 months, the infant can rely on the vestibular, tactile, and proprioceptive modalities during rocking to discriminate rhythmic patterns [74, 75]. Thus, very early during development, the fetus and the infant can detect tempo changes on the basis of one or more sensory modalities and can also detect synchrony between events. These capabilities are essential for the processing of more complex rhythmic stimuli in their social environment.

Language—Spoken language is a rhythmic auditory stimulus to which the infant is exposed before birth. Languages belong to different rhythmic classes (accentual, syllabic, or moraic). Before 2 months of age, infants can discriminate their native language from another one on the basis of prosodic cues that involve rhythmic information [76]. However, newborns fail to discriminate two foreign languages from the same rhythmic class [77]. The multimodal dimension of language is also important. At 8 months, infants detect an audiovisual asynchrony of 666 ms and 500 ms but not of 366 ms, independently of the language they hear (native or unfamiliar) [78, 79]. The native language is an element of transnatal continuity for the infant. The early life experience of native language will provide support for the development of the infant's social and cultural skills.

Songs—Singing is a common parental practice even before birth. Songs, which are frequently sung and sung in the same way by mothers, constitute for the infant a familiar rhythmical situation [80, 81]. The 6-month-old infant's attention is more mobilized by the mother singing than by her speaking [82] perhaps because songs are more rhythmic than speech. Singing enables the 6-month-old infant to reach an intermediate level of arousal, neither too high nor too low [83], and thus contributes to infant emotional regulation.

Music—Music is another rhythmic stimulation often experienced by the fetus. Near-term fetuses can detect changes in musical tempo (when it is one third faster)

[7] Soon after birth, infants can detect the synchrony between events in different sensory modalities [39, 72].

[84]. Newborns can detect differences in rhythmic patterns [85]. Around 2 months of age, infants can detect variations in rhythmic pattern and tempo changes [86–88].

These very early rhythmic abilities, including the ability to synchronize with external rhythms, must facilitate the development of social competences in infants. Toward the age of 4–5 months, infants are more sensitive to the temporal contingency characteristics of maternal behavior compared to those of unfamiliar partners [89] and soon become sensitive to sharing the same rhythm with another person [90]. At 14 months, a toddler who has experienced being in synchrony with an adult through body movement will then tend to cooperate more easily with the adult [91]. Thus, the emergence of prosocial behavior is facilitated by rhythmical synchronization with the partner. As adults, people who are good at discriminating rhythms also tend to be good at distinguishing sentences in a noisy environment [92] and are therefore better at maintaining social connection through conversation.

4.2.2 Influence of Parenting on Infant Rhythms

The infant has an early capacity to process rhythms from the environment. Reciprocally, how can parents support the development of physiological and behavioral rhythmicities in their infants?

The sleep-wake rhythm is known to be strongly influenced by parental practices. For example, although light is the main circadian rhythm synchronizer, it turns out that parents do not usually expose their young infants to well-defined light/darkness cycles: infants (50 days old on average) spend only an eighth of the day exposed to a light intensity of less than 100 lux[8] [5, 93]. However, there is a relationship between the acrophase of exposure to light and activity. Infants with the most robust circadian activity rhythms are those who are exposed the longest to brightness above 100 lux and at a higher amplitude of light intensity over 24 h. Sleep patterns and sleep quality are also impacted by parenting. An analysis of parent diaries of full-term infants showed that infants who sleep better at night are significantly more exposed to light at the beginning of the afternoon [94]. In addition to sufficiently exposing the infant to light during the day, parenting practices regarding light exposure are equally important during the night. Thus, during their waking phases for diaper changing or feeding, mothers use different light sources [95]: parents may turn on a bright light, a soft light, or not use any light. Infants (1 month old) whose parents use a bright light show less robust sleep-wake rhythms during the day [13].

Sleep conditions set up by parents also influence sleep-wake rhythms. Infants can sleep alone in a different room from the parents, share the parents' room, or share their bed. "Co-sleeping" practices are alternately defined as either room-sharing or

[8] 0.5 lux, full moonlight; 10 lux, dusk or candlelight; 20–80 lux, lit city; 100 lux, minimum brightness to read a text; 100–200 lux, home lighting; 300–500 lux, public places; 1000 lux, very well-lit place; 5000 lux, outside when overcast; 10,000 lux, outside in average weather; 20,000 lux, intense artificial light (right next to a 50 W halogen lamp); 50,000–100,000 lux, outside in sunny weather (Source http://www.sirtin.fr/2008/05/28/comment-mesurer-leclairage/).

bed-sharing, where proximity involves physical contact. Studies have shown that these practices (room-sharing and bed-sharing) do not play a crucial role in establishing sleep-wake rhythms (or the melatonin rhythm), although co-sleeping seems to allow more robust sleep-wake rhythms [13]. However, there is a strong individual variability between 1 and 3 months of age.[9] It also seems that the sleep organization of a co-sleeping infant is different from that of an infant sleeping alone[10] [96]. In addition, the presence of the mother during the infant's sleep affects its average heart rate and heart-rate variability. The sympathetic system is activated differently, probably due to different thermoregulations between the two sleeping conditions [97]. Studies that analyze cortisol levels have shown a significant correlation between mothers' and infants' cortisol levels at bedtime specifically when infants are breastfed and not in formula-fed infants [98]. This study emphasizes that synchronized cortisol levels may be related to several factors, such as the transfer of cortisol via breast milk but also through skin-to-skin contact, environmental features, and possibly the level of income. However, 7% of infants have free-running sleep-wake circadian rhythmicity after birth (Shimada et al. 1999) cited in [99]) and the free-running rhythm is not reset by maternal entrainment factors [99].

Another parental practice to consider in establishing infant rhythms is massage. The practice of massage in the perinatal period[11] has an effect on sleep-wake rhythms and melatonin secretion rhythms. It appears to act as a powerful synchronizer, promoting the adjustment of the infant's circadian system to environmental conditions [100].

Parental practices based on rhythmic stimuli can also influence the behavior of infants. Rocking the infant is a common practice in many cultures. However, to our knowledge, no systematic study has addressed the practices and procedures involved in rocking. A few earlier studies have investigated the effects of mechanical rocking on infant behavior. Vrugt and Pederson [63] studied the effect of different frequencies of mechanical vertical rocking in 2-month-old infants. Their results showed that rocking at 1.5 Hz (a tempo of 667 ms) will lull most infants to sleep (compared to other tested frequencies) and lead to less crying. The amplitude and direction of the rocking enhance its soothing effects [62, 101]. These limited data do not explain why rhythmic vestibular stimulations are used fairly universally to lull to sleep or calm infants. The vestibular modality is probably appropriate for infants because it has been widely experienced during gestation and possibly after birth, during holding. It could be hypothesized that these rhythmic stimuli regulate the attentional level from a state of alertness to a controlled state. Moreover, rocking is often coupled to singing or music. Song and music are also rhythmic stimulations, and the infant experiences them through parenting habits. It has been shown that listening to music has a positive effect on the metabolism (in adults at least), particularly on the HPA axis, the endocrine, and the immune system [102]. It would

[9] All infants studied were breastfeeding on demand (in two groups).

[10] Laboratory bed-sharing practices: they sleep less deep sleep (NREM3-4) and more light sleep (NREM1-2).

[11] 14 days from the 10th day of life after term birth.

therefore have a positive effect on overall physiology. In addition, music allows the synchronization of behaviors and shared intentionality and promotes cooperation between individuals. Nowadays, music therapy is used to encourage the development of attachment bonds and to help stabilize premature infants during hospitalization in the NICU [103].

Various parenting practices may therefore influence the infant's rhythms and particularly activity rhythms. This aspect is interesting because the sleep patterns of the infant influence the interactions between the mother and her baby: the infant's sleep time amount would be predictive of synchrony in the interaction between mother and infant [104]. Thus, parenting practices are fundamental to develop appropriate rhythmicity in the caregiver-infant dyad.

4.2.3 Rhythms and Social Interactions

Social interactions in the perinatal period also present rhythmic features. First, physiological rhythms play a role in the interaction behavior in the caregiver-infant dyad. Second, interaction behaviors between the caregiver and the infant present a temporal organization. Thus, a strict definition of rhythm in interaction corresponds to the tempo of the interaction, that is to say the duration of the intervals separating two identical or equivalent behaviors. This concept also encompasses that of synchrony, which corresponds to a state of interaction in which paralinguistic and nonverbal behaviors (volume, pitch, speech speed) of participants are coordinated in their expression and timing [105]; behaving in a synchronous interaction is not actually behaving simultaneously. The notion of synchrony in interaction refers more to the fact that the coordination of behavior between the caregiver and the infant reflects a contingency, not a coincidence. In the context of studying the temporal aspects of social interactions, various terms have been defined and used in everyday language to cover very specific concepts. The following section describes more precisely caregiver-infant interactions and their physiological and behavioral rhythms and sometimes other temporal relationships.

In infants, physiological rhythms are regulated by the coordination of affective behaviors during social interactions [106]. Even before birth, fetal heart rate changes according to the mother's activity, such as resting and silent vs. awake and speaking [107]. The infant's physiological rhythms also support the quality of the mother-infant interaction rhythms [108]. The quality of the interaction is predicted to some extent by changes in the duration of sleep between 6 weeks and 5 months [104]. Thus, there is a real interdependence of physiological rhythms between the infant and the caregiver. It has been shown that the heart rates of the infant and the mother are coordinated with a deviation of less than 1 s [109], while the attentional and awakening micro-rhythms of the infant are regulated by the physical proximity of the mother [110].

Interaction rhythms are also dependent on attentional rhythms. Face-to-face interactions are composed of millisecond oscillations between states of attention and non-attention between partners. The mother may break habituation/monotony by introducing novelty as soon as the infant's attention declines [111] (see the Sect. 4.1.7 and the section below). Thus, rhythmic adjustments occur between the physiological systems of the infant and the caregiver, as well as between their attentional states.

At the behavioral level, rhythmic adjustments occur mostly through synchrony of behavior between partners. After birth, face-to-face interactions present modulations in behavioral rhythm and synchrony. The temporal pattern of interactions often follows a "burst-pause" pattern, which corresponds to an alternation between the periods of activity by one partner and pauses in which the other partner can act in turn. In addition, during interactions, some events appear stochastically; i.e., they are predictable in light of the events that precede them (this does not necessarily mean regular events), and sometimes the events are predictable over time (stochastic cyclicity) because they have a temporal regularity. Thus, it is possible for each partner to anticipate behavior. This anticipation allows a form of synchrony in interactions. Synchrony is a temporal property of the mother-infant behavior system (in the context of social interactions): the behavior of one partner matches the behavior of the other in a time-adjusted manner (i.e., in a short time window). This ability requires the mother and the infant (independently of each other) to anticipate the behavior of the other in order to trigger their own behavior within this time window. Such behaviors are called synchronized behaviors. The ability of infants to synchronize some of their behavior is probably due to their ability to perceive rhythm (see Sect. 4.2.1). Rhythmical interactions allow time-balanced interactions between the partners (Barnard 1987, cited in [112]), and synchronous interactions decrease the stress response in both the mother and the infant [113]. However, the appropriateness and predictability of interactions between the infant and the mother depend not only on periods of synchrony but also on periods of non-synchrony (Tronick et al. 2005, cited in [114]).

Since the 1970s, the temporal patterning of behavior observed in mother-infant interaction has been described as a central characteristic of early communication [115]. Thus, the behavioral patterns of infants are known to be related to the temporal patterns of the mother's movements and expressions [115], and newborns synchronize their body movements with the speech rate of adults [116]. Feeding also involves a well-paced interaction that takes the form of a turn-taking sequence in which mothers respond to signals from their infants [117]. By 3 months, infants and mothers not only take turns when interacting but anticipate each other's vocal turns with great accuracy [118, 119]. Infants' vocal turn-taking involves close matching of expressive sounds such as imitation of the prosodic contours of parental vocalizations [120]. These early experiences of communication are essential for social and cognitive development [121].

Around 5–6 months, infants are even more sensitive to the maternal voice [82]: the more marked rhythmicity in maternal singing supports the attention of the infant more effectively. Singing is a mode of interaction that provides strong evidence of temporal regularity. Mothers use songs in a ritualized way, during particular times such as diaper changing and feeding [122, 123]. The rhythmic pattern remains stable from one iteration to another [80]. When the mother sings to her 6-month-old infant, the cortisol level changes to an intermediate level; if the baseline cortisol level (before singing) is high, it decreases slightly (after 10 min of singing followed by 10 min of interaction), and if the baseline cortisol level is low, it increases slightly. Thus, the rhythmic feature of singing modulates the arousal level of prelinguistic infants [83]. The spoken voice, even with the marked characteristics of infant-directed speech, is more variable and re-engages the attention of the infant [82].

With development, interactive games involving rhythmic organization of behavior become more and more frequent modes of communication. The fun and excitement of these games lie specifically in adults' and infants' sense of the duration of events and of their prediction of the next expected event. It is in fact the interruption of regularity that creates fun and enjoyment [61].

Later, in the course of the first year of life, shared rhythmicity, through music or rhythmic movements, promotes the expression of prosocial behavior [90, 91]. From 2½ years of age, children adjust more precisely their drumming rhythm to a 600 ms tempo (a tempo that is rather difficult to produce spontaneously) in the condition where they can drum jointly with a social partner (rather than when supplied with machine audiovisual stimuli or when alone) [124]. More broadly, the quality of synchrony in interactions between mother and infant at 3 months and at 9 months is predictive of certain social skills, such as greater social regulation at 2 years, a better understanding of morality, and more empathic speech in adolescence [11]. Maternal synchrony is specifically predictive of better social skills in young children and a better ability to take part in positive reciprocal activities with a close friend as a teenager. This type of paternal synchrony is also associated with less aggression in young children and a greater ability to dialogue in conflicting situations at adolescence. The early development of rhythmical interactions is therefore based on physiological rhythms and the infant's ability to perceive temporal regularities. Rhythmic interactions are fundamental to the child's social development. But, it is legitimate to question the influence of cultural practices on the role of rhythm in social interaction.

4.2.4 Cultural Influences

Each culture has its own timing during an interaction. Just as for their native language, infants need to acquire the keys to their culture in order to interpret and synchronize effectively with other individuals (the microcultural rhythm mentioned by Condon 1982, cited in [105]). There are cultural differences in the temporal structure of infant-directed speech and vocal interaction that has been described in interactions with 2- and 3-month-old infants [125]. These differences highlight the cultural differences that may exist in verbal/speech communication as well as at a nonverbal level. Depending on the culture, interacting individuals are not sensitive in the same way to the synchrony of movements. Although differences in the temporal organization of infant-directed speech and turn-taking have been noted across cultures, vocal interaction between mothers and infants also appears to be rhythmically organized around a fairly regular beat [126, 127]. Thus, Western cultures are less sensitive to synchrony than Latin American, African, and Asian cultures (Hall 1976, cited in [105]). During development, the infant must learn, through interactions, these cultural codes of interaction, and it may be that culture-specific rhythm and timing constitute very early forms of cultural learning, ones that precede a "social cognition" [126, 128]. Games are powerful socialization contexts, and indeed, it has been shown that the tempo of triadic interactions (between father, mother, and child) depends on the culture. Thus, Americans interact at a faster tempo than Swedes [129].

4.2.4.1 Music

Music and singing are important experiences through which infants may learn a number of cultural codes. It has been shown that, like adults, infants prefer consonant music and easily detect small changes in the frequency or pitch if the music is consonant rather than dissonant. Though infants can process tempos and rhythms, there is a perceptual narrowing process in musical perception. Six-month-old North American infants can detect changes in a larger number of different rhythms than a North American adult (who in turn is dependent on his/her own rhythmic culture). But at 12 months, infants perform better in the detection of variation in western rhythms and are poorer for foreign rhythms [88]. Unlike the perceptual narrowing in language and in face discrimination that progress with daily experience, the perceptual narrowing in rhythm discrimination progresses without daily experience necessarily.

4.2.4.2 Song

Lullabies used by caregivers to lull the infant to sleep have the same acoustic features in most cultures. These features make them recognizable by adults from another culture (even when filtered so as not to recognize the language) [130]. Nevertheless, there are cultural differences in the practice of the mother singing to her infant. In Western societies, mothers usually install their infants in a separate room, or at least isolate them. Mothers let their infants sleep alone (independently of a bedtime ritual) and rarely sing lullabies to their babies. In these cultures, songs are more frequently used in the context of play, and their features differ because the purpose of these songs is to heighten the infant's attention (e.g., through rhymes). In other cultures, as in India, mothers usually stay with their infants until they fall asleep. During this time, mothers often sing lullabies, which are songs designed to soothe the infant and decrease its level of attention. Lullabies or rhymes, depending on the culture, are a way for the mother to modulate the attention of her infant.

4.2.4.3 Sleep

One study showed that the correspondence between the mother's and the infant's activity rhythms is also found in the lifestyle of traditional cultures, in which infants are fed on demand. In this context, the movements of the mother and the infant are very well synchronized, during both day and night. What is remarkable in relation to what has been stated above is that when the father sleeps with the infant, this synchrony of activities is not found between the father and infant [131]. The socio-economic development of a country does not necessarily impact parenting practices, which are often rooted in the culture. For example, the practice of co-sleeping (discussed above for its possible effects on the development of more robust rhythms) by Japanese mothers has not significantly declined today compared to 40 years ago [132]. Parental practices around sleep also vary across cultural contexts but not nationality: thus, French parents from the city of Lyon in France choose the spoken voice and the music box much more than French parents living in Reunion Island, who prefer to give a feeding bottle, sing songs, rock the infant, or tap rhythmically [133].

To adjust the infant sleeping rhythms by parenting also requires that parents have a good representation of how the sleep of an infant is structured. A study showed that Asian and Caucasian parents have different perceptions of the quality of their infant's sleep [134]. In countries with Caucasian predominance, the definitions of sleep problems are mostly related to sleep variables (number of nocturnal awakenings, sleep latency), whereas in countries with Asian predominance, predictors are more related to demographic variables (age of the infant, parental age, education level of parents).

4.3 Current Clinical Translational Perspectives

The experience of rhythm goes hand in hand with the ability to anticipate events, enabling the individual to predict their occurrences. Thus, infants experience the world not only through actual events, most of which involve multiple sense modalities (the sound of the word is associated with facial movement), but also through the absence of stimulation, perceived as an empty or vacant period (Marcelli, cited in [135]). The experience of rhythm is then an experience of alternation of presence and absence. The appearance of the next event, predicted by the rhythmic sequence of preceding events, enables the infant to accept its absence or lack, precisely because of the certainty of its return. The duration of the separation between the infant and the caregiver is also imposed by the physiological duration between two meals (breast or bottle), which is approximately 3 h: the infant is supposed to meet the caregiver within this maximal period.

According to Ciccone [135], the rhythms experienced by the infant (as early as during fetal life) support the development of thought, including the notion of absence, which is linked to the possibility of anticipating the next event. Ciccone refers to the trauma of separation described by Winnicott and suggests it is possible to measure the duration separation by a proportionality computation: at 3 months, 8 h spent at the nursery is the mathematical equivalent of 44 days for a 30-year-old adult.

Rhythms, and especially motor rhythms, support a form of reinsurance and return to the relaxation state. According to Michel Fain (cited in [136]), rocking an infant is the equivalent of a self-soothing process provided by the mother. In the psychosomatic clinic, self-soothing processes are repeated motor or perceptual activities, rhythmically used to manage excitations that cannot be contained by mental processes or to remove a traumatic reality threatening the integrity [136]. By generating rhythmical patterns and temporal coherence through multimodality and by creating anticipation opportunities, rhythms provide a secure base in the representation of the body placed in the environment.

The following section will address various problems related to the disruption of rhythms experienced by the infant.

4.3.1 Disorders Related to the Disruption of Rhythms

Specifically in the postpartum, sleep phases alternate with awake and attention phases, and sleep patterns are modulated by the internal clock of the infant, by social rhythms, and by parenting practices. Therefore, changes in sleep rhythms affect arousal and attention phases which are necessary for integration of new competencies. Thus, circadian rhythm disorders generally have serious consequences on human health (immune system, cancer, etc.) as well as on cognitive development (for a review, see [137]). Indeed, some authors have shown that the circadian rhythm of sleep at 7 and 19 months has a positive impact on mental development scores at 24 months and on language development scores at 36 months [138]. Moreover, the circadian pattern of perinatal activity is predictive of anxiety level: regular daily activity, as assessed by the Baby Social Rhythm Metric (Baby SRM) at 1 month, significantly predicted the level of school anxiety (between 6 and 13 years). The authors showed that greater regularity was associated with lower school anxiety [139]. The regularity of sleep patterns is also correlated with certain emotional dimensions. Children who demonstrate disorganized attachment (in the strange situation) at 36 months of age also sleep less at night (with more night waking), go to bed later, and spend less time in bed, according to parental report [140]. It also appears that the regulation of attention and synchrony in mother-infant interaction at 3 months are predictive of visual IQ at 2 years [111].

4.3.2 Sudden Infant Death Syndrome (SIDS)

Although no straightforward cause of SIDS has been identified [141], it seems that rhythmic dysregulation may be a causal factor leading to SIDS. Melatonin concentration (in the cerebrospinal fluid) is significantly lower in infants who have died of SIDS than in those who have died from other ailments [142], suggesting that SIDS may be explained, at least in part, by a defect in the organization of circadian physiology. Various data show that SIDS occurs between 1 and 4 months of age, that is to say during a period when the most important changes in sleep patterning occur [45]. Apart from one other known risk factor that is birth weight, children at risk of SIDS have abnormalities in the central nervous system, mainly located in the brainstem and hypothalamus, regions involved in sleep/awake cyclicity and in the central control of respiration and cardiovascular activity. Moreover, in infants at risk of SIDS, the arousal thresholds for respiratory, tactile, visual, or thermal stimuli are higher during sleep. Consequently, these infants are less likely to wake up spontaneously (these data are to be added to those between 1 and 4 months of age; the arousal threshold is higher when the infant sleeps on its belly). These findings highlight the importance of considering the establishment of sleep/awake rhythms and sleep organization in assessing the risk of SIDS.

Another possible source of rhythm disturbance that increases the probability of SIDS is the Earth's geomagnetic activity. A correlational study [143] showed that 50–80% of the variance in monthly SIDS incidence can be explained by a greater number of days spent in weak magnetic fields. This specific variation in geomagnetic activity induces an abnormal decrease in nocturnal melatonin. When these conditions occur, the geomagnetic influence increases during the night (melatonin is synthesized in greater quantity at night) and in winter (melatonin levels are higher). These researches rely on the facts that deaths occur most often between 10 pm and 8 am and that 70% of them occur during the winter and fall. A study carried out near the North Pole, where geomagnetic activity is higher, confirmed that for some variation in geomagnetic field, it is possible to record a decrease in the concentration of salivary melatonin [144].

Although the causes and risk factors for SIDS are complex and not well established, it appears that the disruption of endogenous rhythms may put some infants at higher risk.

4.3.3 Prematurity: Benefits Provided by Rhythms

Rhythmic experiences in utero are a necessary foundation for the establishment of infant-mother bonding. Premature birth interrupts the continuity between prenatal and postnatal rhythmic experience. It is therefore important for practitioners involved in the care of premature infants to consider ways of providing the infant with rhythmic stimuli that bridge pre- and postnatal conditions [145].

Toward the end of gestation, the circadian system of the fetus is not yet mature. In the case of premature birth, the quality of the circadian rhythms (body temperature and heart rate) is influenced by gestational age (i.e., maturation) and by intrauterine growth [9]. It is obviously difficult to show the effect of environmental rhythmicities on the development of premature infants as there are too many factors to control. Nevertheless, it seems that infants born before 31 weeks (postconception) who are exposed to light cycles gain more weight than those exposed to very low light [146].

The rhythmic stimuli that are most clearly lacking in the experience of a premature infant compared to an age-matched fetus in utero are the ones pertaining to vestibular stimulation. Yet, it is known that rhythmic stimulation (rocking, etc.) has a positive impact on the premature infant ([147–150]; see also [39]). The NIDCAP program is aimed at providing individualized care centered on both the infant and its family. It pays particular attention to the role of adaptive environmental rhythms for the preterm infant in order to facilitate the expression of its own behavioral rhythms (rocking, non-nutritive sucking). One often overlooked aspect of this program is the attention paid to the infant's light environment, which is controlled to maintain a level of brightness that is similar to that of the intrauterine environment, with a gradual adaptation to the day-night cycle.

Social interactions are quite naturally affected by premature birth. Generally, preterm mothers are less sensitive to their infant's signals, and premature infants are in turn less responsive to maternal solicitations, perhaps due to the fact that their nervous system is less mature than that of term infants [112]. The quality of mother-infant interactional synchrony has been evaluated via the MISS (Maternal-Infant Synchrony Scale) at the time of feeding between a mother and her premature infant [112]. Mothers of infants born prematurely do not use the same cues as those of term infants in their exchanges during meals, but they are more sensitive to the vocal cues of their infants [117]. Kangaroo care has for a long time provided parents support in caring for their prematurely born infant. In this situation, infants benefit from body temperature regulation, heartbeat synchronization, and movement and posture coordination with the parent who carries them. It has been shown that at term, a prematurely born infant with experience of "kangaroo care" has a more mature and organized sleep-wake rhythm than the controls. Furthermore, at 3 months corrected age, these infants have higher thresholds to negative emotion and more efficient arousal modulation while attending to increasingly complex stimuli. At 6 months corrected age, their attention is longer and faster, and their exploration behavior is more sustained [110].

Finally, a growing body of research has shown that music experience involving rhythm has beneficial effects on the development of preterm infants. Firstly, it was found to increase the effectiveness of feeding; broadcasting music to preterm infants during non-nutritive sucking phases increases the frequency, duration, and endurance of their sucking behavior leading to efficient feeding and earlier discharge from specialized services [151]. However, the effects of music can also be measured through other physiological indicators. Music in NICU units shows strong benefits for premature infants in terms of their heart rate, behavior, oxygen saturation, and sleep [152]. Live music performed by a certified music therapist is even more effective than recorded music. Live singing by the mother has also been found to have immediate beneficial effects on preterm infants' physiological state and arousal [153]. Music also offers the potential for mutual regulation between the caregiver and child. Edwards [103] argues that music therapist interventions support the establishment of attachment behaviors.

4.3.4 Autism

The importance of rhythm, motor synchrony, and emotional interpersonal development in social communication has been highlighted by numerous studies. The role of melatonin in the development of circadian rhythms and in the synchronization of the circadian clock with external rhythms has led to the hypothesis that this hormone may influence motor, emotional, and interpersonal synchrony. Some authors consider that autism spectrum disorders are at least in part an expression of a disturbance of biological rhythms. In fact, various studies have shown that children with autism spectrum disorder (ASD) present disorders of sleep-wake rhythms, cortisol rhythms, and melatonin secretion rhythms (for a recent review, see [154]). Furthermore, congenitally blind children, who consequently have an abnormal melatonin secretion (no circadian synchronization via the retinoic-hypothalamic tract) and who present sleep disorders, are more prone to ASD [154]. Some authors also point out that the prevalence of epileptic disorders in autism is estimated to be higher than in the general population [155]. Indeed in some forms of ASD, rapid sensory stimulation can cause epileptic seizures. The hypothesis put forward by Amos [155] is that a change in sensory stimuli rhythms causes physiological stress (due to an increase in the level of arousal) triggering a seizure. Other studies point out that people with autism recognize social interactions better if their perceptions are slowed down. This has been tested through presentation of slowed down video [156]. Thus, there is a body of evidence highlighting disturbances of different types of rhythms in this population. Since the processing of rhythms at different levels, including social rhythms, seems dependent on the circadian clock, it is possible that children with ASD, who present a circadian system disorder, also have a disorder in processing social rhythms. Some researchers have started investigating the genetic factors involved in the chronobiological and social timing difficulties associated with ASD [157], but more research is needed in this area.

This hypothesis would at least partly explain the difficulty these children have in interpreting social cues, based on a specific timing of interaction. To our knowledge, no studies have considered rhythm disorders in children with ASD, and we are currently investigating the synchronization performances in children with autism.

4.3.5 Maternal Depression and Prenatal Anxiety

It is well established that prenatal stress can have long-term consequences on infant behavior [158]. Stress, anxiety, and depression alter the physiology of the mother by disrupting the hypothalamic-pituitary-adrenal (HPA) axis. In addition, major depressive disorder (MDD) is characterized by shorter telomeres than normal. Both MDD and telomere length are associated with high levels of stress, causing dysfunction of the HPA axis and abnormal cortisol levels. One study showed that children from families at risk of developing MDD have a premature aging of their own telomeres, even before experiencing the onset of depression [159]. Another study showed that sleep disorders in children may in part be related to stress or depression in the mother during pregnancy [160]. Infants of depressed mothers have different physiological and behavioral patterns compared to those of non-depressed mothers, which can be explained by exposure to higher cortisol levels during pregnancy [161]. Infants born to mothers who were depressed during pregnancy also have greater right frontal EEG activity and lower vagal tone compared to infants of non-depressed mothers [162]. Antenatal maternal anxiety is predictive of behavioral and emotional disorders in preschoolers and children aged 8–9 years and of changes in the activation of HPA axis.

Depressed mothers demonstrate fewer marked rhythms in their motor behavior and in their interaction. Consequently, some rhythm disturbances in infants or in the dyads have been reported in the context of maternal depression. Mothers with depressive disorders generally have fewer attuned interactions synchronized with the behavior of their 3-month-old infant [163]. Moreover, the effect of music and lullabies is lower when the mother is depressed. Thus, infants of mothers with depressive symptoms (usually associated with obstetric complications) are more aroused when hearing music or a lullaby [164], contradicting their soothing effect. One study showed the value of using different rhythmic stimuli, such as music, singing, or rocking, to support the quality of intersubjectivity in the mother-infant dyad when the mother presents postpartum depression [165]. Furthermore, it appears that maternal sensitivity is an important factor in modulating the effect of anxiety and depression [162].

Thus, maternal depression in the perinatal period may impact the physiology of the infant via disturbances in cortisol secretion rhythms as well as through interaction rhythms.

4.4 Next Steps…

This broad review highlights the importance and pervasiveness of biological, physiological, and behavioral rhythms in the perinatal period as a framework for the harmonious development of the fetus and infant. It also provides arguments in support of the idea that rhythms expressed at different levels, such as in gene expression, physiology, behavior, and spontaneous behaviors, are connected with those that pervade the infant's physical and social environments. It is indeed conceivable that a hierarchical relationship exists between the various kinds of rhythms discussed in the chapter. But more research is called for in order to clarify the complex relations between them, both in healthy development and in atypical trajectories. Circadian rhythms could influence behavioral rhythms, which could in turn support attentional processes and the development of the crucial social skills and socio-cognitive abilities that underlie the major achievements that mark early human development.

References

1. Roenneberg T, Kuehnle T, Juda M, Kantermann T, Allebrandt K, Gordijn M, Merrow M (2007) Epidemiology of the human circadian clock. Sleep Med Rev 11(6):429–438. https://doi.org/10.1016/j.smrv.2007.07.005
2. Simpkin CT, Jenni OG, Carskadon MA, Wright KPJ, Akacem LD, Garlo KG, LeBourgeois MK (2014) Chronotype is associated with the timing of the circadian clock and sleep in toddlers. J Sleep Res 23(4):397–405. https://doi.org/10.1111/jsr.12142
3. Serón-Ferré M, Torres-Farfan C, Forcelledo ML, Valenzuela GJ (2001) The development of circadian rhythms in the fetus and neonate. Semin Perinatol (6):363–370
4. Reppert SM, Weaver D, Rivkees SA, Stopa E (1988) Putative melatonin receptors in a human biological clock. Science 242(4875):78–81. https://doi.org/10.1126/science.2845576

5. Tsai S-Y, Thomas KA, Lentz MJ, Barnard KE (2012) Light is beneficial for infant circadian entrainment: an actigraphic study. J Adv Nurs 68(8):1738–1747. https://doi.org/10.1111/j.1365-2648.2011.05857.x
6. Mirmiran M, Kok JH, Boer K, Wolf H (1992) Perinatal development of human circadian rhythms: role of the foetal biological clock. Neurosci Biobehav Rev 16(3):371–378. https://doi.org/10.1016/S0149-7634(05)80207-6
7. Korte J, Hoehn T, Siegmund R (2004) Actigraphic recordings of activity-rest rhythms of neonates born by different delivery modes. Chronobiol Int 21(1):95–106
8. McGraw K, Hoffmann R, Harker C, Herman JH (1999) The development of circadian rhythms in a human infant. Sleep 22(3):303–310. https://frodon.univ-paris5.fr/url?http://search.ebscohost.com/login.aspx?direct=true&db=psyh&AN=1999-05089-003&lang=fr&site=ehost-live
9. Mirmiran M, Ariagno RL (2000) Influence of light in the NICU on the development of circadian rhythms in preterm infants. Semin Perinatol 24(4):247–257
10. Germain AM, Valenzuela GJ, Ivankovic M, Ducsay CA, Gabella C, Serón-Ferré M (1993) Relationship of circadian rhythms of uterine activity with term and preterm delivery. Am J Obstet Gynecol 168(4):1271–1277. https://doi.org/10.1016/0002-9378(93)90379-W
11. Feldman R (2015) Sensitive periods in human social development: new insights from research on oxytocin, synchrony, and high-risk parenting. Dev Psychopathol 27(2):369–395. http://journals.cambridge.org/abstract_S0954579415000048
12. Warren WS, Cassone VM (1995) The pineal gland: photoreception and coupling of behavioral, metabolic, and cardiovascular circadian outputs. J Biol Rhythm 10(1):64–79. https://doi.org/10.1177/074873049501000106
13. Burnham MM (2007) The ontogeny of diurnal rhythmicity in bed-sharing and solitary-sleeping infants: a preliminary report. Infant Child Dev 16(4):341–357
14. Kennaway DJ (2000) Melatonin and development: physiology and pharmacology. Semin Perinatol 24(4):258–266. https://doi.org/10.1053/sper.2000.8594
15. Ivars K, Nelson N, Theodorsson A, Theodorsson E, Ström JO, Mörelius E (2015) Development of salivary cortisol circadian rhythm and reference intervals in full-term infants. PLoS One 10(6):e0129502. https://doi.org/10.1371/journal.pone.0129502
16. Guilleminault C, Leger D, Pelayo R, Gould S, Hayes B, Miles L (1996) Development of circadian rhythmicity of temperature in full-term normal infants. Neurophysiol Clin 26(1):21–29
17. de Vries JIP, Visser GHA, Prechtl HFR (1982) The emergence of fetal behaviour. I. Qualitative aspects. Early Hum Dev 7(4):301–322. https://doi.org/10.1016/0378-3782(82)90033-0
18. de Vries JIP, Visser GHA (1987) Diurnal and other variations in fetal movement and heart rate patterns at 20–22 weeks. Early Hum Dev 15(6):333–348. http://www.sciencedirect.com/science/article/pii/0378378287900296
19. Watanabe K, Iwase K, Hara K (1973) Visual evoked responses during sleep and wakefulness in pre-term infants. Electroencephalogr Clin Neurophysiol 34(6):571–577
20. Porges S (1994) Le tonus vagal: indicateur du stress et de la vulnérabilité au stress chez l'enfant. Médecine & Enfance, octobre, 494
21. Van Puyvelde M, Loots G, Meys J, Neyt X, Mairesse O, Simcock D, Pattyn N (2015) Whose clock makes yours tick? How maternal cardiorespiratory physiology influences newborns' heart rate variability. Biol Psychol 108(April 2015):132–141. https://doi.org/10.1016/j.biopsycho.2015.04.001
22. Thelen E (1979) Rhythmical stereotypies in normal human infants. Anim Behav 27:699–715. https://doi.org/10.1016/0003-3472(79)90006-X
23. Thelen E (1981) Kicking, rocking, and waving: contextual analysis of rhythmical stereotypies in normal human infants. Anim Behav 29(1918):3–11. https://doi.org/10.1016/S0003-3472(81)80146-7
24. Zentner M, Eerola T (2010) Rhythmic engagement with music in infancy. Proc Natl Acad Sci U S A 107(13):5768–5773. https://doi.org/10.1073/pnas.1000121107
25. Eerola T, Luck G, Toiviainen P (2006) An investigation of pre-schoolers' corporeal synchronization with music. 9th international conference on music perception and cognition, pp 472–476

26. de Vries JIP, Fong BF (2006) Normal fetal motility: an overview. Ultrasound Obstet Gynecol 27(6):701–711. https://doi.org/10.1002/uog.2740
27. Wolff PH (1968) Sucking patterns of infant mammals. Brain Behav Evol 1:354–367
28. Wright P, Fawcett J, Crow R (1980) The development of differences in the feeding behaviour of bottle and breast fed human infants from birth to two months. Behav Process 5(1):1–20. https://doi.org/10.1016/0376-6357(80)90045-5
29. Crook CK, Lipsitt LP (1976) Neonatal nutritive sucking: effects of taste stimulation upon sucking rhythm and heart rate. Child Dev 47(2):518–522. https://doi.org/10.2307/1128812
30. DeCasper AJ, Fifer WP (1980) Of human bonding: newborns prefer their mothers' voices. Science 208(4448):1174–1176. https://doi.org/10.1126/science.7375928
31. Bobin-Bègue A, Provasi J, Marks A, Pouthas V (2006) Influence of auditory tempo on the endogenous rhythm of non-nutritive sucking. Rev Eur Psychol Appl 56(4):239–245
32. Bobin-Bègue A, Provasi J (2008) Régulation rythmique avant 4 ans: effet d'un tempo auditif sur le tempo moteur. Annee Psychol 108(04):631–658. https://doi.org/10.4074/S000350330800403X
33. Drake C, Jones MR, Baruch C (2000) The development of rhythmic attending in auditory sequences: attunement, referent period, focal attending. Cognition 77:251–288
34. Provasi J, Bobin-Bègue A (2003) Spontaneous motor tempo and rhythmical synchronization in 21/2- and 4-year-old children. Int J Behav Dev 27(3):220–231
35. Vanneste S, Pouthas V, Wearden JH (2001) Temporal control of rhythmic performance: a comparison between young and old adults. Exp Aging Res 27(1):83–102. https://doi.org/10.1080/036107301750046151
36. Moussay S, Dosseville F, Gauthier A, Larue J (2002) Circadian rhythms during cycling exercise and finger-tapping task. Chronobiol Int 19(6):1137–1149. https://doi.org/10.1081/CBI-120015966
37. Cohen RA, Barnes HJ, Jenkins M, Albers HE (1997) Disruption of short-duration timing associated with damage to the suprachiasmatic region of the hypothalamus. Neurology 48(6):1533–1539. https://doi.org/10.1212/WNL.51.3.919-b
38. Wolff PH (1969) The natural history of crying and other vocalizations in infancy. In: Foss BM (ed) Determinants of infant behavior IV. Methuen, London, pp 81–111
39. Provasi J, Anderson DI, Barbu-Roth MA (2014) Rhythm perception, production, and synchronization during the perinatal period. Front Psychol 5(September):1–16. https://doi.org/10.3389/fpsyg.2014.01048
40. Brennan M, Kirkland J (1982) Classification of infant cries using descriptive scales. Infant Behav Dev 5(2–4):341–346. https://doi.org/10.1016/S0163-6383(82)80044-1
41. Wermke K, Mende W (2009) Musical elements in human infants' cries: in the beginning is the melody. Music Sci 13(2 Suppl):151–175. https://doi.org/10.1177/1029864909013002081
42. Mampe B, Friederici AD, Christophe A, Wermke K (2009) Newborns' cry melody is shaped by their native language. Curr Biol 19(23):1994–1997. https://doi.org/10.1016/j.cub.2009.09.064
43. Provasi J, Barbu-Roth MA (2009) Motor synchronization to tempo in newborns. In Proceeding of the 12th international symposium on rhythm perception and production. Workshop, distored Time and motor control. Proceeding of the 12th international symposium on rhythm perception and production. Workshop, distored time and motor control, Lille, France
44. Louis J, Cannard C, Bastuji H, Challamel M-J (1997) Sleep ontogenesis revisited: a longitudinal 24-hour home polygraphic study on 15 normal infants during the first two years of life. Sleep 20(5):323–333
45. Mirmiran M, Maas YGH, Ariagno RL (2003) Development of fetal and neonatal sleep and circadian rhythms. Sleep Med Rev 7(4):321–334. https://doi.org/10.1053/smrv.2002.0243
46. Grigg-Damberger M, Gozal D (2007) The visual scoring of sleep and arousal in infants and children. J Clin Sleep Med 3(2):201–240
47. Galland BC, Taylor BJ, Elder DE, Herbison P (2012) Normal sleep patterns in infants and children: a systematic review of observational studies. Sleep Med Rev 16(3):213–222. https://doi.org/10.1016/j.smrv.2011.06.001

48. Schwichtenberg AJ, Anders TF, Vollbrecht M, Poehlmann J (2011) Daytime sleep and parenting interactions in infants born preterm. J Dev Behav Pediatr 32(1):8–17. https://doi.org/10.1097/DBP.0b013e3181fa57e4
49. Nishihara K, Horiuchi S, Eto H, Uchida S (2002) The development of infants' circadian rest-activity rhythm and mothers' rhythm. Physiol Behav 77(1):91–98
50. Wulff K, Dedek A, Siegmund R (2001) Circadian and ultradian time patterns in human behavior: part 2: social synchronisation during the development of the infant's diurnal activity-rest pattern. Biol Rhythm Res 32(5):529–546. https://doi.org/10.1076/brhm.32.5.529.1295
51. Thomas KA, Burr RL, Spieker S, Lee J, Chen J (2014) Mother-infant circadian rhythm: development of individual patterns and dyadic synchrony. Early Hum Dev 90(12):885–890. https://doi.org/10.1016/j.earlhumdev.2014.09.005
52. Schaal B, Orgeur P, Rognon C (1995) Odor sensing in the human fetus: anatomical, functional, and chemoecological bases. http://psycnet.apa.org/psycinfo/1995-98392-008
53. Bakeman R, Adamson LB (1984) Coordinating attention to people and objects in mother-infant and peer-infant interaction. Child Dev 55(4):1278–1289. https://doi.org/10.2307/1129997
54. Robertson SS, Bacher LF, Huntington NL (2001) The integration of body movement and attention in young infants. Psychol Sci 12(6):523–526. http://www.ncbi.nlm.nih.gov/pubmed/11760142
55. Brackbill Y (1973) Continuous stimulation reduces arousal level: stability of the effect over time. Child Dev 44:43–46
56. Feldman R, Mayes LC (1999) The cyclic organization of attention during habituation is related to infants' information processing. Infant Behav Dev 22(1):37–49. https://doi.org/10.1016/S0163-6383(99)80004-6
57. Jones MR (1974) Cognitive representations of serial patterns. Human information processing. http://scholar.google.fr/scholar?q=mari+riess+jones+1974&btnG=&hl=fr&as_sdt=0%2C5#0
58. Martin T, Egly R, Houck JM, Bish JP, Barrera BD, Lee DC, Tesche CD (2005) Chronometric evidence for entrained attention. Percept Psychophys 67(1):168–184. https://doi.org/10.3758/BF03195020
59. Perra O, Gattis M (2012) Attention engagement in early infancy. Infant Behav Dev 35(4):635–644. https://doi.org/10.1016/j.infbeh.2012.06.004
60. Stroganova TA, Orekhova EV, Posikera IN (1998) Externally and internally controlled attention in infants: an EEG study. Int J Psychophysiol 30(3):339–351
61. Parrott WG, Gleitman H (1989) Infants' expectations in play: the joy of peek-a-boo. Cognit Emot 3(4):291–311
62. Pederson DR, Vrugt DT (1973) The influence of amplitude and frequency of vestibular stimulation on the activity of two-month-old infants. Child Dev 44(1):122–128
63. Ter Vrugt D, Pederson DR (1973) The effects of vertical rocking frequencies on the arousal level in two-month-old infants. Child Dev 44(1):205–209
64. Wichniak A, Tracik F, Geisler P, Ebersbach G, Morrissey SP, Zulley J (2001) Rhythmic feet movements while falling asleep. Mov Disord 16(6):1164–1170
65. Mistlberger RE, Skene DJ (2004) Social influences on mammalian circadian rhythms: animal and human studies. Biol Rev Camb Philos Soc 79(3):533–556. https://doi.org/10.1017/S1464793103006353
66. Cito G, Luisi S, Mezzesimi A, Cavicchioli C, Calonaci G, Petraglia F (2005) Maternal position during non stress test and fetal heart rate patterns. Acta Obstet Gynecol Scand 84(4):335–338. https://doi.org/10.1111/j.0001-6349.2005.00644.x
67. Lecanuet J-P, Jacquet A-Y (2002) Fetal responsiveness to maternal passive swinging in low heart rate variability state: effects of stimulation direction and duration. Dev Psychobiol 40(1):57–67
68. Kisilevsky BS, Muir DW (1991) Human fetal and subsequent newborn responses to sound and vibration. Infant Behav Dev 14(1):1–26. https://doi.org/10.1016/0163-6383(91)90051-S
69. Kisilevsky BS, Hains SMJ, Lee K, Xie X, Huang H, Ye HH, Zhang K, Wang Z (2003) Effects of experience on fetal voice recognition. Psychol Sci 14(3):220–224. https://doi.org/10.1111/1467-9280.02435

70. Bertoncini J, Nazzi T, Cabrera L, Lorenzi C (2011) Six-month-old infants discriminate voicing on the basis of temporal envelope cues (L). J Acoust Soc Am 129(5):2761–2764. https://doi.org/10.1121/1.3571424
71. Granier-Deferre C, Ribeiro A, Jacquet A-Y, Bassereau S (2011) Near-term fetuses process temporal features of speech. Dev Sci 14(2):336–352. https://doi.org/10.1111/j.1467-7687.2010.00978.x
72. Lewkowicz DJ (2000) The development of intersensory temporal perception: an epigenetic systems/limitations view. Psychol Bull 126(2):281–308. https://doi.org/10.1037/0033-2909.126.2.281
73. Bahrick LE, Lickliter R, Castellanos I, Todd JT (2015) Intrasensory redundancy facilitates infant detection of tempo: extending predictions of the intersensory redundancy hypothesis. Infancy:1–28. https://doi.org/10.1111/infa.12081
74. Phillips-Silver J, Trainor LJ (2005) Feeling the beat: movement influences infant rhythm perception. Science 308(5727):1430. https://doi.org/10.1126/science.1110922
75. Phillips-Silver J, Trainor LJ (2008) Vestibular influence on auditory metrical interpretation. Brain Cogn 67(1):94–102. https://doi.org/10.1016/j.bandc.2007.11.007
76. Mehler J, Christophe A (1994) Language in the infant's mind. Philos Trans R Soc Lond Ser B Biol Sci 346(1315):13–20. https://doi.org/10.1098/rstb.1994.0123
77. Nazzi T, Bertoncini J, Mehler J (1998) Language discrimination by newborns: toward an understanding of the role of rhythm. J Exp Psychol Hum Percept Perform 24(3):756–766. https://doi.org/10.1037/0096-1523.24.3.756
78. Hains SMJ, Muir D (1996) Effects of stimulus contingency in infant-adult interactions. Infant Behav Dev 19(1996):49–61. https://doi.org/10.1016/S0163-6383(96)90043-0
79. Pons F, Lewkowicz DJ (2014) Infant perception of audio-visual speech synchrony in familiar and unfamiliar fluent speech. Acta Psychol 149:142–147. https://doi.org/10.1016/j.actpsy.2013.12.013
80. Bergeson TR, Trehub SE (2002) Absolute pitch and tempo in mothers' songs to infants. Psychol Sci 13(1):72–75
81. Delavenne A, Gratier M, Devouche E (2013) Expressive timing in infant-directed singing between 3 and 6 months. Infant Behav Dev 36:1–13
82. Nakata T, Trehub SE (2004) Infants' responsiveness to maternal speech and singing. Infant Behav Dev 27(4):455–464. https://doi.org/10.1016/j.infbeh.2004.03.002
83. Shenfield T, Trehub SE, Nakata T (2003) Maternal singing modulates infant arousal. Psychol Music 31(4):365–375. https://doi.org/10.1177/03057356030314002
84. Kisilevsky BS, Hains SMJ, Jacquet A-Y, Granier-Deferre C, Lecanuet J-P (2004) Maturation of fetal responses to music. Dev Sci 7(5):550–559. https://doi.org/10.1111/j.1467-7687.2004.00379.x
85. Winkler I, Háden GP, Ladinig O, Sziller I, Honing H (2009) Newborn infants detect the beat in music. Proc Natl Acad Sci U S A 106(7):2468–2471. https://doi.org/10.1073/pnas.0809035106
86. Baruch C, Drake C (1997) Tempo discrimination in infants. Infant Behav Dev 20(4):573–577. https://doi.org/10.1016/S0163-6383(97)90049-7
87. Demany L, McKenzie B, Vurpillot E (1977) Rhythm perception in early infancy. Nature 266:718–719. https://doi.org/10.1038/266718a0
88. Hannon EE, Trehub SE (2005) Metrical categories in infancy and adulthood. Psychol Sci 16(1):48–55. https://doi.org/10.1111/j.0956-7976.2005.00779.x
89. Bigelow A (1998) Infants' sensitivity to familiar contingencies in social interaction. Infant Behav Dev 21:298. https://doi.org/10.1016/S0163-6383(98)91511-9
90. Tunçgenç B, Cohen E, Fawcett C (2015) Rock with me: the role of movement synchrony in infants' social and nonsocial choices. Child Dev 86(3):976–984. https://doi.org/10.1111/cdev.12354
91. Cirelli LK, Einarson KM, Trainor LJ (2014) Interpersonal synchrony increases prosocial behavior in infants. Dev Sci:1–9. https://doi.org/10.1111/desc.12193

92. Slater J, Kraus N (2016) The role of rhythm in perceiving speech in noise: a comparison of percussionists, vocalists and non-musicians. Cogn Process 17(1):79–87. https://doi.org/10.1007/s10339-015-0740-7
93. Rivkees SA (2004) Emergence and influences of circadian rhythmicity in infants. Clin Perinatol 31(2):217–228. , v–vi. https://doi.org/10.1016/j.clp.2004.04.011
94. Harrison Y (2004) The relationship between daytime exposure to light and night-time sleep in 6-12-week-old infants. J Sleep Res 13(4):345–352. https://doi.org/10.1111/j.1365-2869.2004.00435.x
95. McBean AL, Montgomery-Downs HE (2015) What are postpartum women doing while the rest of the world is asleep? J Sleep Res 24(3):270–278. https://doi.org/10.1111/jsr.12265
96. Mosko SS, Richard C, McKenna J, Drummond S (1996) Infant sleep architecture during bedsharing and possible implications for SIDS. Sleep 19(9):677–684
97. Richard CA, Mosko SS (2004) Mother-infant bedsharing is associated with an increase in infant heart rate. Sleep 27(3):507–511
98. Benjamin Neelon SE, Stroo M, Mayhew M, Maselko J, Hoyo C (2015) Correlation between maternal and infant cortisol varies by breastfeeding status. Infant Behav Dev 40:252–258. https://doi.org/10.1016/j.infbeh.2015.06.005
99. Nishihara K, Horiuchi S, Eto H, Kikuchi S, Hoshi Y (2012) Relationship between infant and mother circadian rest-activity rhythm pre- and postpartum, in comparison to an infant with free-running rhythm. Chronobiol Int 29(3):363–370. https://doi.org/10.3109/07420528.2012.657762
100. Ferber SG, Laudon M, Kuint J, Weller A, Zisapel N (2002) Massage therapy by mothers enhances the adjustment of circadian rhythms to the nocturnal period in full-term infants. J Dev Behav Pediatr 23(6):410–415
101. Pederson DR (1975) The soothing effect of rocking as determined by the direction and frequency of movement. Can J Behav Sci 7(3):237–243
102. Yamasaki A, Booker A, Kapur V, Tilt A, Niess H, Lillemoe KD, Warshaw AL, Conrad C (2012) The impact of music on metabolism. Nutrition 28(11–12):1075–1080. https://doi.org/10.1016/j.nut.2012.01.020
103. Edwards J (2011) The use of music therapy to promote attachment between parents and infants. Arts Psychother 38(3):190–195. https://doi.org/10.1016/j.aip.2011.05.002
104. de Graag JA, Cox RFA, Hasselman F, Jansen J, de Weerth C (2012) Functioning within a relationship: mother-infant synchrony and infant sleep. Infant Behav Dev 35(2):252–263. https://doi.org/10.1016/j.infbeh.2011.12.006
105. Kim YY (2015) Achieving synchrony: a foundational dimension of intercultural communication competence. Int J Intercult Relat 48:27–37. https://doi.org/10.1016/j.ijintrel.2015.03.016
106. Moore GA, Calkins SD (2004) Infants' vagal regulation in the still-face paradigm is related to dyadic coordination of mother-infant interaction. Dev Psychol 40(6):1068–1080. https://doi.org/10.1037/0012-1649.40.6.1068
107. Voegtline KM, Costigan KA, Pater HA, DiPietro JA (2013) Near-term fetal response to maternal spoken voice. Infant Behav Dev 36(4):526–533. https://doi.org/10.1016/j.infbeh.2013.05.002
108. Feldman R (2006) From biological rhythms to social rhythms: physiological precursors of mother-infant synchrony. Dev Psychol 42(1):175–188. https://doi.org/10.1037/0012-1649.42.1.175
109. Feldman R, Magori-Cohen R, Galili G, Singer M, Louzoun Y (2011) Mother and infant coordinate heart rhythms through episodes of interaction synchrony. Infant Behav Dev 34(4):569–577. https://doi.org/10.1016/j.infbeh.2011.06.008
110. Feldman R, Weller A, Sirota L, Eidelman AI (2002) Skin-to-skin contact (kangaroo care) promotes self-regulation in premature infants: sleep-wake cyclicity, arousal modulation, and sustained exploration. Dev Psychol 38(2):194–207. https://doi.org/10.1037/0012-1649.38.2.194
111. Feldman R, Greenbaum CW, Yirmiya N, Mayes LC (1996) Relations between cyclicity and regulation in mother-infant interaction at 3 and 9 months and cognition at 2 years. J Appl Dev Psychol 17(3):347–365. https://doi.org/10.1016/S0193-3973(96)90031-3

112. Reyna BA, Brown LF, Pickler RH, Myers BJ, Younger JB (2012) Mother-infant synchrony during infant feeding. Infant Behav Dev 35(4):669–677. https://doi.org/10.1016/j.infbeh.2012.06.003
113. Feldman R, Singer M, Zagoory O (2010) Touch attenuates infants' physiological reactivity to stress. Dev Sci 13(2):271–278. https://doi.org/10.1111/j.1467-7687.2009.00890.x
114. Van Puyvelde M, Loots G, Vinck B, De Coster L, Matthijs L, Mouvet K, Pattyn N (2013) The interplay between tonal synchrony and social engagement in mother-infant interaction. Infancy 18(5):849–872. https://doi.org/10.1111/infa.12007
115. Trevarthen C (1979) Communication and cooperation in early infancy: a description of primary intersubjectivity. In: Before speech: the beginning of interpersonal communication. Cambridge University Press, Cambridge
116. Condon WS, Sander LW (1974) Synchrony demonstrated between movements of the neonate and adult speech. Child Dev 45(2):456–462. https://doi.org/10.2307/1127968
117. Stevenson MB, Roach MA, Ver Hoeve JN, Leavitt LA (1990) Rhythms in the dialogue of infant feeding: preterm and term infants. Infant Behav Dev 13(1):51–70. https://doi.org/10.1016/0163-6383(90)90005-S
118. Dominguez S, Devouche E, Apter G, Gratier M (2016) The roots of turn-taking in the neonatal period. Infant Child Dev 25(3):240–255. https://doi.org/10.1002/icd.1976
119. Nomikou I, Leonardi G, Radkowska A, Rączaszek-Leonardi J, Rohlfing KJ (2017) Taking up an active role: emerging participation in early mother–infant interaction during peekaboo routines. Front Psychol 8:1656. https://doi.org/10.3389/fpsyg.2017.01656
120. Gratier M, Devouche E (2011) Imitation and repetition of prosodic contour in vocal interaction at 3 months. Dev Psychol 47(1):67–76. https://doi.org/10.1037/a0020722
121. Jaffe J, Beebe B, Feldstein S, Crown CL, Jasnow MD, Rochat P, Stern DN (2001) Rhythms of dialogue in infancy: coordinated timing in development. Monogr Soc Res Child Dev 66(2):i–viii, 1-132.
122. Gudmundsdottir HR, Trehub SE (2012) Mothers as singing mentors for infants. In: Graham Welch JN, Howard DM (eds) The Oxford handbook of singing. Oxford University Press, Oxford, pp 2013–2015. https://doi.org/10.1093/law/9780199599752.003.0065
123. Rock AML, Trainor LJ, Addison TL (1999) Distinctive messages in infant-directed lullabies and play songs. Dev Psychol 35(2):527–534
124. Kirschner S, Tomasello M (2009) Joint drumming: social context facilitates synchronization in preschool children. J Exp Child Psychol 102(3):299–314. https://doi.org/10.1016/j.jecp.2008.07.005
125. Keller H, Otto H, Lamm B, Yovsi RD, Kärtner J (2008) The timing of verbal/vocal communications between mothers and their infants: a longitudinal cross-cultural comparison. Infant Behav Dev 31(2008):217–226. https://doi.org/10.1016/j.infbeh.2007.10.001
126. Gratier M (2003) Expressive timing and interactional synchrony between mothers and infants: Cultural similarities, cultural differences, and the immigration experience. Cogn Dev 18(2003):533–554. https://doi.org/10.1016/j.cogdev.2003.09.009
127. Trevarthen C (2000) Musicality and the intrinsic motive pulse: evidence from human psychobiology and infant communication. Music Sci 1999:155–215. https://doi.org/10.1177/10298649000030S109
128. Gratier M, Trevarthen C (2008) Musical narrative and motives for culture in mother-infant vocal interaction. J Conscious Stud (10):122–158
129. Hedenbro M, Shapiro AF, Gottman JM (2006) Play with me at my speed: describing differences in the tempo of parent-infant interactions in the Lausanne triadic play paradigm in two cultures. Fam Process 45(4):485–498
130. Trehub SE, Unyk AM, Trainor LJ (1993) Maternal singing in cross-cultural perspective. Infant Behav Dev 16:285–295. https://doi.org/10.1016/0163-6383(93)80036-8
131. Siegmund R, Tittel M, Schiefenhövel W (1994) Time patterns in parent-child interactions in a trobriand village (Papua New Guinea). Biol Rhythm Res 25(3):241–251. https://doi.org/10.1080/09291019409360299

132. Shimizu M, Park H, Greenfield PM (2014) Infant sleeping arrangements and cultural values among contemporary Japanese mothers. Front Psychol 5:718. https://doi.org/10.3389/fpsyg.2014.00718
133. Louis J, Govindama Y (2004) Troubles du sommeil et rituels d'endormissement chez le jeune enfant dans une perspective transculturelle. Arch Pediatr 11(2004):93–98. https://doi.org/10.1016/j.arcped.2003.11.012
134. Sadeh A, Mindell JA, Rivera L (2011) "My child has a sleep problem": a cross-cultural comparison of parental definitions. Sleep Med 12(5):478–482. https://doi.org/10.1016/j.sleep.2010.10.008
135. Ciccone A (2005) L'expérience du rythme chez le bébé et dans le soin psychique. Neuropsychiatr Enfance Adolesc 53(1–2 Special Issue):24–31. https://doi.org/10.1016/j.neurenf.2005.01.002
136. Duclos K (2002) Au sujet d'une modalité particulière de recours à l'activité physique : les procédés autocalmants. Philos Sci 6(1):93–103. https://eudml.org/doc/103670
137. Golombek DA, Casiraghi LP, Agostino PV, Paladino N, Duhart JM, Plano SA, Chiesa JJ (2013) The times they're a-changing: effects of circadian desynchronization on physiology and disease. J Physiol Paris 107(4):310–322. https://doi.org/10.1016/j.jphysparis.2013.03.007
138. Dearing E, McCartney K, Marshall NL, Warner RM (2001) Parental reports of children's sleep and wakefulness: longitudinal associations with cognitive and language outcomes. Infant Behav Dev 24(2):151–170. https://doi.org/10.1016/S0163-6383(01)00074-1
139. Monk TH, Burk LR, Klein MH, Kupfer DJ, Soehner AM, Essex MJ (2010) Behavioral circadian regularity at age 1 month predicts anxiety levels during school-age years. Psychiatry Res 178(2):370–373. https://doi.org/10.1016/j.psychres.2009.09.020
140. Pennestri M-H, Moss E, O'Donnell K, Lecompte V, Bouvette-Turcot A-A, Atkinson L, Minde K, Gruber R, Fleming AS, Meaney MJ, Gaudreau H (2015) Establishment and consolidation of the sleep-wake cycle as a function of attachment pattern. Attach Hum Dev 17(1):23–42. https://doi.org/10.1080/14616734.2014.953963
141. Simpson JM (2001) Infant stress and sleep deprivation as an aetiological basis for the sudden infant death syndrome. Early Hum Dev 61(1):1–43. https://doi.org/10.1016/S0378-3782(00)00127-4
142. Sturner WQ, Lynch HJ, Deng MH, Gleason RE, Wurtman RJ (1990) Melatonin concentrations in the sudden infant death syndrome. Forensic Sci Int 45:171–180
143. O'Connor RP, Persinger MA (1997) Geophysical variables and behavior: LXXXH. A strong association between sudden infant death syndrome and increments of global geomagnetic activity - possible support for the melatonin hypothesis. Percept Mot Skills 84(2):395–402
144. Weydahl A, Sothern RB, Cornélissen G, Wetterberg L (2000) Geomagnetic activity influences the melatonin secretion at latitude 70° N. Biomed Pharmacother 55:s57–s62. https://doi.org/10.1016/S0753-3322(01)90006-X
145. Maiello S (2003) The rhythmical dimension of the mother-infant relationship – transcultural considerations. J Child Adolesc Ment Health 15(2):81–86. https://doi.org/10.2989/17280580309486552
146. Brandon DH, Holditch-Davis D, Belyea M (2002) Preterm infants born at less than 31 weeks' gestation have improved growth in cycled light compared with continuous near darkness. J Pediatr 140(2):192–199. https://doi.org/10.1067/mpd.2002.121932
147. Barnard KE, Bee HL (1983) The impact of temporally patterned stimulation on the development of preterm infants. Child Dev 54(5):1156–1167. https://doi.org/10.2307/1129671
148. Groswasser J, Sottiaux M, Rebuffat E (1995) Reduction in obstructive breathing events during body rocking: a controlled polygraphic study in preterm and full-term infants. Pediatrics 96(1 Pt 1):64–68
149. White-Traut RC, Nelson MN (1988) Maternally administered tactile, auditory, visual, and vestibular stimulation: relationship to later interactions between mothers and premature infants. Res Nurs Health 11(1):31–39. https://doi.org/10.1002/nur.4770110106

150. White-Traut RC, Nelson MN, Silvestri JM, Vasan U, Littau S, Meleedy-Rey P, Gu G, Patel M (2002) Effect of auditory, tactile, visual, and vestibular intervention on length of stay, alertness, and feeding progression in preterm infants. Dev Med Child Neurol 44(2):91–97. https://doi.org/10.1111/j.1469-8749.2002.tb00293.x
151. Standley JM (2012) A discussion of evidence-based music therapy to facilitate feeding skills of premature infants: the power of contingent music. Arts Psychother 39(5):379–382. https://doi.org/10.1016/j.aip.2012.06.009
152. Loewy J, Stewart K, Dassler A-M, Telsey A, Homel P (2013) The effects of music therapy on vital signs, feeding, and sleep in premature infants. Pediatrics 131(5):902–918. https://doi.org/10.1542/peds.2012-1367
153. Filippa M, Devouche E, Arioni C, Imberty M, Gratier M (2013) Live maternal speech and singing have beneficial effects on hospitalized preterm infants. Acta Paediatr 102(10). https://doi.org/10.1111/apa.12356
154. Tordjman S, Davlantis KS, Georgieff N, Geoffray M-M, Speranza M, Anderson GM, Xavier J, Botbol M, Oriol C, Bellissant E, Vernay-Leconte J, Fougerou C, Hespel A, Tavenard A, Cohen D, Kermarrec S, Coulon N, Bonnot O, Dawson G (2015) Autism as a disorder of biological and behavioral rhythms: toward new therapeutic perspectives. Front Pediatr 3(February). https://doi.org/10.3389/fped.2015.00001
155. Amos P (2013) Rhythm and timing in autism: learning to dance. Front Integr Neurosci 7(April):1–15. https://doi.org/10.3389/fnint.2013.00027
156. Charrier A, Tardif C, Gepner B (2016) Amélioration de l'exploration visuelle d'un visage par des enfants avec autisme grâce au ralentissement de la dynamique faciale: une étude préliminaire en oculométrie. L'Encéphale. https://doi.org/10.1016/j.encep.2016.02.005
157. Wimpory D, Nicholas B, Nash S (2002) Social timing, clock genes and autism: A new hypothesis. J Intellect Disabil Res 46(4):352–358. https://doi.org/10.1046/j.1365-2788.2002.00423
158. Weinstock M (2008) The long-term behavioural consequences of prenatal stress. Neurosci Biobehav Rev 32(6):1073–1086. https://doi.org/10.1016/j.neubiorev.2008.03.002
159. Gotlib IH, LeMoult J, Colich NL, Foland-Ross LC, Hallmayer J, Joormann J, Lin J, Wolkowitz OM (2014) Telomere length and cortisol reactivity in children of depressed mothers. Mol Psychiatry:1–6. https://doi.org/10.1038/mp.2014.119
160. Armstrong KL, O'Donnell H, McCallum R, Dadds M (1998) Childhood sleep problems: association with prenatal factors and maternal distress/depression. J Paediatr Child Health 34(3):263–266. https://doi.org/10.1046/j.1440-1754.1998.00214.x
161. Field TM (2011) Prenatal depression effects on early development: a review. Infant Behav Dev 34(1):1–14. https://doi.org/10.1016/j.infbeh.2010.09.008
162. Kaplan L a, Evans L, Monk C (2008) Effects of mothers' prenatal psychiatric status and postnatal caregiving on infant biobehavioral regulation: can prenatal programming be modified? Early Hum Dev 84(4):249–256. https://doi.org/10.1016/j.earlhumdev.2007.06.004
163. Zárate-Guerrero G, Devouche E, Espinosa-Gómez MC, Apter G (2014) Évaluer les difficultés interactives entre une mère déprimée et son bébé de 3 mois au moyen de l'échelle GRMII de Fiori-Cowley et Murray. Neuropsychiatr Enfance Adolesc 62(1):47–52. https://doi.org/10.1016/j.neurenf.2013.08.003
164. Hernandez-Reif M, Maluga M, Field T (2012) Maternal depression and infant birth measures relate to how neonates respond to music. Infant Behav Dev 35(4):655–661. https://doi.org/10.1016/j.infbeh.2012.07.004
165. Van Puyvelde M, Rodrigues H, Loots G, Coster L, De D, Ville K, Matthijs L, Simcock D, Pattyn N (2014) Shall we dance? Music as a port of entrance to maternal–infant intersubjectivity in a context of postnatal depression. Infant Ment Health J 35(3):1–12. https://doi.org/10.1002/imhj.21431

Part II

At Risk-Interactions

Impact of Immediate Peripartum Psychopathology and Parental Psychiatric Disorders

5

Marc Poget, Marie-Camille Genet, and Gisèle Apter

Perinatal psychiatric disorders are far from exceptional. Pregnancy is probably the period during which women, are at highest risk for psychopathology, receive the most attention, care, interest, and monitoring. It is also a time when individual and family psychological upheavals are most intense and might lead to the exacerbation of a psychiatric disorder, the outbreak of a latent one, or the appearance of specific pregnancy-related disorders. These concerns have finally gained interest from mainstream research after decades of false beliefs that psychiatric disorders disappeared or could not emerge during the peripartum [1–4].

The number of studies focusing on perinatal psychiatry and infant mental health has been on the rise in recent years, even though essentially centered on mood disorders for the majority of them. Less than half of what would be expected given the number of studies on mood disorders focus on schizophrenia during pregnancy and ten times fewer than expected on personality disorders [5]. The numbers show the overwhelming interest in depressive mood and peripartum depression notwithstanding the prevalence ratios of other pathologies.

We are now critically aware that psychiatric illness is pervasive in the peripartum in connection with a variety of risk factors and should therefore be included in a comprehensive peripartum health-care plan [6]. Yet, there remain important controversies on the specificity of psychiatric disorders during the peripartum. Notwithstanding this debate, which goes beyond the scope of this chapter, we need to acknowledge the existence of this form of psychopathology and consider its impact on the infant and its interactions with its environment through early development [2, 4, 7, 8].

M. Poget
Centre Hospitalier de la Polynésie française, Tahiti, French Polynesia

M.-C. Genet
Formatrice COPES, Unité Aubier, EPS Erasme, Antony, France

G. Apter (✉)
Groupe Hospitalier du Havre, Université de Rouen Normandie, Rouen, France

© Springer Nature Switzerland AG 2019

G. Apter et al. (eds.), *Early Interaction and Developmental Psychopathology*,
https://doi.org/10.1007/978-3-030-04769-6_5

Obtaining reliable epidemiological data during the peripartum is not easy, because of both the particular features of certain puerperal disorders and the dearth of specific tools to evaluate their prevalence. Psychiatric disorders during pregnancy and the immediate postpartum can be described as either preexisting conditions or de novo disorders. Both of these circumstances will be studied here with parenthood, parent-infant interactions, and infant emotional development in mind. After a brief overview of psychiatric issues possibly affecting mothers during the peripartum and what is known of their impact on offspring, we will describe the most common negative outcome for the infant, i.e., consequences of neglect and neglectful interactions during the first months postpartum. Directions for the future encompassing parental mental health and infant welfare including interactive processes will be offered.

5.1 Preexisting Maternal Mental Health Disorders

5.1.1 Schizophrenia

Schizophrenia affects around 1% of the population, and the number of pregnant women presenting this type of disorder appears to have grown in recent years. This can be explained by improvements in health care, which aim to stabilize these patients and improve their socio-professional circumstances. It thus appears natural for all these women to engage in lasting relationships and plan a family. Epidemiological studies still remain rare, with small population groups and therefore low levels of statistical power, undermining results.

In order to at least partially address this lack of data, Hameed and Lewis [9] recently published a systematic review of 46 papers presenting the results of 18 longitudinal studies on the developmental outcomes of children whose parents were affected by severe mental illness, i.e., schizophrenia with one or both parents affected. The authors concluded that notwithstanding the methodological issues in the studies, in general, children were at very high risk for poor development and heightened risk for all mental health disorders. They concluded by recommending that *specific intervention models to support their {offspring} development be further developed and evaluated.* The fact that women affected with schizophrenia and by other major psychiatric disorders are at much higher risk for pregnancy and birth complications such as preeclampsia, prematurity, and small for gestational age (SGA) should in fact attract much greater attention than it actually does and should promote multidisciplinary management of such clinical cases including perinatal psychiatry and interaction-focused interventions [10, 11]. In fact, as with most psychiatric conditions, treatment of women during pregnancy is recommended, while absence of treatment is often more deleterious than not [12].

With regard to interaction, the most recent effort at reviewing data has come up with an analysis of 27 papers concluding that again, notwithstanding small numbers and methodological issues, mother-infant interaction during the first year of life with mothers affected by schizophrenia is characterized by less sensitivity to infant cues and impaired quality of mutuality. The authors recommend that: "Further research should investigate both sources of resilience and risk in the development of offspring of parents with a diagnosis of schizophrenia and psychosis" [13].

5.1.2 Bipolar Disorder and Recurrent Major Depressive Disorder

Due to higher prevalence and the more numerous studies on severe mood disorders, bipolar depression, specifically its treatment during pregnancy, has interested psychiatrists from early on [14]. Again, as in parents affected with schizophrenia, the risks for psychiatric disorders in offspring of parents affected by bipolar disorder are high. In a recent study, outcome could be differentiated between offspring of the former compared to the latter with children of parents with bipolar disorder at higher risk for affective and mood disorders versus ADHD in those of parents with schizophrenia [15]. When considering pregnancy and birth outcomes as well as parent-infant interaction, pregnancy and childbirth are at higher risk in the case of mothers affected with bipolar disorder [16].

Parent-infant interaction in the case of bipolar disorder is again seldom studied in part due to the fact that depression and mood disorders have been the major focus of mother-infant interaction studies and that the two have not always been clearly teased apart. Looking strictly at developmental milestones of young infants, results show that motor skills are affected to some extent in infants of treated mothers compared to non-treated ones, with no global developmental risk in either the treated or the non-treated group [17]. However, researchers did not assess the quality of interactions or emotional regulation. When maternal sensitivity and mutuality of interactions were assessed at 1 year postpartum, a negative trend in the group whose parents were affected with bipolar depression was found, pointing to the need for more data on the first months of life [18]. Specific issues and existence of social support when available have been argued as actually the most useful elements to guide tailored clinical management in these complex situations [19].

5.1.3 Addiction and Substance Abuse Disorders

Addiction and substance abuse disorders have obvious dramatic consequences during the perinatal period, owing to the fetotoxicity of drugs and their impact on gestation, birth weight, and the newborn's behavior (abstinence syndrome and sequelae of prenatal exposure). These consequences, as well as parental behaviors, may differ somewhat with each drug under consideration. Moreover, in the case of illegal drug abuse, the environment is often inadequate for infant care. There again, epidemiological data about drug abuse are unreliable or incomplete. Direct and indirect infant outcome measures are still in need. Very recently, epidemiological data focusing on the unreported rates of fetal alcohol syndrome hit the headlines, exposing to the public what has been known for over a century but has tended to go unnoticed [20]. Warning against the use of cannabis has also been highlighted as having a very high negative impact on the fetus and newborn even though its use during pregnancy has considerably increased in recent years [21, 22]. Parent-infant interaction in the case of substance abuse is however more often linked to other issues underlying the addiction (personality disorders, mood disorders, emotional regulation disorder) rather than to a single type of toxic drug per se. Often, in the case of addiction and use of behavior-modifying substances, the risk of violence is heightened, thus adding a possibility of negative relationships and trauma to infant and caregiver. Infants of parents with substance abuse in addition to psychiatric disorders present the highest degree of negative developmental outcome when studied longitudinally [23, 24].

5.1.4 Eating Disorders

Symptoms of eating disorders such as anorexia and bulimia tend to lessen during pregnancy. However, early interactions appear to be disrupted in 20% of cases by an unreasonable preoccupation with food [25]. Again, there is a paucity of research and data on these issues. Another problem during pregnancy is that consequence of hyperemesis gravidarum, which the DSM does not recognize as a disorder, whereas the ICD-10 does, has not been studied. Whether this highly stressful and impairing condition during the prepartum has an impact on parenthood, the newborn, and parent-infant interaction is still unknown.

5.1.5 Cognitive Deficit

Cognitive deficit (mental retardation) is generally not considered a psychiatric disorder per se, but depending on its severity and the fact that it is often comorbid with psychiatric disorders, thus enhancing the negative impact of mental disorder, it can require intervention and specific professional care for parenthood to emerge as adaptable to a newborn and infant. It may hinder maternal learning, adapting, anticipating, and reflexive functioning capacities. Unfortunately, this field is still largely unexplored during the perinatal period.

5.1.6 Borderline Personality Disorders

Last but not least, borderline personality disorder may appear as the least studied nosographic entity among those researched during the perinatal period. Its prevalence is thought to range from 1% to 6% depending on studies, and the disorder represents a major portion of the clinical populations referred to psychiatric services. Their clinical characteristics result in a major impact on the mother-baby interactive system. The risk of chronic depression and history of trauma are high in borderline personality disorder; therefore, the symptomatology may be confusing, either due to the depressive aspect being on the forefront or to referral to social services as chaotic relationships and major negative life events are predominant [5, 26, 27]. As with other mental health issues, pregnancy and birth represent very high-risk contexts due to associated substance abuse, to smoking (and other substances), and to chaotic access to health care during pregnancy [28, 29].

5.1.7 Mood and Anxiety Disorders

Mood and anxiety disorders are the most common and most prevalent disorders (see paragraph below). They can be preexisting and exacerbated by pregnancy and the postpartum. They are essentially studied during pregnancy (their impact on) or after birth, as this period heightens the risk of appearance of depressive disorders and exacerbation of anxiety traits due to the stress of recent parenthood and the responsibilities it involves.

5.2 Peripartum-Related Maternal Mental Health Disorders

5.2.1 Perinatal Psychoses

Perinatal psychoses affect 1–2 in 1000 births even if they are still difficult to quantify, especially as their designation, conception, and diagnostic criteria differ, making the disorder a controversial entity [30]. In any case, whatever its origin, the associated symptoms are strong and marked by severe delirium and a dissociative syndrome. Most authors consider that perinatal psychosis is in fact a manifestation of a mood or affective disorder. This might be a reason why, in fact, once again there are no specific studies available on interactions of mothers having been affected with puerperal psychosis with their infants or on their infants' early development. Information is included in mother-baby unit studies but often provides little insight and at a macrolevel at best, essentially using such outcome measures as reaching major motor development milestones and maternal mental health at hospital discharge with sometimes sparse follow-up data in rare studies of in-patient programs [31, 32].

5.2.2 Peripartum Depression

During the antenatal period, depression is estimated to affect between 10 and 12% of future mothers (EPDS cut-off > 13) [33, 34]. A meta-analysis carried out by Dayan et al. [35] points out a number of risk factors:

- Social factors: low educational level, unemployment, lack of social support, and low socioeconomic status.
- Negative life events, especially when numerous, such as conjugal violence and work-related stress.
- History of psychiatric episodes.

However, in this meta-analysis, Dayan reports that confounding factors are rarely taken into account and highlights the lack of prospective studies.

Concerning postnatal depression, there is a great variability in the results of epidemiological studies. This can be explained firstly by the absence of specific diagnostic evaluation tools (tools are either for screening such as the Edinborough Postpartum Depression Scale (EPDS) or for depression notwithstanding the peripartum) and secondly by a variation in the postnatal period when the evaluation took place. Its prevalence is estimated to be around 10%.

Some specialists are in favor of considering depression during this period to be a specific clinical condition. Cooper and Murray [36], for instance, highlighted clinical symptoms dominated by anxiety, irritability, and phobias. Suicide seemed to be exceptionally rare until quite recently, and the feeling of usefulness may appear as a protective factor. Indirect and specific signs such as intolerance to the baby's complaints or even iterative consultations for the baby without a specific motive should be triggers raising the question for such a diagnostic risk as peripartum depression.

More recently, a consortium to study postpartum depression called the Postpartum Depression: Action Towards Causes and Treatment (PACT) Consortium has formed with the aim to better circumvene this specific pathology. It has most notably already highlighted the heterogeneity of this disorder, its existence in different cultural contexts, and the important consequences this has on its diverse symptomatology and the various aspects of depression when linked to anxiety disorders [8, 37, 38].

Whatever its origin and its associated symptomatology, peripartum depression (PPD) takes its toll on infant, toddler, and childhood development. For close to 20 years, Lynne Murray and her team have studied the offspring of mothers affected with PPD [39, 40]. At each of her outcome studies, age 2, 5 and ongoing, she found higher risk of externalized and internalized behavioral disorders with a strong gender effect. Goodman et al. [41] have confirmed this negative impact in a recent review of the literature. (For an extensive micro-view on parent-infant interaction in the case of maternal depression, see Part 2 Chap. 4.)

Mood and anxiety disorders are among the most frequent negative outcomes found in offspring of mothers with PPD during all of childhood and adolescence and up to adulthood [42, 43].

5.2.3 Anxiety Disorders

Anxiety may be normal around birth. In fact, it has an adaptive function fostering healthy parental preoccupation for the infant. During the prenatal period, it focuses on the birth, potential disability, or even the appearance of the future baby [44]. During the postnatal period, anxiety focuses instead on the anticipation of separation [45] or the needs of the baby [46]. Studies have shown a prevalence of generalized anxiety of 6–8% (20% when clinical symptoms are incomplete [47]). Women presenting an obsessive compulsive disorder (OCD) have a tendency to see their symptoms soften or stabilize during pregnancy, only to see them become aggravated in the postpartum. The emergence of impulsion phobias (complusive thoughts of fear of harming the baby) is quite frequent, and, without being specific, they characterize this period. PTSDs are found in 1–6% of women (6–24% when clinical symptoms are incomplete).

5.3 From Parental Psychiatric Disorders to Infant Mental Health

Many authors have raised the question of the transgenerational transmission of psychiatric disorders and the mechanisms underlying their impact on child development.

From a clinical perspective, it could be hypothesized that children are influenced by their mother's mental health condition through disturbances of mother-baby interaction. Among mothers with schizophrenia, visual interactions are characterized by mutual avoidance; corporeal interactions are described as chaotic, vocal interactions as poor, and emotional tuning and adjustment as asynchronous and discordant [48, 49]. Among depressed mothers, the verbal address frequency [50], voice quality [51], eye-to-eye contact [52], emotional expression, and quality of answer [53] are likely candidates for altered communication.

Recent studies in epigenetics place the environment at the core of debates concerning transmission. Genetic discoveries have fueled hopes explaining many diseases, but research results are disappointing so far. Note that it is remarkable that many of these studies forget to explore the perinatal period! Yet, Epigenetics enables us to refocus on the peripartum via gene-environment interactions. Even though the results to date are modest, animal studies have already proposed models for more extensive research on behavioral epigenetics [54–57]. Even when taken with caution, it is possible to incorporate epigenetics research within an integrative and multidimensional model of child disorder genesis.

Devlin et al. [58] suggest that prenatal depression impacts gene expression in the newborn. The stress model has been the most considered: many studies have shown an impact of maternal stress on the hypothalamo-pituitary axis regulation of the baby, via epigenetic mechanisms. More recently, Zucchi et al. [59] have shown that maternal stress induces epigenetic changes in genes involved in schizophrenia and bipolar disorder. Though they do not have obvious causal links, these results show the extent of environmental effects on issues of pathogeny of psychiatric disorders.

It should be remembered here that gene-behavior-environment interactions are at the very least bi-directional. Psychiatric disorders, especially chronic ones, can come with and/or favor a fragile environment or even a harmful one for the mother and the baby. For example, the quality of spouse support has a major influence on the qualitative and quantitative impact of maternal disorders on the interaction. In general terms, environmental risk factors that might favor the occurrence of a psychiatric disorder need to be considered as vulnerability factors for the whole family. However, a psychiatric disorder is in itself a risk factor for environmental instability, leading to a negative loop from which the family struggles to escape. Clearly, when there are several of these factors, vulnerability grows exponentially. Particular attention must thus be paid to all the negative elements that may hinder parental interactions and lead to poorer relations, where the most deleterious consequence is neglect and child abuse.

5.3.1 Neglect as a Psychopathological Paradigm: Direct Effects of Parental Mental Health on Infant Emotional Development?

Neglect, a negative form of abuse and its correlate, maltreatment, can be observed in diverse contexts. Its influence on development is now well documented, and knowledge on its negative consequences seems to continuously unfold as more research on epigenetics during pregnancy and early childhood is made available [60]. Impact on lifelong health issues notwithstanding, mental health is also in the forefront [61]. Pregnancies that are met with neglectful behavior whether it be due to maternal mental health issues or to environmental insults are followed by heightened risk of negative outcomes including intrauterine growth retardation, premature birth, increased risk of maternal and infant mortality, and multiple disorders found in early childhood [62].

The diagnosis of neglect is difficult. Over and above the fact that it is not always considered a medical issue or is often denied due to the potential pejorative judgment it delivers on parents, it is demanding since it requires both precise training in the observation of the baby and a capacity to observe parent-infant interactive sensitivity non-judgmentally. Often, parents' issues take center stage and monopolize the attention of professionals. The more or less insensitive, even neglectful, interactions that may be observed are too often attributed to parental stress and their distraught reaction to negative circumstances. Yet, however true this analysis may be, it should not mask the insufficient response to infants' needs that are unfortunately its consequences. In addition, observation of a nonverbal infant, even in the case of an objective scale such as the neonatal behavior assessment scale (NBAS) or other observation tools (see Part 3 Chap. 2; also see in the specific case of neglect the Steinhauer Guide[1] [63]), requires a capacity to accept identification to the infant's emotions and to enter the infant's intersubjective world (see Trevarthen this volume).

The first clinical signs of neglect can appear very early in infants, even in the first months of life. They are subtle and nonspecific but yet evocative in their given contexts. Their essential and primary signs are that the infant takes refuge in sleep, sleeps more than the average age-related duration, and/or falls suddenly into sleep (forsaking the drowsiness stage of the NBAS), and/or does not directly gaze at parent/look in their eyes (averts gaze eyes and face, whereas visual interaction is possible with a stranger), and/or does not babble or chirp, with a paucity or absence of

[1] http://hdl.handle.net/2268/165697
http://observatoiremaltraitance.ca/Documents/Guide%20d'%C3%A9valuation%20des%20capacit%C3%A9s%20parentales_25-09-2014.pdf

vocalizations. In summary, there is a lack of what could be considered positive emotional expression both during interaction and at rest.

Autonomic nervous system disorders are common and suggest an absence of environmental regulation underlying the interactive dysfunction. The infant may seem physically unkempt or "grayish" and unadjusted to physical interactive behaviors, i.e., the infant may actively invite the parent to be more intrusive and hyperstimulation while paradoxically averting gaze and arching away. Hypervigilance, i.e., acute constant "glued" gaze and stressful hypertonia during such habitual actions as feeding and changing, is also a clue to dysregulated interactive initiatives and responses from the environment.

Early signs of neglect are often visible through disorders of the muscle tone system: too much body tonus and the infant is too rigid, with central axis as tense as peripheral (limb) tone, whereas too little body tonus implies loose and unresponsive (flabby) limbs. Thus, one may identify a tonicity disorder, whether it be one of hypertonicity (the baby rearing up, with tense limbs) or of hypotonicity (baby like a rag doll). Such infants also often cling to a single functional modality, such as gaze. They will turn their gaze to a light source and maintain it locked on the source, keeping their fists closed and their toes hooked (in a gripping reflex type reaction; see NBAS chapter for detail). At times, they stiffen around their vertical axis and arch their bodies backward. This will consequently create tension around their digestive axis often causing reflux which can at times be so adverse that it will require medical treatment. Crying is more frequent than would be expected usually, triggered by being laid horizontally in their cots. Only holding it vertically seems to soothe the infant. In such a situation, indeed, infants often express and seek a form of rocking movement that in reality corresponds to a series of repeated up and down moves. These babies actually actively refuse reclining rocking and the more curled up position it affords. They seem to avoid any nesting or rooting behavior.

5.3.2 Body Movements and Motor Skills

The motor skills of these neglected babies are poor, and they lack self-body exploration. Their hand movements are rare and atypical when these should be accompanied by vocalizations, especially after the age of 6 months. The neglected infant looks for excitatory stimulation or a temporarily secure grip but has little respite for relaxation or for engaging in mutual exchanges, amodal perceptions, manipulations, and object exploration. The games put at his disposal are often bright and noisy and are often associated with screen time, with screens placed too close and conveying too high an intensity, ill adapted to developmental age through sound and light.

The infant's body language during social interaction as well as when he is alone shows poor expressivity, the two hemi-bodies are not brought together in the first months of life, and the lower body is not self-explored or used. The baby often has delay in its walking and sometimes gives the impression of having a muscular or neurological disorder that calls for investigations. The vocalizations of the baby are not modulated; the movements are stiff. When the infant awakens, it does not come progressively out of sleep but arouses with a jolt. It is important to understand that the overall condition of a neglected baby is variable and affords many individual differences. But some of the most significant signs are atypical tonus, low levels of excitability and lack of self-regulation, and distorted interactive patterns: those of gaze, gestures, exchanges, play, care, and sleep.

5.3.3 Emotional Regulation

These neglected babies therefore show strong signs of emotional regulation disturbance. They have difficulty containing their emotions and transforming them. Since they do not have access to their parent's sensitivity for emotional regulation, they may use their own body to try to reduce excitability. Infants thus may present expressions of disorganization and anger. They may also use mechanisms of emotional withdrawal that can be evaluated, through screening and observational tools. Emotional displays are disproportionate and inappropriate with respect to fear and anger and interactively difficult to predict. These children struggle to recognize their own emotions and tend to avoid situations of intimacy. They then, unfortunately rapidly become poor interactive initiators, thus themselves creating emotionally dysregulated patterns of interaction.

Neglect leads to a greater likelihood for the child to develop an insecure or disorganized attachment that persists over time. These children do not perceive themselves as worthy of being loved and have an image of others as unavailable or rejecting. Secondary cognitive signs exist. In general, these children are less enthusiastic about learning, have little or no initiative, appear more frustrated, and may express anger when no clear cause can be identified; they are also difficult to console. Thus they become difficult to care for and will more often than not, when seen at a later developmental stage, be at risk of rejection due to their disrupted behaviors.

In terms of the processes of attachment construction, the neglected child reacts to separation from the parent either by showing very little distress or, on the contrary, by being utterly inconsolable. Attachment theory considers the bonds that the young child establishes with a neglectful parent as templates for later relationships. In this case, the child expects that other people will not satisfy his needs and therefore does not elicit them. He discourages those who come to him for help or who try to relate with him.

It is important to realize that even if emotional neglect from an attachment figure is the subtlest form of psychological abuse, its effects are as devastating as those of other forms of maltreatment [64].

5.3.4 General Consequences

Developmental sequelae directly attributable to neglect will thus be found in the following four areas:

- Mutual engagement and communication.
- Expression and regulation of affect.
- Attachment and representations of oneself and others.
- Exploratory capacities and neurocognitive development.

Needless to say, these major impacts show the requirement for substantial preventive measures when possible, as well as adapted longitudinal care in order to preserve infants' developmental potentialities and to enhance developmental trajectories. Specialized, sensitive care for these infants may preserve both, infants from the ill-effects of neglect, and their parents from the dysregulated interactions that they unfortunately spontaneously propose when they are themselves at loss. Parents often involuntarily respond inadequately to their infants' needs; nonetheless, this is detrimental to their child. It will therefore be their aptitude and the possibility to address their child's issues and access/acceptance of environmental support that will be an essential element for care and long-term outcome.

5.4 Clinical Implications and Care of Parents with Mental Health Disorders During the Peripartum

5.4.1 During Pregnancy

In order to best support parents and specifically women, it is essential to address peripartum illness as early as possible. This reduces stress and trauma. Acknowledgment during the peripartum as part of usual ob-gyn medical care should include maternal and infant psychiatric care. This avoids stigma and provides early care when managing known chronic psychiatric as well as de novo clinical situations. It requires a high level of interaction between the obstetrics department and adult (women's when available) psychiatric and child psychiatric services. The former, obstetrics specialists, are in the front line and need to refer patients as quickly as possible at the earliest warning sign. Systematic referral and network care promote destigmatization and therefore acceptance of treatment. Depending on assessment outcomes, various therapeutic measures need to be taken according to resources and patient compliance. We list here some that have been documented. The list is not complete but addresses large groups of therapeutic approaches. These are not mutually exclusive; on the contrary, more than one type of therapeutic approach will quite often be useful:

- *Parenthood/adult-oriented psychotherapeutic outpatient consultations*: Time is limited during pregnancy; therefore, therapeutic consultations need to be sparse and efficient. One program that shows potential is the one developed by the Swiss Geneva team consisting of a limited number of sessions during pregnancy to prevent postnatal depression in case of risk factors or of the presence of antenatal depression [65].

- *Proposals for drug treatments*: The benefit-risk balance takes on a completely different dimension during pregnancy and lactation. For each drug prescription, it is necessary to question its impact on the interaction and therefore on the baby. When indicated, it is not always easy to convince parents of such a prescription. For some mothers, taking medication is an active and potentially toxic procedure for the fetus or baby, while not taking it allows them to put themselves in a passive position that seems less dangerous from their point of view. It is up to professionals and prescribers to support them and show them that caring for themselves, seeking to mitigate the effects of a psychiatric disorder on their child, is a way for them to be a parent despite their psychiatric illness. Medication, when adequately prescribed, and at clinically relevant doses, can be prescribed during pregnancy with a benefit/risk balance, always taking into account the risk of nonprescription as well as the risk of prescription for fetus and mother [12, 66–68].
- *Integrated preparation for childbirth and adapted maternity ward stays including* adapting medication in the case of behavioral problems, a longer stay in the maternity ward, sequential periods of mother-child separation to allow each of them to rest while the infant is in the nursery, psychiatric and psychological assessment and support, sustained nursing care by midwives and nurses, neonatal surveillance (especially in the case of impregnation and abstinence syndrome of the baby, etc.) with kangaroo unit-type care, and organization of postnatal mother baby unit care when available.
- *Hospitalization in a psychiatry unit* that has expertise in parenthood issues.
- *Hospitalization in high-risk pregnancy unit* with perinatal psychiatry consultation liaison.
- Request for *environmental assessment and intervention of child welfare services in high-risk situations* or extremely negative social environments.

The precise indications of these various orientations have yet to be more widely studied, as most tailored mental health management has not been rigorously assessed through randomized controlled trials. Such studies are indeed difficult to conduct. For example, the effects of a prolonged hospital stay for at-risk mothers, receiving appropriate psychiatric care on quality of mother-infant interaction over a significant period of time, are difficult and costly to assess. In Australia, a collaborative approach to infant, maternal, and community-based treatment has shown positive results even if numbers are still small [69]. They have recently made it a point to include parent-infant relationship in their comprehensive therapeutic model in addition to maternal and infant separate care [70].

Having a well-specified temporal framework is highly exclusive to the peripartum. The infant's timing is not the same as the adult's. Not only might the parental psychiatric disorders have a major impact on interactions and the emotional, physical, and psycho-affective development of the baby from birth, but the infant's rapid development is itself a double risk factor. It can negatively impact maternal mental health due to the overwhelming perinatal biologically driven upheavals, and it can increase a sense of imbalance by imposing interaction between a swiftly changing infant in need of an adaptable parent whose psychiatric disorder will be slow to resolve. It is essential to take into account the rhythm of general psychiatric care for adults, which is generally slow relative to the infant's rapid evolution [71]. These considerations reinforce the need for new practices addressing the urgency of assessment and early intervention. This requires a monitoring and guidance system by an available and reactive multidisciplinary team. It can be illustrated by the following example:

Clinical vignette*: why include interactions and parental development in addition to psychiatric diagnostic assessment.*

Ms. A and Ms. B both gave birth at approximately the same time of year, same gestational age infant and comparable pregnancy health outcome measures. Both mothers are affected by a severe depressive episode during the first weeks postpartum. In both cases, mother-baby interactions are marked by maternal depressive mood, and at 2 months of age, both infants show early signs of dysregulation. However, when faced with acknowledging both their own and their infant's symptomatology, Ms. A and Ms. B strongly differ.

Ms. A refuses help from the care providers for her and her baby since she does not recognize that she requires treatment for her depressive disorder. Personality disorder was not assessed for either patients, and family support though available for Ms. A was shunned by her. She does not recognize or acknowledge that the infant may have dysregulated interactive reactions.

Ms. B at first also reluctant to accept parent-infant outpatient care admits that it would be a benefit for the infant's needs, even if she still refuses to fully acknowledge her mood disorder and therefore that her own condition requires treatment.

It seems in this case essential to assess parenting disorders and interactive disorders independently from psychiatric pathology. Manzano et al. [72] developed the concept of "narcissistic scenarios of parenthood" and that of developmental bereavement [73] in order to access parenthood status. They surmise that in order to access full maternal (parental preoccupation to quote Winnicott), parents must put their infant's needs first before their own and therefore to be able to identify with the infant's reality, here and now. This means acknowledging differences between their own emotions and that of their infant, accepting that they will eventually have to seek the support of others to respond as best as necessary, to the developmentally challenging growing infant, the more challenging that their own psychopathology obstructs their everyday life.

This differentiation is essential because it will of course considerably modify the care plan.

Studies, unfortunately, even when undertaken longitudinally, continue to underscore the negative impact of maternal mental health issues on offspring's developmental outcomes [27, 74, 75], partly due to lack of power and partly due to lack of precise data [76].

5.5 Conclusion

We propose that in order to move forward, perinatal and infant psychiatry need to systematically look at the following, tryptic, maternal (parental/caregiver) mental health, infant mental health, and parent-infant interaction in order to address the issue of infant development and its boomerang impact on parental aptitudes. It has been argued that integrating a cumulative pathway through a complex system's theory developmental model could be a more effective and pragmatic clinical approach [74, 77].

This implies more integrative and translational research in order to address the main public health issue of mental health of infants and children whose parents are unfortunately affected or meet with mental disorders. To better tackle these essential issues, research questions and designs should be informed by pragmatic mental health interactive clinical issues. They could offer a window to exploring the infant and its parent through a framework where modifying the system will prove more effective than aiming for change in either of its participants alone.

References

1. Howard LM, Molyneaux E, Dennis CL, Rochat T, Stein A, Milgrom J (2014) Non-psychotic mental disorders in the perinatal period. Lancet 384(9956):1775–1788
2. Jones I, Chandra PS, Dazzan P, Howard LM (2014) Bipolar disorder, affective psychosis, and schizophrenia in pregnancy and the post-partum period. Lancet 384(9956):1789–1799
3. Khalifeh H, Brauer R, Toulmin H, Howard LM (2015) Perinatal mental health: what every neonatologist should know. Early Hum Dev 91(11):649–653
4. Stein A, Pearson RM, Goodman SH, Rapa E, Rahman A, McCallum M, Howard LM, Pariante CM (2014) Effects of perinatal mental disorders on the fetus and child. Lancet 384(9956):1800–1819
5. Sved Williams A, Apter G (2018). Working with women with borderline personality disorder and their infants. 16th Waimh World Congress Rome May 27–31
6. Howard LM, Piot P, Stein A (2014) No health without perinatal mental health. Lancet 384(9956):1723–1724
7. Herrman H (2015) Protecting the mental health of women in the perinatal period. Lancet Psychiatry 2(2):116–118
8. Putnam K, Robertson-Blackmore E, Sharkey K, Payne J, Bergink V, Munk-Olsen T, Deligiannidis K, Altemus M, Newport J, Apter G, Devouche E (2015) Heterogeneity of postpartum depression: a latent class analysis. Lancet Psychiatry 2(1):59–67
9. Hameed MA, Lewis AJ (2016) Offspring of parents with schizophrenia: a systematic review of developmental features across childhood. Harv Rev Psychiatry 24(2):104–117
10. Schneid-Kofman N, Sheiner E, Levy A (2008) Psychiatric illness and adverse pregnancy outcome. Int J Gynecol Obstet 101(1):53–56
11. Vigod SN, Kurdyak PA, Dennis CL, Gruneir A, Newman A, Seeman MV, Rochon PA, Anderson GM, Grigoriadis S, Ray JG (2014) Maternal and newborn outcomes among women with schizophrenia: a retrospective population-based cohort study. BJOG Int J Obstet Gynaecol 121(5):566–574
12. Robinson GE (2012) Treatment of schizophrenia in pregnancy and postpartum. J Popul Ther Clin Pharmacol 19(3):e380–e386
13. Davidsen KA, Harder S, MacBeth A, Lundy JM, Gumley A (2015) Mother–infant interaction in schizophrenia: transmitting risk or resilience? A systematic review of the literature. Soc Psychiatry Psychiatr Epidemiol 50(12):1785–1798
14. Viguera AC, Nonacs R, Cohen LS, Tondo L, Murray A, Baldessarini RJ (2000) Risk of recurrence of bipolar disorder in pregnant and nonpregnant women after discontinuing lithium maintenance. Am J Psychiatr 157(2):179–184
15. Sanchez-Gistau V, Romero S, Moreno D, de la Serna E, Baeza I, Sugranyes G, Moreno C, Sanchez-Gutierrez T, Rodriguez-Toscano E, Castro-Fornieles J (2015) Psychiatric disorders in child and adolescent offspring of patients with schizophrenia and bipolar disorder: a controlled study. Schizophr Res 168(1–2):197–203

16. Rusner M, Berg M, Begley C (2016) Bipolar disorder in pregnancy and childbirth: a systematic review of outcomes. BMC Pregnancy Childbirth 16(1):331
17. Santucci AK, Singer LT, Wisniewski SR, Luther JF, Eng HF, Sit DK, Wisner KL (2017) One-year developmental outcomes for infants of mothers with bipolar disorder. J Clin Psychiatry 78(8):1083–1090
18. Logsdon MC, Mittelberg M, Jacob AE, Luther JF, Wisniewski SR, Confer A, Eng H, Wisner KL (2015) Maternal–Infant interaction in women with unipoloar and bipolar depression. Appl Nurs Res 28(4):381–383
19. Battle CL, Weinstock LM, Howard M (2014) Clinical correlates of perinatal bipolar disorder in an interdisciplinary obstetrical hospital setting. J Affect Disord 158:97–100
20. May PA, Chambers CD, Kalberg WO, Zellner J, Feldman H, Buckley D, Kopald D, Hasken JM, Xu R, Honerkamp-Smith G, Taras H (2018) Prevalence of fetal alcohol spectrum disorders in 4 US communities. JAMA 319(5):474–482
21. Brown QL, Sarvet AL, Shmulewitz D, Martins SS, Wall MM, Hasin DS (2017) Trends in marijuana use among pregnant and nonpregnant reproductive-aged women, 2002-2014. JAMA 317(2):207–209
22. Jansson LM, Jordan CJ, Velez ML (2018) Perinatal marijuana use and the developing child. JAMA 320(6):545–546
23. Siqveland TS, Moe V (2014) Longitudinal development of mother–infant interaction during the first year of life among mothers with substance abuse and psychiatric problems and their infants. Child Psychiatry Hum Dev 45(4):408–421
24. Siqveland TS, Haabrekke K, Wentzel-Larsen T, Moe V (2014) Patterns of mother–infant interaction from 3 to 12 months among dyads with substance abuse and psychiatric problems. Infant Behav Dev 37(4):772–786
25. Stein A, Woolley H, Senior R, Hertzmann L, Lovel M, Lee J et al (2006) Treating disturbances in the relationship between mothers with bulimic eating disorders and their infants: a randomized, controlled trial of video feedback. Am J Psychiatr 163(5):899–906
26. Apter G, Devouche E, Gratier M, Valente M, Le Nestour A (2012) What lies behind postnatal depression: is it only a mood disorder. J Personal Disord 26(3):357–367
27. Genet MC, Golse B, Devouche E, Apter G (2014) Psychopathologie, attachement et devenir des enfants de mères présentant un trouble de personnalité borderline/état-limite: une revue de la littérature. Psychiatr Enfant 57(1):259–329
28. Blankley G, Galbally M, Snellen M, Power J, Lewis AJ (2015) Borderline personality disorder in the perinatal period: early infant and maternal outcomes. Australas Psychiatry 23(6):688–692
29. Pare-Miron V, Czuzoj-Shulman N, Oddy L, Spence AR, Abenhaim HA (2016) Effect of borderline personality disorder on obstetrical and neonatal outcomes. Womens Health Issues 26(2):190–195
30. Dayan J, Andro G, Dugnat M (2014) Psychopathologie de la périnatalité et de la parentalité. Elsevier-Masson, Issy-Les-Moulineaux
31. Glangeaud-Freudenthal NM, Howard LM, Sutter-Dallay AL (2014) Treatment–mother–infant inpatient units. Best Pract Res Clin Obstet Gynaecol 28(1):147–157
32. Kenny M, Conroy S, Pariante CM, Seneviratne G, Pawlby S (2013) Mother–infant interaction in mother and baby unit patients: before and after treatment. J Psychiatr Res 47(9):1192–1198
33. Andersson L, Sundstrom-Poromaa I, Wulff M, Astrom M, Bixo M (2004) Implications of antenatal depression and anxiety for obstetric outcome. Obstet Gynecol 104:467–476
34. Wu J, Viguera A, Riley L, Cohen L, Ecker J (2002) Mood disturbance in pregnancy and the mode of delivery. Am J Obstet Gynecol 187:864–867
35. Dayan J, Creveuil C, Dreyfus M, Herlicoviez M, Baleyte JM, O'Keane V (2010) Developmental model of depression applied to prenatal depression: role of present and past life events, past emotional disorders and pregnancy stress. PLoS One 5(9):e12942
36. Cooper PJ, Murray L (1995) Course and recurrence of postnatal depression. Evidence for the specificity of the diagnostic concept. Br J Psychiatry 166:191–195
37. Di Florio A, Putnam K, Altemus M, Apter G, Bergink V, Bilszta J, Brock R, Buist A, Deligiannidis KM, Devouche E, Epperson CN (2017) The impact of education, country,

race and ethnicity on the self-report of postpartum depression using the Edinburgh postnatal depression scale. Psychol Med 47(5):787–799
38. Putnam KT, Wilcox M, Robertson-Blackmore E, Sharkey K, Bergink V, Munk-Olsen T, Deligiannidis KM, Payne J, Altemus M, Newport J, Apter G, Postpartum Depression: Action Towards Causes and Treatment (PACT) Consortium (2017) Clinical phenotypes of perinatal depression and time of symptom onset: analysis of data from an international consortium. Lancet Psychiatry 4(6):477–485
39. Murray L, Arteche A, Fearon P, Halligan S, Croudace T, Cooper P (2010) The effects of maternal postnatal depression and child sex on academic performance at age 16 years: a developmental approach. J Child Psychol Psychiatry 51(10):1150–1159
40. Murray L, Arteche A, Fearon P, Halligan S, Goodyer I, Cooper P (2011) Maternal postnatal depression and the development of depression in offspring up to 16 years of age. J Am Acad Child Adolesc Psychiatry 50(5):460–470
41. Goodman SH, Rouse MH, Connell AM, Broth MR, Hall CM, Heyward D (2011) Maternal depression and child psychopathology: a meta-analytic review. Clin Child Fam Psychol Rev 14(1):1–27
42. Gonçalves H, Pearson RM, Horta BL, González-Chica DA, Castilho E, Damiani M, Lima RC, Gigante DP, Barros FC, Stein A, Victora CG (2016) Maternal depression and anxiety predicts the pattern of offspring symptoms during their transition to adulthood. Psychol Med 46(2):415–424
43. Weissman MM, Wickramaratne P, Gameroff MJ, Warner V, Pilowsky D, Kohad RG, Verdeli H, Skipper J, Talati A (2016) Offspring of depressed parents: 30 years later. Am J Psychiatr 173(10):1024–1032
44. Huizink AC, Mulder EJ, Buitelaar JK (2004) Prenatal stress and risk for psychopathology: specific effects or induction of general susceptibility? Psychol Bull 130(1):115–142
45. Hock E, Shirtzinger MB (1992) Maternal separation anxiety: its developmental course and relation to maternal mental health. Child Dev 63:93–102
46. Winnicott DW (1971) Playing and reality. Tavistock, London
47. Van Batenburg-Eddes, T., de Groot, L., Huizink, A.C., Steegers, E.A., Hofman, A., Jaddoe, V.W., et al. (2009). Maternal symptoms of anxiety during pregnancy affect infant neuromotor development: the Generation R study. Dev Neuropsychol, 34(4), 476–493
48. Lamour M (1985) Des nourrissons avec leurs mères psychotiques. Rev Pédiatr 7:327–334
49. Lamour M (1989) Les nourrissons de parents psychotiques. In: Lebovici S, Weil-Halpern F (eds) Psychopathologie du bébé. PUF, Paris, pp 655–673
50. Teasdale JD, Fogarty S, William JM (1980) Speech rate as a measure of short-term variation in depression. Br J Clin Psychol 19:271–278
51. Sherer KR (1986) Vocal affect expression: a review and a model for future research. Psychol Bull 99:143–165
52. Beebe B, Badalamenti A, Jaffe J, Feldstein S, Marquette L, Helbraun E et al (2008) Distressed mothers and their infants use a less efficient timing mechanism in creating expectancies of each other's looking patterns. J Psycholinguistic Res 37(5):293–307
53. Libert J, Lewinsohn P (1973) The concept of social skill with special reference to the behavior of depressed persons. J Consult Clin Psychol 40:304–312
54. Champagne FA (2010) Early adversity and developmental outcomes: interaction between genetics, epigenetics, and social experiences across the life span. Perspect Psychol Sci 5(5):564–574
55. Champagne FA, Meaney MJ (2006) Stress during gestation alters postpartum maternal care and the development of the offspring in a rodent model. Biol Psychiatry 59(12):1227–1235
56. Lester BM, Tronick E, Nestler E, Abel T, Kosofsky B, Kuzawa CW, Marsit CJ, Maze I, Meaney MJ, Monteggia LM, Reul JM (2011) Behavioral epigenetics. Ann N Y Acad Sci 1226(1):14–33
57. Szyf M, Weaver I, Meaney M (2007) Maternal care, the epigenome and phenotypic differences in behavior. Reprod Toxicol 24(1):9–19

58. Devlin AM, Brain U, Austin J, Oberlander TF (2010) Prenatal exposure to maternal depressed mood and the MTHFR C677T Variant affect SLC6A4 Methylation in infants at birth. PLoS One 5(8):1–8
59. Zucchi FC, Yao Y, Ward ID, Ilnytskyy Y, Olson DM, Benzies K, Kovalchuk I, Kovalchuk O, Metz GA (2013) Maternal stress induces epigenetic signatures of psychiatric and neurological diseases in the offspring. PLoS One 8(2):1–9
60. Provençal N, Binder EB (2015) The effects of early life stress on the epigenome: from the womb to adulthood and even before. Exp Neurol 268:10–20
61. Taylor SE, Way BM, Seeman TE (2011) Early adversity and adult health outcomes. Dev Psychopathol 23(3):939–954
62. Apter G, Genet MC, Alecian M, Devouche E (2017) Interactions précoces: modèles et recherches en psychopathologie développementale. EMC Psychiatr/Pédopsychiatrie 14(4):1–9
63. Degraux C, Pelsser V (2011) La grille de Steinhauer: explications, utilisations et limites dans l'accompagnement
64. Garret-Gloanec N., Gloanec Y. (2007) De la psychiatrie périnatale à la psychiatrie néonatale. EMC (Elsevier Masson SAS, Paris), Psychiatrie/Pédopsychiatrie, 37-200-B-25
65. Moayedoddin A, Moser D, Nanzer N (2013) The impact of brief psychotherapy centred on parenthood on the anxio-depressive symptoms of mothers during the perinatal period. Swiss Med Wkly 143:w13769
66. Apter G, Devouche E (2013) The multifaceted question of the prescription of antidepressants during pregnancy. Shanghai Arch Psychiatry 25(5):317
67. Apter G, Devouche E, Becquemont L (2015) Impact of pregnancy on psychotropic medication prescription: a French cohort study. Therapie 70(3):251–257
68. Langan R, Goodbred AJ (2016) Identification and management of peripartum depression. Am Fam Physician 93(10):852–858
69. van der Ham J, Berry K, Hoehn E, Fraser J (2013) A collaborative approach to perinatal and infant mental health service delivery in Australia. Australas Psychiatry 21(4):371–375
70. Lee VWW, Newman LK (2018) A model for the provision of integrated perinatal and infant mental health services in regional settings. Australas Psychiatry 6(5):531–533
71. Williams AS, Apter G (2017) Helping mothers with the emotional dysregulation of borderline personality disorder and their infants in primary care settings. Aust Fam Physician 46(9):669
72. Manzano J, Palacio Espasa F, Zilkha N (1999) Les scenarios narcissiques de la parentalité. PUF, Paris
73. Manzano J, Righetti-Veltema M, Perreard EC (1997) Le syndrome de dépression du prépartum. Résultat d'une recherche sur les signes précurseurs de la dépression du post-partum. Psychiatr Enfant 40(2):533–552
74. Apter G, Bobin A, Genet MC, Gratier M, Devouche E (2017) Update on mental health of infants and children of parents affected with mental health issues. Curr Psychiatry Rep 19(10):72
75. Prenoveau JM, Craske MG, West V, Giannakakis A, Zioga M, Lehtonen A et al (2017) Maternal postnatal depression and anxiety and their association with child emotional negativity and behavior problems at two years. Dev Psychol 53(1):50
76. Lipscomb ST, Leve LD, Harold GT, Neiderhiser JM, Shaw DS, Ge X, Reiss D (2011) Trajectories of parenting and child negative emotionality during infancy and toddlerhood: a longitudinal analysis. Child Dev 82(5):1661–1675
77. Masten AS, Cicchetti D (2010) Developmental cascades. Dev Psychopathol 22(3):491–495

Parental Psychiatric Disorders and Early Interaction: Dysregulation and Repair

6

Gisèle Apter and Emmanuel Devouche

Interactions between a mother/caregiver and her/their infant can be modeled as a three-dimensional triptych: with each partner linked to the interactive experience that constitutes a third dimension, where they meet and which can be thought of as existing both between and around each of them. The status of parenthood is a partly constructed condition, its development essential to the adult-infant communication system, often straining and stressful for the new parent. The emergence of novel "properties," i.e., parental capacities adapted to the system's better functioning, is difficult to predict. Conditions and properties of the system, i.e., parental pathology/infant condition need to be analyzed in order to better describe the system's evolution. Parental preexisting pathology per se has been examined in Chaps. 5 and 8. Here, we aim to study the disruptions and dysregulations that can afflict the system itself, and we go on to suggest how to address these issues clinically when parental guidance is an option.

6.1 Parent-Infant Early Interactions: An Open and Evolving System

Interactions are dynamic and coordinated in time. They need to be examined both microanalytically and in a diachronic manner. We now know that each behavior tends to continue and potentially enhance the one that precedes it. Rhythmicity and synchrony are the main properties that support mutuality and coherence of interactive behaviors in small narrative meaning-matching and meaning-making episodes [1].

G. Apter (✉)
Groupe Hospitalier du Havre, Montivilliers, France

Université de Rouen Normandie, Rouen, France

E. Devouche
Paris Descartes University, Paris, France

© Springer Nature Switzerland AG 2019

G. Apter et al. (eds.), *Early Interaction and Developmental Psychopathology*,
https://doi.org/10.1007/978-3-030-04769-6_6

Over time, their messiness, errors, and repairs amidst mutual adult-infant motivation to communicate and expand are enriched by infant and parent development and its necessary adjustment. Thus the dyadic system is an open system that is constantly expanding and nourished by the caregiver-infant intersubjective world [2].

An unwell caregiver progressively includes the pathological intersubjective patterns of thought and behavior that are part of its functioning into the dyadic system he/she forms with the infant, and the system will, as best as it can, organize and reorganize with the caregiver's (mother's) properties whatever they may be (as well as the infant's; see Chap. 7 for the cases of prematurity and low birth weight specifically). And in fact, the imposed properties of this three-part system, stemming from the necessity for the infant of an intersubjective relationship, can be considered the main attribute of the said system. The system will thus have the capacity to disorganize and modify each partner's condition, including the parent's characteristics. It is indeed interesting for the field of perinatal psychiatry to realize that working at the interaction level may lead to significant intrapersonal change in the adult also.

We have seen that the dyadic system is based on a continuous flow of meaning-matching and meaning-making interactions. Yet, because of their inherent messiness associated with the difference between two asymmetrically developed individuals (i.e., an adult and a helpless but competent neonate or infant), mutually regulated and harmonious interactions occur for only a third of the time during which adults and infants are engaged with each other. The rest of time is spent preparing and repairing the inevitable misunderstandings and interruptions of everyday exchange. These micro-breaks mostly go unnoticed in healthy and well-attuned dyads, thanks to the general smoothing-over provided by proto-narrative processes within the flow of co-regulated behavior [3]. It is the observation and analysis of the construction of this intersubjective temporal coherence, unique to each dyadic system, that is of particular interest to us. It provides insight into how and where the interruption and dysregulation unbalances the temporal flow of togetherness, resulting in distorted interactive rhythms, themselves linked to further disorganization of behavioral patterns for the infant, including a risk of loss of the sense of agency and of adapted regulated emotional motivation.

6.1.1 The Dyad: Regulation and Repair

The observation of the phases of interactive breakdown and repair gives us access, on the one hand to what happens "spontaneously" during an ecological observation and, on the other hand, to interactive changes following laboratory interventions such as the still-face procedure or therapeutic interventions in the course of parent-child psychotherapy.

The concept of repair is associated to that of "breakdown" in the synchrony and mutuality of an interaction. Through microanalytic observation of an interaction, with second-by-second or even frame-by-frame precision, it becomes possible to identify specific moments when one of the two partners exerts a pressure on the system through behavior that is non-synchronous and/or mis-attuned, leading to a breakdown of mutuality. This failing can occur at two levels, separately or jointly. In theory, the loss of connection can be primarily temporal-based on mismatched quantitative aspects, as when one of the two partners interrupts its action (gesture, vocalization, gaze) or accelerates an action in a way that does not match the previous established pattern. The loss of connection can also stem from qualitative aspects, as when one of the two partners responds to the other with an emotionally incongruent emotion or with inappropriate intensity. The mother can, for example, modify the rate at which she presents an object to her infant or leave too long a break after the baby's vocalization in relation to their previous exchange. The lag may also consist in a qualitative "un"tuning; one of the two partners interrupts and/or transforms a planned and consistent action into a different register than expected. The infant can solicit its mother by a vocalization, and she will react by the proposal of an object, but without a vocal response adapted to that of the infant. In practice, most micro-breaks are complex and all the more difficult to disentangle as they do not last long and are thus often overlooked. These micro-breaks become real dissonances, and the repair mechanisms have to be actived at the same level in order to be successful. It is interesting to note that micro-breaks are frequent and that they give rise to no less frequent repairs [4–8].

It is the macro-breaks that usually interest psychopathologists the most, as well as how the dyad will be able to cope with the unevenness of parental solicitation and response. This concern is related to the ever-present focus, for clinicians, on finding adequate and as early as possible therapeutic approaches. It is noteworthy that most interactions lead to a cycle of breakdowns and repairs that do not cause particular trouble, provided that the style and tempo have a form of regularity and therefore a form of predictability. As a result, the infant can vary and improvise within a sufficiently flexible framework that serves as a scaffold for the temporal sequence of the interaction [9, 10]. What needs to be studied more closely are the shifts in tempo and unpredictability of rhythm that can impede infants' capacity to adapt within an interactive framework that involves working together with awareness and sensitivity for the partner.

6.1.2 The Dyad: Balanced and Yet on the Move

Interactive disorder only appears if too much variation occurs in the interactive patterns. It is easy to understand that modifying a single aspect of an interaction will have little effect. Recurrent patterns involving either too much or too little stimulation conversely constitute a context of risk for the development of disorders. Too few interactive solicitations, i.e., a paucity of stimuli or interactive neglect, entail major shortcomings known to cause significant development delays. Sequelae can be definitive if neglect is lasting and occurs at key moments of development [11]. In contrast, too much solicitation and stimulation are associated with infant hypertonia and hypervigilance. The question of subtler distortions, such as lagging, increased repetitiveness, and failed or intrusive stimulations (even when not neglectful), all form complex patterns that will give shape to stabilized interaction styles, often strongly constraining the responses of the infant and inducing situations with unpredictable resolutions.

It is the study of these complex patterns which, among other things, occupies the field of clinical psychopathology. Indeed, clinically oriented researchers aim to develop models of understanding which interactive patterns are most often associated with harmonious development. These are interactive styles that can accommodate degrees of variation with improvisational quality, both structured and "attuned," and that are well suited to buffer all sorts of environmental stressors. Interactive "errors" and "tolerable false notes" could thus be distinguished from breakdowns and dissonances. This would enable a distinction to be drawn between issues of to whom intervention is aimed and of how to propose interactive preventive therapeutic support. The aim of therapists would be to restore the improvisational quality of adapted and adaptive parent-infant interaction.

Breakdowns and distortions can be schematically described along three different trajectories, they are based on a model integrating Masten and Cichetti's developmental cascades hypothesis and our own cumulative assumption as concerns developmental courses [12–14]:

- Brief and sporadic dissonances will not be memorized like patterns and configurations in the long run. They are not frequent enough to be embedded in the synaptic durable pathways that are built in during the first months of life [15]. They represent the unpredictability of existence that ends up merging into the daily lot of temporal micro-variations, the level of negative activity of which is insufficient to lead to one of the following two courses.
- If durable and regular, interactive breaks give rise to styles which, when repeated, are and remain predictable for the child. This style is constructed out of the interactive breaks and dysregulations, linked to pathological environmental circumstances and/or parental psychopathological disorder. These multiple breaks, if they are organized, may represent compensations for otherwise life-threatening situations (trauma, war, catastrophe, parental hospitalization, etc.).
- If durable but unpredictable, major breakdowns and distortions come together in a chaotic and inherently unstable system where the slightest disturbance causes the system to derail, failing to achieve a new balance and lacking the ability to build on any solid relation with past experiences. The main concern in this case is the difficulty to act on both partners and/or for both partners to be active without reinforcing their shared instability. Since all parts of the system are involved in the disruptive causes and in how the momentary interactive style comes to be built, how to intervene to both stabilize and repair the system at the same time becomes a major challenge.

It is this last interactive style in particular which has massive deleterious consequences for the infant. Because of its emotional, motor, and psychic immaturity, the infant can only process interactive information in a raw manner.

6.2 When the Evolving Balance of the Interactive System Is Threatened

6.2.1 The Case of Postpartum Depression (PPD)

6.2.1.1 Too Much Predictability, Less Availability

Postnatal depression has mobilized particular interest from psychiatrists and psychologists because of the negative impact it has on the development of offspring during infancy and through childhood. Indeed, infants of parents who have postpartum depression are at higher risk of developing psychological and behavioral disorders during early and late childhood [16, 17]. They also tend to show lower levels of secure attachment than infants of non-depressed parents, both in the short term (infancy) and in the long term (adolescence), as shown by several longitudinal studies on depressed mothers [18]

Most studies report a high prevalence of maternal postnatal depression ranging from 10% to 20% according to epidemiological data [19, 20] and 13% on average in the seminal meta-analysis of O'Hara and Swain [21]. More recent studies, according to Dayan and Baleyte [22], observe a variation of prevalence according to the severity of depression ranging from 2% to 10%. Other studies find the same rates, between 10% to 15%, and show that the risk is significantly higher in "high-risk populations," in particular, because of socioeconomic difficulties in low- and middle-income countries [23–25]. While these rates approximate the proportion of depression observed in a population of women without children aged less than 1 year, the risk of experiencing a depressive episode during the peripartum is three times higher than at any other time of life [26]. According to the recent meta-analysis of Paulson and Bazemore [27], paternal prenatal and postpartum depression is prevalent in close to 10% of men in the reviewed studies and appears relatively higher in the 3- to 6-month postpartum period. Paternal depression also shows a moderate positive correlation with maternal depression [28]. Interestingly, most of the studies conducted on the impact of parental perinatal depression on infant focused only on one parent, mainly the mother, leading to two separated literatures [29].

Among the numerous studies that focus on the effects of parental postnatal depression on behavioral and affective interactions with the baby, the one conducted by Field [30] has been the one to most clearly show how maternal depression entails maternal emotional unavailability toward the infant. The mother is supposed to act as an important modulator of the infant's emotional regulation and to offer optimal stimulation, as well as synchronous interactions. When she is unavailable psychologically, this sensitivity to synchrony is often lost. The infant then finds itself trying to synchronize to a non-contingent partner. Depending on its preexisting regulatory capacities (see NBAS for evaluation, Part 3 Chap. 2), it will thus be at risk for emotional dysregulation. This phenomenon generates changes in the behavior, emotions, and physiological states of the infant. Indeed, the baby basically needs interpersonal and intersubjective regulation for its homeostasis and may show signs of emotional and behavioral disorganization when the mother (the father or other attachment figure) is physically or psychologically "unavailable," especially in the case when this is totally involuntary and related to maternal mental disorders. By observing the proto-conversations between a depressed mother and her infant, one can perceive that it is not the "failures," inevitable and inherent to any interaction, that are the most harmful to the interaction but the parental unavailability that makes it impossible for temporary inherent "failures" to be repaired. In this situation, the caregiver is then not only unable to validate infant emotions and behaviors but also, due to this unavailability, unable to engage with the motivation of the infant for social interaction. Thus this repetitive non-repair and non-contingency or unavailability becomes the usual way in which the infant learns and interacts within its social environment.

Studies conducted on paternal depression also reveal a clear tendency for "parental" unavailability. In their meta-analysis, Wilson and Durbin [31] emphasize that paternal postpartum depression leads to a decrease in positive emotions, tenderness, sensitivity, and social engagement and to an increase in hostility towards the baby, thus impacting its capacity for interaction. Authors point out that paternal depression has a significant and negative effect on parenting behaviors by fathers and speak to the importance of continuing to include fathers and other significant others in research on child development and the family environment. Mezulis et al. [32] observed, in 350 father-infant dyads, that paternal depression during a child's infancy exacerbated the effect of maternal depression. They also noticed that this potentializing effect was limited to depressed fathers spending medium to high amounts of time caring for their infants. Authors emphasize the moderating role fathers may play in reducing or exacerbating the adverse long-term effects of maternal depression during a child's infancy on behavioral problems developing in childhood. The negative impact would be all the more important if both parents were affected by perinatal depression [33].

6.2.1.2 Impact on the Interactive Dynamics

As an open system evolving in time, parent-infant interactive organization is likely to follow different trajectories depending on how each part of the system, parent and infant and their patterns, evolve. The system is indeed dynamic, and one risk is that the pathological behavioral pattern that the parent addresses to the baby during daily interactive episodes leads to actual infant adaptation to the system as the least adverse way in which the infant can relate leading in turn to a sustained relational pattern. In other words, the risk is to enter a negative loop in which the dysregulated (for the infant) interactive system is self-sustaining. When, from birth the parent already presents with an existing depression, then the question arises to what extent antenatal maternal depression might have already had a negative impact on the developing fetus and how, in turn, this influences the parent-infant relationship from birth through implicit neonatal and postnatal characteristics [12, 34].

Although numerous studies have been conducted on interactive models and patterns of dyadic interaction, few have explored interactions per se between affected parents and offspring or focused on outcome measures for these interactions. The mutual influence parents and infants have on each other includes models of mutual regulation and primary intersubjectivity supporting a system theory approach that looks at social development as a dyadic dynamic flow of matching, mismatching, and repair [7, 16, 30, 35]. Some studies have found that in the first semester, in case of maternal depression, interactions are dysregulated, and their main finding is that these infants and parents cannot mutually "connect." Using the global rating scales, Zarate-Guerrero et al. [36] observed that mothers diagnosed with depression without any comorbid personality disorder were less actively engaged, less sensitive, and less responsive in comparison with "control" mothers. Authors did not however observe significant differences on both scales dedicated to 3-month-old infants' behaviors, although all scores were higher in control infants. This study confirms Murray and Cooper's [35] observations that already at this age, interactive patterns reorganize into rigid configurations too tight for improvisation or too chaotic and loose for regulation. Thus infants are unable to establish a sense of agency and are at risk for current and later emotional dysregulation.

Early manifestations of the wanting interactive system in the context of parental depression are already visible from the first months of life in both partners' behavioral patterns even though all studies did not find a specific behavioral pattern in infants (for an extended exploration of PPD and interaction, see Chap. 8). This supports the idea that the impact of postpartum depression on early interaction is not linear. PPD alone is far from sufficient to predict a single negative impact on interactive dynamics. More recently, the heterogeneity of postpartum depression and its frequent comorbidity with personality disorders and/or anxiety disorders have raised more questions than they have provided answers on the manner in which PPD and its diversity of underlying pathologies may affect children's mental health [13, 37].

6.2.2 The Case of Borderline Personality Disorder

6.2.2.1 Too Little Predictability, Chaotic Communication

Borderline personality disorder (BPD) is characterized by a pervasive pattern of instability in affect regulation, impulse control, interpersonal relationships, and self-image. Mothers with BPD frequently feel overwhelmed by relationships per se. In case of parenthood, the inherent needs of their infants may add to more intense feelings of being overwhelmed. Indeed, the infant's constant yet necessary demands may be hard to tolerate for BPD mothers. Due to identity issues, and intense emotional personal dysregulation, these mothers may either totally "absorb" their infant's needs as their own or become blind to their specific needs and behaviors overlooking in both cases the creative-individual aspects of their infant's expressions.

"Borderline" mothers thus oscillate between extreme and intense mood variations and between idealization of relationships and anger and rejection. When the partner receiving these emotions is a developing infant, the fear and weight of the responsibility involved may be overpoweringly devastating, precipitating maternal self-esteem to even lower levels and reinforcing depressive symptoms. Risk of rejection in order to avoid such fear and risk of collapse also put the relationship in a dangerous zone of over- and under-involvement, alternating between intrusiveness and abandonment, mirroring the parent's own experience of parenting that it is, tragically, aiming to avoid or to repair.

The concept of continuity/discontinuity is particularly helpful to understand infant emotional development and to create a model in order to apprehend the infant's capacity for representation and memory of small narrative snips [38]. On the one hand, there is a need for potential discontinuity, i.e., sporadic glitches in the interactive patterns at the micro-level, in order for repairable macro-levels of improvisation to occur; and, on the other hand, chaotic unpredictability, i.e., major diverse nonlinear disturbing or destabilizing effects, totally incapacitates the infant whose developmental potential is undermined.

When infant's self and interactive regulation systems are overwhelmed, their capacity to "experience a continuity of being" as Winnicott [39] put it many decades ago is greatly hindered. It is becoming clear how important it is, at a macro-level, for the infant to be understood within its own reality, for its own sake, that is to say to perceive as closely as possible its own developing aptitudes reflected in the predictability of parental behavior. Indeed, for example, if waiting time (for a bottle at a macro-level or for a vocal response at a micro-level) constantly exceeds the infant's individual capacity to anticipate upcoming events, it will be unable to cope or to remain available or, in other words, to establish an emotionally fulfilling relationship, on the sole basis of its own creative representational world. The risk is then for the infant to be dislocated from the interactive space and to cascadingly be less and less able to self-regulate. Intrusiveness at a macro-level such as touching and precipitated vocal stimulation may mask an inappropriate micro-level unresponsiveness. Close observation and analysis of timeliness, quality, and quantity of all modalities of interactions (gazing, vocalizing, touching, caregiving, repositioning, etc.) are necessary in order to correctly understand where and how distortions occur.

6.2.2.2 Interactions Less Predictable for Infants and Their Caregivers

To date we know very little about the interactions between borderline mothers and their infants. The first small-scale study to explore this was conducted on eight mothers affected with BPD and showed that although they were more insensitively intrusive with their 2-month-old infants after an interactive disruption (the still-face [SF]), the infants themselves did not significantly differ in their behavior from controls before the interruption [40]. Patterns and negative infant emotional configurations among infants of 17 mothers with BPD were then qualitatively described [41]. In general, studies are too sparse on BPD parenting, but in older infants, a negative impact of maternal psychopathology on the status of attachment (i.e., more disorganized attachment) has been found.

Two separate studies on vocal interaction, one comparing 6 BPD mothers and their 3-month-olds with 6 control dyads [10] and the other comparing 17 BPD and control dyads [42] show atypicalities in the speech mothers' with BPD address to their infants. The first study suggests that these mothers' speech is highly repetitive both in terms of its verbal content and its prosody. Both studies show that mothers with BPD produce more unvoiced sound, whistles, and whispers, with frequent changes in perceived timbre or voice quality (e.g., from breathy to creaky). Both studies also show that although BPD mothers talk to their infants as much as control mothers and although their utterances are, on average, of equal duration, they interrupt their speech for much longer periods and in a more erratic fashion than control mothers. Interactions between mothers with BPD and their 3-month-old infants were found to include less infant participation, longer interruptions, more repetition, and unvoiced sounds, leading to a temporal organization of the speech of mothers with BPD that is less predictable for the infant [43].

Apter et al. [44] conducted a study on 19 mothers diagnosed with BPD and 41 controls with no history of psychopathology. They were observed with their 3-month-old infants using Tronick's Face-to-Face Still-Face paradigm. The authors found that infants whose mothers have BPD express less positive vocalizations and less non-autonomic self-regulation than infants of mothers with no psychopathology. The stress of the SF episode affects their gaze and self-regulation behaviors more strongly than those of infants of controls. The Reunion episode seems particularly challenging for mothers with BPD, who show fewer smiles and an increase in intrusive behavior. In their conclusion, the authors emphasize the importance of observing distortions in the early caregiving relationship of mothers with BPD and their infants. Considering what we already know about the negative impact of dysregulation on attachment and child psychopathology, it seems essential to take into account the impact of disturbed regulatory behavior that is observed between mothers and initially healthy infants as early as 3 months postpartum. This calls for attempts to intervene very early on, much earlier than has been envisaged up until now.

6.3 Repairing the Interactive Co-regulation Process in Case of Major Distortions

The question of emotional regulation and how to promote it includes issues of temperament and behavior through the functions of emotional expression, intersubjectivity, attachment, and psychopathological manifestation [45–47]. The question of the regulation of negative emotions (crying, protestations, fear, anguish, shame, alarm, or distress and anger) is at the center of attachment theory [48, 49]. In addition, the regulation of positive and negative emotions has common neuropsychological mechanisms [46, 50].

Two models exist with regard to this regulation within intersubjective exchanges. As concerns positive emotions, the infant may go from a moment of disorganization to one of positive emotional exchange, thus experiencing positive moments of regulation, thanks to maternal regulation. This would give it a sense of elation and dyadic expansion of consciousness, as described in Tronick's model [2, 6]. In this state, the emotional developmental achievement enhances the infant's sense of control over its own intentions and goals, promoting its sense of agency, in turn scaffolded by parental self and mutual regulation [9].

Concerning negative emotions, the baby is also in direct need of interpersonal regulatory mechanisms. Caregiving is a motivational system, recently studied by the theory of attachment, which is one of the dimensions of parental care. Response to needs for both closeness and exploration are the elements that build Attachment patterns [51]. Interpersonal regulation is therefore one of the functions of the caregiving system. Hence, maternal sensitivity is linked to the construction of the baby's attachment style. The mother needs to respond appropriately (depending on the characteristics of the interaction) to the baby's signals in order to comfort it [52]. Moreover, the concepts of mentalization and parental reflexive function developed by Fonagy and Target [53] have shed light on the notion of maternal sensitivity. It is essential for the mother to be able to reflect, contain, interpret, and regulate the negative emotions of the baby. This capacity can only develop if the mother apprehends her baby as having its own states of mind, i.e., intentions and mental states that are different from her own [48, 54]. This ability to recognize the infant's mental state is the basis of the baby's emotional regulation potentialities and must be solicited even when the mother is in a state of stress. Yet, this is particularly difficult for mothers with psychopathology, specifically with BPD [18], or for mothers who have experienced "unelaborated trauma." It can also be hindered by maternal depression and emotional flatness, due to lack of energy and low self-esteem. Moreover, the lack of quality of reflexive maternal functioning is hypothesized as the manner in which parental disorganized attachment is often transmitted to the child [53].

This reflexive function is necessary in order for the parent to exercise specific affective attunement to the infant's negative emotions allowing it to be recognized through its entire emotional repertoire [48]. It is this reflexive aptitude that allows the mother to be the "mirror" of her baby's emotions [55, 56]. In this manner, the parent, faced with signals of distress or alarm from the baby, responds at the same infraverbal emotional level (by coherent attuned facial expression and prosody) by both accentuating (recognition and visible translation) and temporally reorganizing (slowing and buffering) negative infant feelings [57]. This allows the baby to physically experience being "validated" in the sensing of its negative emotion, together with being understood without being overwhelmed by the negative emotion the mother is expressing: because the expression is mirroring with alteration, this means the mother is not being overpowered by it but yet understands and is able to have access to a bearable representation.

The caregiving interactive system is a model for an interpersonal mechanism of stress regulation organization. This is now considered a component of the theory of attachment [48, 58]. It is this interpersonal regulation that allows the infant to regulate its own negative emotions or what has been called "the fearful arousal" [59]. This macro-level of regulation allows the infant to be organized and to develop predictable patterns of emotional regulation. Thus, the regulation of negative emotions is primarily an interpersonal phenomenon and only secondarily becomes internal, depending on the subject's own internalizing competencies [48, 60]. If the regulation of negative emotions in the adult therefore seems an individual capacity, it is in fact embodied and built upon interpersonal experience [48]. In case of environmental insult and parental psychopathology, the manner in which it will unfold may be partly or totally impeached.

6.3.1 The Case of BPD

The clinical management of mothers with BPD with their babies highlights the impact of BPD on parenting. These repercussions have been described by Le Nestour et al. [61] and Apter et al. [44]. These authors relied on DSM-IV criteria (see Table 6.1). Clinicians' daily work aim to design interventions to help mothers who have often experienced major life stressors or trauma and are afflicted with BPD, to interact more effectively with their infants and to allow infants born in traumatic and traumatized environments to move forward towards the best developmental trajectories possible.

Very recently, Sved Williams and Apter [62] and Apter and Sved Williams [63] proposed a review of relevant information on current knowledge of BPD and its management when mothers with BPD are caregivers to an infant and when infants

Table 6.1 The nine diagnostic criteria for borderline personality disorder

A pervasive pattern of instability of interpersonal relationships, self-image, and affects and marked impulsivity beginning by early adulthood and present in a variety of contexts, as indicated by five (or more) of the following:
1. Frantic efforts to avoid real or imagined abandonment
2. A pattern of unstable and intense interpersonal relationships characterized by alternating between extremes of idealization and devaluation
3. Identity disturbance: markedly and persistently unstable self-image or sense of self
4. Impulsivity in at least two areas that are potentially self-damaging
5. Recurrent suicidal behavior, gestures, threats, or self-mutilating behavior
6. Affective instability due to a marked reactivity of mood (e.g., intense episodic dysphoria, irritability, or anxiety usually lasting a few hours and only rarely more than a few days)
7. Chronic feelings of emptiness
8. Inappropriate anger or difficulty controlling anger (e.g., frequent displays of temper, constant anger, recurrent physical fights)
9. Transient, stress-related paranoid ideation or severe dissociative symptoms

Reprinted with permission from the Diagnostic and Statistical Manual of Mental Disorders, Fourth Edition, Text Revision. Copyright 2000 American Psychiatric Association are examined in distorted parenting environmental context. These authors provide useful guidelines for primary care practitioners, such as:

- Keeping the diagnosis in mind.
- Openly discussing BPD diagnosis where relevant.
- Providing psychoeducational material and ongoing support to the woman and her family.
- Referring to specialized services for BPD.
- Referring to standard maternal-child health services and specialized infant mental health services.
- Ongoing communication with other services and supervision for the practitioner.
- Infant safety must remain a priority alongside sensitive care of the mother.
- Preferring a timely intervention as infants develop rapidly and their needs are urgent.
- Involving child protection services when necessary.

6.4 Care and Prevention Measures in the Postnatal Period

Immediate postnatal interventions are becoming increasingly difficult due to lack of funding, shorter lengths of stay for women in maternity wards, absence of social and family support, and diversity of local mental health systems and resources even in high-income countries. Prenatal and peripartum care then becomes all the more important as it will make it possible to prepare and refer for appropriate care. This may have several objectives:

- Give the mother and child time to meet in a safe environment.
- Allow the mother to rest and ensure a relatively good quality of sleep.
- Allow professionals to assess the quality of interactions and the clinical condition of baby and mother.
- Allow social assessment.
- Monitor possible early signs of postpartum decompensation.

This requires, however, availability of a multidisciplinary team. Depending on the clinical assessment and evolution, several therapeutic orientations are possible:

- Baby−/parent-oriented outpatient care, home visit by a specialized mobile team, and specialized care for the baby.
- Maternal hospitalization in a psychiatric unit and baby fostered by the family or the child welfare services if necessary, when MB units are not available or maternal symptoms are too prevalent and put infant at life risk.
- Hospitalization in a mother-baby unit.
- No mother-child follow-up but continuation of adult psychiatric follow-up.
- No follow-up at all.

- Reporting of a child at risk.
- Network with primary care and prevention services.

All these orientations are not exclusive and can be mixed. Studies are rare and do not provide a consensus on specific care indications. Moreover, the means available in terms of trained professionals are very heterogeneous from one place to another, yet the needs are significant and must take into account social and demographic contexts. In any case, interventions must be implemented as early on as possible and developed and tailored to needs as quickly as possible by an experienced transdisciplinary team.

6.5 Perspectives

As pointed out, there are many approaches for general practitioners to help infants and mothers with significant emotional dysregulation, and helping the mother also helps the developing infant and for that matter the whole family.

Through this brief summary of interactions with parents suffering from psychopathology in the perinatal period, it appears that what we do not know far exceeds what we do know. For the time being, research has concentrated mainly on maternal depression, but too little on the infant and even less on their interactions. Although the analysis of the interaction components enables us to describe the impact of some psychiatric disorders, this approach remains insufficient. A systemic approach with multidirectional interactions with the environment is essential. We urgently need to emerge from an adult-centered position. The unexplored fields of research are colossal but the stakes are such that they must become a priority of the public authorities. Rather than being frightened by the magnitude of the task, it is up to us to galvanize ourselves to deal with the many possible challenges involved.

We need to implement therapeutic interventions designed to develop more robust and resilient repair patterns in mutual regulatory efforts. Longitudinal outcome studies should help us to better understand both derailing mechanisms and their potential for repair.

References

1. Delavenne A, Gratier M, Devouche E (2013) Expressive timing in infant-directed singing between 3 and 6 months. Infant Behav Dev 36(1):1–13
2. Tronick EZ, Brushweller-Stern N, Harrison AM, Lyons-Ruth K, Morgan AC, Nahum JP et al (1998) Dyadically expanded states of consciousness and the process of therapeutic change. Infant Ment Health J 19:290–299
3. Gratier M, Trevarthen C (2008) Musical narrative and motives for culture in mother-infant vocal interaction. J Conscious Stud 15(10–11):122–158
4. Tronick EZ (1989) Emotions and emotional communication in infants. Am Psychol 44(2):112
5. Tronick EZ (2003) Things still to be done on the still-face effect. Infancy 4:451–473

6. Tronick EZ (2004) Why is connection with others so critical? Dyadic meaning making, messiness and complexity governed selective processes which co-create and expand individuals' states of consciousness. Emotional Dev:293–315
7. Tronick EZ (2007) The neurobehavioral and social-emotional development of infants and children. Norton, New York
8. Tronick EZ, Beeghly M (2011) Infants' meaning-making and the development of mental health problems. Am Psychol 66:107–119
9. Bruner JS (1990) Acts of meaning, vol 3. Harvard University Press, Cambridge
10. Gratier M, Apter-Danon G (2008) The improvised musicality of belonging: repetition and variation in mother-infant vocal interaction. In: Malloch S, Trevarthen C (eds) Communicative musicality: narratives of expressive gesture and being human. Oxford University Press, Oxford, pp 301–328
11. Enlow MB, Egeland B, Blood EA, Wright RO, Wright RJ (2012) Interpersonal trauma exposure and cognitive development in children to age 8 years: a longitudinal study. J Epidemiol Community Health 66(11):1005–1010
12. Apter G, Bobin A, Genet MC, Gratier M, Devouche E (2017) Update on mental health of infants and children of parents affected with mental health issues. Curr Psychiatry Rep 19(10):72
13. Apter G, Devouche E, Gratier M, Valente M, Le Nestour A (2012) What lies behind postnatal depression: is it only a mood disorder. J Personal Disord 26(3):357–367
14. Masten AS, Cicchetti D (2010) Developmental cascades. Dev Psychopathol 22(3):491–495
15. Shonkoff JP (2011) Protecting brains, not simply stimulating minds. Science 333(6045):982–983
16. Murray L (1992) The impact of postnatal depression on infant development. J Child Psychol Psychiatry 8(1):37–55
17. Murray L, Halligan SL, Goodyer I, Herbert J (2010) Disturbances in early parenting of depressed mothers and cortisol secretion in offspring: a preliminary study. J Affect Disord 122:218–223
18. Lyons-Ruth K, Yellin C, Melnick S, Atwood G (2005) Expanding the concept of unresolved mental states: Hostile/Helpless states of mind on the adult attachment interview are associated with disrupted mother–infant communication and infant disorganization. Dev Psychopathol 17:1–23
19. Kumar R, Robson KM (1984) A prospective study of emotional disorders in childbearing women. Br J Psychiatry 144:35–47
20. O'Hara MW, Zerovski EM, Phillips LH (1990) Controlled prospective study of postnatal mood disorders: comparison of childbearing and non-childbearing women. J Abnorm Psychol 99:3–15
21. O'Hara MW, Swain A (1996) Rates and risk of post-partum depression-a meta-analysis. Int Rev Psychiatry 8:37–54
22. Dayan J, Baleyte J-M (2008) Dépressions périnatales. In: Dayan J (ed) Les dépressions périnatales. Evaluer et traiter, Coll. Médecine et psychothérapie, Paris/Masson, pp 21–43
23. Gelaye B, Rondon MB, Araya R, Williams MA (2016) Epidemiology of maternal depression, risk factors, and child outcomes in low-income and middle-income countries. Lancet Psychiatry 3(10):973–982
24. Harvey ST, Pun PK (2007) Analysis of positive Edinburgh depression scale referrals to a consultation liaison psychiatry service in a two-year period. Int J Ment Health Nurs 16:161–167
25. Reck C, Struben K, Backenstrass M (2008) Prevalence, onset and co-morbidity of postpartum anxiety and depressive disorders. Acta Psychiatr Scand 118:459–468
26. Cox JL, Holden J (1994) Perinatal psychiatry. Use and misuse of the Edinburgh post-natal depression scale. Gaskel, London
27. Paulson JF, Bazemore SD (2010) Prenatal and postpartum depression in fathers and its association with maternal depression: a meta-analysis. JAMA 303(19):1961–1969
28. Serhan N, Ege E, Ayrancı U, Kosgeroglu N (2013) Prevalence of postpartum depression in mothers and fathers and its correlates. J Clin Nurs 22(1–2):279–284

29. Fredriksen E, von Soest T, Smith L, Moe V (2018) Parenting stress plays a mediating role in the prediction of early child development from both parents' perinatal depressive symptoms. J Abnorm Child Psychol:1–16
30. Field T (1994) The effects of mother's physical and emotional unavailability on emotion regulation. Monogr Soc Res Child Dev 59:208–227
31. Wilson S, Durbin CE (2010) Effects of paternal depression on fathers' parenting behaviors: a meta-analytic review. Clin Psychol Rev 30(2):167–180
32. Mezulis AH, Hyde JS, Clark R (2004) Father involvement moderates the effect of maternal depression during a child's infancy on child behavior problems in kindergarten. J Fam Psychol 18(4):575
33. Gressier F, Tabat-Bouher M, Cazas O, Hardy P (2015) Dépression paternelle du post-partum: revue de la littérature. Presse Med 44(4):418–424
34. Vameghi R, AKBARI SAA, Sajedi F, Sajjadi H, ALAVI H (2016) Path analysis association between domestic violence, anxiety, depression and perceived stress in mothers and children's development. Iran J Child Neurol 10(4):36
35. Murray L, Cooper PJ (1997) The role of infant and maternal factors in postpartum depression, mother-infant interaction and infant outcomes. In: Murray L, Cooper e PJ (eds) Postpartum depression and child development. The Guilford Press, New York/London, pp 111–135
36. Zárate-Guerrero G, Devouche E, Espinosa-Gómez MC, Apter G (2014) Évaluer les difficultés interactives entre une mère déprimée et son bébé de 3 mois au moyen de l'échelle GRMII de Fiori-Cowley et Murray. Neuropsychiatr Enfance Adolesc 62(1):47–52
37. Putnam K, Robertson-Blackmore E, Sharkey K, Payne J, Bergink V, Munk-Olsen T et al (2015) Heterogeneity of postpartum depression: a latent class analysis. Lancet Psychiatry 2(1): 59–67
38. Nagy E, Molnar P (2004) Homo imitans or homo provocans? Human imprinting model of neonatal imitation. Infant Behav Dev 27(1):54–63
39. Winnicott DW (1960) The theory of the parent-infant relationship. Int J Psychoanal 41:585–595
40. Crandell LE, Patrick MP, Hobson RP (2003) Still-face'interactions between mothers with borderline personality disorder and their 2-month-old infants. Br J Psychiatry 183(3):239–247
41. Apter-Danon G, Candilis D (2005) A challenge for perinatal psychiatry: therapeutic management of maternal borderline personality disorder and their very young infants. Clin Neuropsychiatry 2(5):302–314
42. Delavenne A, Gratier M, Devouche E, Apter-Danon G (2008) Phrasing and fragmented time in "pathological" mother-infant vocal interaction. Mus Sci, Special Issue:47–70
43. Gratier M, Devouche E, Dominguez S, Apter G (2015) What words can't tell. Emotion Lang 10:399
44. Apter G, Devouche E, Garez V, Valente M, Genet MC, Gratier M, Dominguez S, Tronick E (2016) The still face: a greater challenge for infants of borderline mothers. J Pers Disord 30:1–14
45. Cole PM, Michel MK, Teti LO (1994) The development of emotion regulation and dysregulation: A clinical perspective. Monogr Soc Res Child Dev 59:73–100, 250–283
46. Apter G (2004) De l'intersubjectivité à l'intrapsychique. Etude des interactions précoces des mères borderline et de leur bébé de trois mois. Thèse de doctorat en psychologie sous la direction de M. Bydlowski. Université Paris 7 Diderot
47. Apter G, Devouche E, Gratier M (2011) Perinatal mental health. J Nerv Ment Dis 199(8):575–577
48. Guédeney N (2011) Les racines de l'estime de soi: apports de la théorie de l'attachement. Dev Dent 23(2):129–144
49. Kobak R (1999) The emotional dynamic of disruptions in attachment relationships. Implications for theory, research, and clinical implications. In: Cassidy J, Shavers P (eds) Handbook of attachment: theory, research and clinical applications. Guildford Press, New York, pp 21–43
50. Heller W (1993) Neuropsychological mechanisms of individual differences in emotion, personality, and arousal. Neuropsychology 7:476–489

51. Bowlby J (1980) Attachment and loss, Loss, sadness and depression, vol 3. Hogarth Press, London
52. Ainsworth MDS, Blehar MC, Waters E, Wall S (1978) Patterns of attachment: a psychological study of the strange situation. Lawrence Erlbaum Associates, Hillsdale, NJ
53. Fonagy P, Target M (2005) Bridging the transmission gap: an end to an important mystery of attachment research? Attach Hum Dev 7:333–343
54. Meins E, Fernyhough C, Wainwright R, Das Gupta M, Fradley E, Tuckey M (2002) Mind-mindedness and attachment security as predictors of theory of mind understanding. Child Dev 73:1715–1726
55. Winnicott DW (1967) Mirror-role of the mother and family in child development. In: Lomas P (ed) The predicament of the family: a psycho-analytical symposium. Hogarth Press, London, pp 26–33
56. Winnicott DW (1971) Playing and reality. Tavistock, London
57. Fonagy P, Gergely G, Jurst M, Target M (2002) Affect regulation, mentalization and the development of the self. Other Press, New York, pp 145–201
58. Gunnar MR (2003) Attachment and press in early development, does attachment add to the potency of social regulators of infant stress? In: Carter CS, Ahnert L, Grossmann KE, Hrdy SB, Lamb ME, Porges SW, Sachser N (eds) Attachment and bonding a new synthesis. The MIT Press, Cambridge, pp 245–255
59. Lyons-Ruth K (2005) L'interface entre attachement et intersubjectivité: perspectives issues de l'étude longitudinale de l'attachement désorganisé. Psychothérapies 25:223–234
60. Sroufe LA, Waters E (1977) Attachment as an organisational construct. Child Dev 48:1184–1199
61. Le Nestour A, Apter-Danon G, Héroux C, Mourgues B, Patouillot-Slatine I (2007) Parentalités limites et prises en charge thérapeutiques. Psychiatr Enfant 50(1):125–177
62. Williams AS, Apter G (2017) Helping mothers with the emotional dysregulation of borderline personality disorder and their infants in primary care settings. Aust Fam Physician 46(9):669
63. Apter G, Williams AES (2018) Infants of emotionally dysregulated or borderline personality disordered mothers. Aust J Gen Pract 47(4):203

7 Parent-Preterm Infant Interaction

Joëlle Provasi

7.1 Consequence of Premature Birth

Premature birth is defined as birth at less than 37 weeks gestational age (GA). It is defined by the number of weeks spent in utero but also by the correlated infant weight at birth. The premature infant is called late preterm and also low birth weight (LBW), if born between 32 and 36 weeks of pregnancy with a weight of less than 2500 g (5 pounds 8 ounces); moderately preterm or very low birth weight (VLBW), if the infant is born between 28 and 32 weeks of pregnancy with a weight of less than 1500 g (3 pounds 5 ounces); and very preterm or extremely low birth weight (ELBW), if the premature infant is born at less than 28 weeks of pregnancy with a weight of less than 1000 g (2 pounds 3 ounces). When the weight is not correlated to the gestational age, it is called a baby small for gestational age or intrauterine growth retardation (IUGR). Preterm infants are a very heterogeneous population. They vary considerably on the basis of perinatal risk factors (e.g., gestational age, birth weight, infection and pulmonary illness, neurological impact, etc.) [1].

7.1.1 Separation Between the Mother and Preterm Infant

The first major consequence of premature birth for mother-infant relationship is that it is associated with prolonged maternal separation [2]. The medical treatment of premature infants generally causes an immediate severance of mother and child after birth [3]. This interruption is medically imposed in order to enhance survival and is recognized by the mother and (parents in general) as being in the best interest of the child, notwithstanding the risk of maternal mortality [4]. However, early and

J. Provasi (✉)
CHArt, Ecole Pratique des Hautes Etudes (EPHE), Paris Sciences Lettres (PSL), Paris, France
e-mail: joelle.provasi@ephe.psl.eu

© Springer Nature Switzerland AG 2019

G. Apter et al. (eds.), *Early Interaction and Developmental Psychopathology*,
https://doi.org/10.1007/978-3-030-04769-6_7

prolonged infant hospitalization gives parents the impression of being dispossessed of their parental role. They feel passive, helpless, and powerless [5]. This has a major impact on maternal behavior when interacting with her infant. As a matter of fact, the lack of physical contact obstructs a cascade of neurobiological changes and mental states required for mother-infant bonding [6]. The authors suggest that in mothers of VLB premature infants (<1500 g), oxytocin concentration never reaches the level necessary to activate the development of usual maternal behavior. Therefore, it does not play the facilitating role it should for caregiving. This leaves the mother with hampered psychological resources and therefore at heightened risk for other vulnerabilities. As the premature infant, in turn, spends most of the time without maternal physical contact, which adds to the difficulties in bonding and attachment [7], premature infants and their mothers often miss out on crucial interactions during the first days (even weeks) of life. This prevents the infant from being held, and caressed, resulting in very little physical and skin to skin contact [8]. This medically forced separation goes against the emotional need of any mother/parent to be close to her/their child [9]. Most mothers will describe the fact that they have to spend the night at home while their child remains hospitalized as a very trying experience. Mothers of hospitalized preterm infants feel a strong need to be close to their baby, whatever the circumstances. Unfortunately, parents are often unable to stay with their infants round-the-clock during the infant's stay in the NICU [10]. This increases stress for both parents and infants.

At the same time, it is known that continuous proximity between mother and baby is absolutely not mandatory in the first weeks of life in order to create a secure quality of attachment [9]. A baby cannot survive on its own, so it is vital that the adult in charge feels invested with his/her own protective role as soon as possible.

Interestingly, perinatal hospitalization and the separation it entails between mother and child actively intensify maternal caregiving. Infant vulnerability and the potential life-threatening conditions to which it is subjected can represent a powerful activator of parental caregiving, enabling major protective care [11]. Flacking, Ewald, Hedberg Nyqvist, and Starrin [12] describe a strategy frequently observed in mothers of very premature babies; they insist on being close to their infants and staying at their bedside. Restoring proximity with the infant is in fact a spontaneous caregiving reaction. Failing to respect this need for closeness only heightens a mother's motivation to seek proximity to the distressed baby. Although early attachment processes may be disrupted for parents of very preterm children because of separation during a lengthy hospitalization and invasive medical procedures, parents can be reassured that they retain the capacity to positively influence their child's development through infancy and early childhood [13].

7.1.2 Maternal Psychological Distress During Neonatal Hospitalization of Preterm Infants

Due to the fact that pregnancy is interrupted before its expected duration, parents are often inadequately prepared for their new role. Therefore, they are at increased risk for anxiety, stress, unresolved grief, and depression [3]. Mothers of preterm infants experience marked psychological distress during infant hospitalization [14], which can average 100 days for children born very preterm [15]. Different types of maternal psychological distress have been listed, such as parenting stress and state anxiety, post-traumatic stress symptoms, and depressive symptoms.

State Anxiety: Many parents of premature infants experience high levels of stress. The unfamiliar environment of the NICU is an additional source of stress. Life-support equipment, monitors, intravenous and nasogastric tubes, oxygen cannulas, isolettes, and alarms all contribute to creating an unfamiliar and threatening environment [8]. In the NICU, the most stressful features for parents are the appearance and behavior of their infant [16]. This negatively impacts their parental role [17]. In fact, parents report more stress for infants with lower gestational ages and lower birth weights [18]. In the same way, mothers of high-risk, VLBW children reported higher levels of perceived stress in comparison with mothers of low-risk, VLBW children [19]. What is perceived as very stressful by parents is what is related to separation, child's pain, respiratory problems, and unresponsiveness [17]. The sense of powerlessness and impairment often alters what parents conceive as their essential role and is therefore likely to increase anxiety, helplessness, frustration, guilt, and anger [20].

Researchers have found that, after the birth of their child, both mothers and fathers of preterm babies were more tired and felt less strong than mothers and fathers of full-term babies [21]. Loss of maternal role has been found to be the greatest source of stress for mothers [22]. Many mothers of preterm infants continued to have high levels of anxiety for months after infant hospital discharge [23]. Indeed, research shows that many mothers must deal with negative feelings such as guilt but also anger toward their child [24], feeling responsible for their babies being in NICU [25]. Another study shows that the mother's vision of herself as the protective caregiver for her baby is upset [4]. Parenting stress remains important in mothers of high-risk infants within the first year of life compared with full-term infants [26].

Post-Traumatic Stress: For parents, the premature birth of a child usually represents a traumatic event by definition, one for which they are poorly prepared. Studies show a clear link between the severity of post-traumatic stress symptoms and parent's perception of the degree of perinatal risk for the child, taking into account gestational age, birth weight, and severity of medical complications during hospitalization [27]. Premature birth is not a single traumatic event but implies a sequence of events, particularly during hospitalization. Immediately after the premature birth of their child, mothers have higher levels of stress and traumatic symptoms than fathers [21]. Mothers show significantly higher levels of post-traumatic stress symptoms such as avoidance, intrusion, and hyper-arousal [28]. Traumatic events can be repeated and reactivated or even increase in frequency during the second year of the child's life [29].

Depressive Symptoms: Mothers of preterm infants are at higher risk for depression than mothers of full-term infants during the immediate postpartum [7]. A Canadian study reported a close relationship between level of prematurity and depressive symptoms: Higher depression scores were observed in mothers of infants born before 33 weeks GA than in mothers of infants born between 33 and 35 weeks of gestation and mothers of full-term infants. Holditch-Davis et al. [14] grouped mothers into five latent classes: low distress, moderate distress, high stress, high depressive and anxiety symptoms, and extreme distress. Mothers in the high depressive and anxiety symptoms and in the extreme distress groups had the sickest infants. In the extreme distress class, mothers had the highest levels of anxiety about their infants, and infants of these mothers had the greatest number of medical issues in the NICU, with the longest duration of respiratory assistance, and the highest rates of surgery, and infections.

It must be noted that stress alone is considered to have a negative influence on the quality of parental care offered to premature infants [8]. Parenting stress is clearly linked to adult functioning, quality of parent-child relationships, and child functioning [30]. Traumatic perinatal experience in mothers can be considered as a major factor influencing quality of mother-child interactions over time, with a potentially long-lasting effect of maternal emotional experience on the infant's interactional behavior [31]. Perceived parenting stress reflects the degree of stressfulness that parents experience through the demands of daily parenting tasks and has been shown to affect both parents and children's behavior [32]. High parenting stress and distress adversely affect early maternal sensitivity and parent-child relationships in the context of preterm birth. Mothers with a strong traumatic experience are more controlling and respond less frequently to infant signals [33]. Moreover, a parent who experiences a stressful event is less available and less sensitive to the needs of the child [34, 35]. The more anxious the parents, the less they touch and talk to their child before leaving the hospital [23]. Finally, maternal depressive symptoms are positively correlated to less affectionate touch at 3 months of age [6].

In sum, how trauma linked to premature birth can interfere with interactive parental behavior is complex and not totally elucidated [36]. Caring for a premature infant requires additional efforts in order to cope with the infant's difficulties and immaturities, thus heightening risk for both mother and infant emotional development.

7.1.3 Are Preterm Infants Already Equipped to Interact with Parents?

The directly observable behavioral interactions between mothers and babies call upon various registers, such as the kinetic, olfactory, vocal, and visual modalities. Preterm infants are a heterogeneous group. They vary considerably due to major differences in the conditions of their birth (weight, GA, and the existence of clinical complications) [1]. Overall, it is the neurobehavioral immaturity of prematurely born infants that impacts early socio-emotional life the most [36]. Adaptive behavior in premature babies is much more disorganized than in full-term infants [37].

It is thus more difficult for a preterm infant to reach a stable calm and alert state. Therefore periods of emotionally positive interaction are less frequent, less lasting, and more difficult to set up [38]. Preterm infants' medical condition may be unstable, their behavioral states therefore less predictable, and their sleep patterns disorganized [39]. In addition, when the baby is awake, he/she tends to be hypervigilant [27]. This adds to instability by overwhelming the infant with stimuli he/she is unable to select and filter for salient information. The hypervigilance state entails fatigue in the premature infant [40, 41] which in turn impedes emotionally positive communication.

In fact, stress responses are specifically altered during the neonatal period in premature infants. The hypothalamic-pituitary-adrenal (HPA) axis, which regulates cortisol production and the body's response to stress, displays decreased HPA regulation reflected by lower basal cortisol levels between birth and 3 months of age [42]. Absolute cortisol levels are significantly lower in preterm infants than in their full-term counterparts. This decrease seen during the neonatal period may persist into early infancy [43]. The cortisol difference between preterm and full-term infants is reflected in delayed maturation of areas involved in learning. In fact, the decreased HPA axis regulation may be a protective factor for children born premature [44]. These authors compared preterm infants with high cortisol response to stressors to those who did not respond strongly to stress. Between the ages of 18 and 60 months, children who demonstrated the highest increase were reported to have greater problems with attention, emotional reactivity, anxiety, and depression than children who did not react as much to a potential stressor.

7.1.3.1 Sleep State

The respiratory sinus arrhythmia is an index of cardiac vagal tone. Doussard-Roosevelt, Porges, and McClenny [45] recorded active and quiet sleep and respiratory sinus arrhythmia (RSA) in 33, 34, and 35 GA VLBW preterm neonates. Lower baseline of RSA indicated a less functional autonomous nervous system. Higher-risk neonates spent more sleep session time in active sleep than healthier preterm neonates. Vagal maturation measured by age-related increases in the amplitude of RSA was associated with less active sleep overall. Cardiac vagal tone matures between 33 and 35 weeks GA. Those neonates exhibiting greater vagal maturation, operationally defined by an increase in the amplitude of RSA from 33 to 35 weeks, spent less time in active sleep averaged across sessions. Follow-up data of 30 of the neonates indicated that greater vagal maturation was associated with better mental processing and gross motor skills at 3 years. Vagal maturation during this critical period (33–35 weeks GA) is assumed to reflect maturation of the neural circuits monitoring and regulating heart rate via the vagal nerve. Vagal maturation is a reflection of neural integrity. The vagal system, monitored in this study via measurements of RSA, is involved in the regulation and coordination of sucking, swallowing, breathing, and vocalizing [46]. Measurement of vagal tone (via the RSA) is proposed as a method to assess, on an individual basis, both stress and vulnerability to stress. The vagal system is involved not only in the adjustment of behaviors in stressful situations but also in the formation of social bonds such as attention, orientation, and maintaining a calm and attentive state of alertness [27]. Monitoring the vagal system may provide an important assessment window to the clinical status and developmental outcome of the high-risk infant [47].

7.1.3.2 Self-Regulation

The premature baby struggles to attain the physiological and behavioral regulation capabilities that enable active involvement with the partners in an emotional social context [27]. Due to their neurological immaturity, preterm infants do not give clear signals when they need to pause or when they feel there is too much or not enough stimulation, thus decreasing their own social responsiveness to others [48]. Preterm infants are less attentive and alert than full-term ones and show more difficulties in providing well-defined cues to their caregiver [49]. Therefore, high-risk premature infants with lower autonomic maturity are less able to elicit maternal engagement [6]. They are described as less rewarding social partners, spending less time in alert states, and producing unclear and difficult to read signals [50]. Overstimulation and withdrawal behavior are very often observed. When overstimulated, the infant cannot reply to parental solicitations. The infant then disconnects from the interaction, and the risk of escalating stimulations in order to reengage heightens [20]. The premature infant is constantly confronted with demands that are too difficult to fulfill. When very prematurely born newborns were observed at 29–32 weeks GA during face-to-face encounters, their first response to simple forms of visual, auditory, and tactile stimulation was withdrawal. In fact, touch and vocal stimuli are strongly aversive and could be hypothesized to be related to a memory of negative intensive care incurred by the baby. “Shutting out stimulation” or “withdrawal” might be considered a manner for these born-too-early infants avoid to “distress” [50]. These moments of relational withdrawal are also accompanied by gaze avoidance.

At about 33–34 weeks GA, neonates begin to respond more discriminately to different forms of social stimulation. They open their eyes more, and attentive gaze increases. Nevertheless, the authors conclude that very immature premature newborn first need to master physiological and motor regulation in order to be able to engage with the external social environment. Interactions with people constitute genuine social experiences enabling the premature infant to manifest itself as an attentive partner to others [51]. The infant’s innate capacity for social engagement and self-regulation plays an essential role in these encounters [6]. Infants who are able to elicit maternal attention are more likely to spend more time interacting with parents.

7.1.3.3 Interactive Capacitites

Preterm infants in the NICU are not necessarily deprived of auditory stimulation [52]. However, sounds are not specifically directed to the infant, they occur randomly in the environment. Thus, the infant may have opportunities to develop basic auditory abilities through general auditory stimulation but not necessarily in an adapted manner that is related to specific vocal and language-processing skills [53]. The NICU has a high level of general noise, which in fact buffers the vast majority of human conversations, leaving the infant deprived of a meaningful language-enriched environment. Thus, preterm infants are missing crucial opportunity to process speech sounds as they would otherwise be able to in utero. Caskey, Stephens, Tucker, and Vohr [54] determined the sound environment of preterm infants cared for in a NICU at 32 and 36 weeks GA. They found that this sound environment was mostly composed of monitor and background noise. Infant exposure to language as a percentage of time was very small, between 2 and 5% of all auditory stimuli. Nevertheless, this percentage increased significantly between 32 and 36 weeks. It has been known that between 17 and 37 days of life, and with average gestational age of 28 weeks, premature babies respond attentively to certain social stimuli including the human voice [38]. In the Caskey et al. study, infant vocalizations (coos, babbles, squeals, or growls) were audible as early as 32 weeks and increased significantly by 36 weeks of GA. More interestingly, exposure to parental language was a significantly stronger predictor of infant vocalizations and conversational turns compared with language from other adults: the more parents talked to their preterm infant in the NICU, the greater the number of reciprocal vocalizations the infant produced. The number of preterm infant vocalizations increased as much as 129% in case of parental presence compared with only hospital nursing staff caring for the infant [55]. In a systematic review of parental vocal interventions, Filippa et al. [56] pointed out that recorded or live maternal voice has beneficial effects on preterm infants' general medical health involving higher levels of oxygenation, fewer critical respiratory events, and fewer episodes of bradycardia and apneas. In addition live addressed speech increases the proportion of quiet alert states [57]. Using a functional optical imaging technique, another study has shown that at 28- to 32-week GA, preterm infants discriminate the phoneme "ba" from the phoneme "ga" and a male voice from a female one [58]. All these results highlight the abilities of the preterm child to process linguistic information and, more generally, information related to communication.

The premature newborn can thus interact with its environment and extract invariants from it [41]. Its ability to associate events, to become habituated to external stimulation, and to discriminate between two stimuli proves that the preterm infant is not only receiving environmental input but also fully active in an interactive system. The premature baby has the sensorimotor capacity to extract regularities from the environment. Preterm infants are able to extract this regularity based on the coherence and redundancy of the sensory flows. It is therefore essential that the different sensory stimulations (smell, voice, kinesthetic contact, and visual stimulus) pertaining to the same event (e.g., his mother interacting with him) give the infant a coherent and multimodal sense of a unified interaction. Each of the different sensory canals must be synchronized with each other [59]. A stable and coherently structured interaction within a human setting offers the child a way to progressively understand his environment. As the search for contingency is a principle of infant behavior, the ability to formulate consistent responses, preferably by the primary caregivers, is a major asset [3].

To conclude on the interactive abilities of the preterm infant, one might first recall that it is more difficult for premature infants to interact with their parents from the very start [3]. Indeed, premature infants are exposed to multiple stressors inherent to the highly technological NICU, enduring 10–16 painful procedures a day as well as excessive noise, light, and handling. However, learning and memory already enable the very young infant to communicate and interact with the primary caregivers.

7.1.4 Are Parents Prepared to Understand or Respond to Their Infants' Signals?

The ability of parents to recognize and give meaning to their child's signals and to adapt their attitudes to their needs is of particular importance as it may compensate the influence of biological risk factors on the development of their prematurely born children [23, 31]. Parents of prematurely born infants find it difficult to interpret and adapt to the immature expressions of their infant. All mothers describe the feeling of being unprepared for the premature delivery and the sight of her baby in the NICU [25]. In turn, the infants' cues are more challenging for parents and harder to interpret [60]. The gap between normal parental expectations and infant expressive capacities needs to be reduced following the birth of a preterm child [61]. The absence of coordinated behaviors and clear cues leads to a difficulty for parents to understand and respond to their infant' needs [8]. Parents may feel that their medically fragile preterm infant is unavailable to them [25]. Maternal perceptions act as mediators between birth and bonding: the more the mother perceives her child to be difficult, the more difficult the bonding will be [62]. Full-term infants are perceived more positively by their mothers.

Parental psychological suffering can generate problematic parental representations of the child. In connection with these representations or with other sorts of beliefs, a priori and/or stereotyped representations, especially concerning the vulnerability of the child, can have an impact on the construction of a relationship with the child [27]. A higher prevalence of unrealistic fears for the infant's safety is in line with results showing more overprotection [2]. On the other hand, parents may tend to minimize the effects of prematurity. This defensive perception of their child will deprive them of a sufficiently attentive look and hinder their adaptation to the child [27].

Mothers often feel they do not understand their child, do not know how to help him, and suffer from seeing him so fragile. They may feel that the child is indifferent to their presence, sometimes even that he does not like them, and that he is more attached to nurses than to them. Sometimes, they may even avoid visiting their child at the NICU [31]. Many studies have shown how mother-preterm infant interactions differ from those with a term infant [2, 63, 64]. In interaction, not only do mothers look, smile, talk, and touch their children born prematurely less than mothers of children born at term, but they also appear less able to coordinate their responses with the brief moments of their infants' calm alert states [65]. Mothers were reported to be overstimulating, more active, and more intrusive compare with mothers of full-term infants [4]. Recently, these differences have been confirmed [66]. This high level of maternal stimulation could be seen as a way to compensate the infants' lack of reactivity. Intrusive mothers are described as being more insensitive to the signals of their children and in particular less respectful of the temporality of their answers [67]. Responses that are random, absent, chaotic, or inappropriate disrupt the interactive process. Contingent responses are vital for successful social events. Mutual gaze, gestures, body movement, and facial expression are key elements of interaction. Based on temporal pattern, predictable response, and reinforcement from their mothers, infants learn positive expressions of emotion [68]. Is this quality of infant-mother interactions available in the NICU?

Mothers of premature infants and premature infants themselves interact differently than full-term infants [28]. Crawford [69] and Greene, Fox, and Lewis [70] demonstrated that mothers of preterm infants exhibit more positive interaction, spend more time engaged in caretaking behaviors, and provide more stimulation to their infants during free play than mothers of full-term infants. They also tend to hold their infants more and demonstrate a higher frequency of affectionate behavior than mothers of full-term infants. Mothers of premature infants were found to be more active than mothers of full-term infants during feeding [71]. They are also more active in the relationship even without a response from their infant. They need to carry the major load of the interaction by vocalizing and smiling more and by trying to engage their infants, because infant levels of reactivity are still lower than full-term infants [68]. For example, the mother who provides a high level of stimulation to her premature infant might receive a lower response rating from the child. Nevertheless she would still meet the needs of her preterm infant more appropriately than one who does not stimulate enough [72]. They are more receptive to their child's signals.

In sum, the first moments of encounter with their premature infant, so small, ill, and apparently fragile, with so few means of communication and interaction, are more challenging for parents to respond to. Intuitive maternal competency represents an important prerequisite for attachment and subsequent bonding. It is essential that parents recognize, understand, and respond to their infant's signs as early as possible [25].

7.1.5 Sensitive Period

Studies on human populations suggest there is a sensitive period shortly after birth which appears to have long-lasting effects on maternal attachment and which may ultimately affect the development of the child [73]. A maternal sensitive period is a period after delivery when mothers form a special attachment to their infant based on emotional reaction to their states and behavior. This period of sensitivity usually begins within the first 12h after delivery. In VLBW preterm infants, close physical contact between mother and child is not usually possible in the hours or days following birth. Mehler et al. [74] investigated the existence of a sensitive period in the case of VLBW preterm infants. They found that infants who had been seen by their mothers within 3 h after birth showed more secure attachment patterns at the age of 12 to 18 months corrected age, than infants whose mothers only visited NICU on the second day of life. Moreover, mothers who had seen and touched their baby within 3 h after birth had a higher rate of secure attachment patterns than those who had only seen them. This finding supports the hypothesis that the first hours after birth are indeed a "sensitive period" for the development of attachment behavior [74]. Moreover, this "sensitive period" has an effect not only on maternal bonding but also on the development of paternal bonding [6].

7.1.6 Parental Closeness

Philosophical, psychological, and neuroscientific arguments justify the presence of the family in the neonatal intensive care unit [75]. A growing body of evidence suggests several benefits of parent-infant closeness during hospital care [1]. Affectionate involvement with the preterm infant can be expressed through close body contact and affectionate gestures such as caresses, kisses, light tapping, cuddling, and other non-utilitarian physical contact [9]. The role of immediate and sustained mother-child contacts after birth is essential. For example, preterm infants held by their mothers during a painful intervention exhibited less crying and grimacing than a control group of infants who were swaddled in the crib for the same procedure [76]. More prolonged and frequent presence of parents in the NICU is associated with less stress and greater neurobehavioral stability in preterm infants [77, 78]. Parenting behavior is believed to be an important mediator between biological risk and developmental outcome. Greater visitation and higher holding frequencies are associated with motor patterns involving better quality of movement, less hypertonia, and more hypotonia [78]. Infants who are visited and held more frequently are calmer, more relaxed, content, and have more fluid body movements. Infant holding is thus associated with less infant stress. Holding is also associated with less excitability, which can help the infant in maintaining states that facilitate movement and interaction. Frequent visits were associated with lower levels of arousal which implies that an infant is calmer when being handled [79]. Infants with low excitability scores are less irritable and have fewer state changes and startles. Moreover, frequency of the mother's visits to the NICU was associated with long-term behavioral and emotional developmental outcomes for the child [80]. The impact of the mother's visit was stronger than the impact of gestational age, birth weight, or the medical risks of the infant.

To summarize, during sensitive periods, certain skills, entailing even small inputs, have a major effect [39]. Parent closeness is essential and has a major impact on infant development. Skin-to-skin contact and kangaroo care are two excellent examples of parent closeness proposed in the NICU (see Sect. 7.3).

7.2 Attachment

Researchers study attachment by observing infants' reaction to stress in the strange situation paradigm, where the stressful trigger is the departure of the mother and the arrival of an unfamiliar person. Being alone and faced with an unknown person triggers attachment behavior and puts an end to exploration behavior. The mother's return constitutes the signal for extinction of the attachment behavior. With this paradigm, researchers have been able to assess the child's reactions at the time of the mother's departure, the stranger's arrival, and the mother's return enabling a classification of attachment styles into three categories: secure, insecure, and disorganized.

7.2.1 Secure Attachment

Secure attachment is the optimal attachment style. Maternal sensitivity during the first year of life is a strong predictor of secure attachment [81]. Maternal sensitivity and responsiveness are of particular importance for preterm infants to develop a secure attachment and may be considered as protective for the child's development [74]. Mothers of children who develop a secure attachment pattern have higher sensitivity scores than the mothers of insecure children [67]. Secure attachment of preterm infants to responsive mothers reduces behavioral disorders in later life. Secure mothers seem capable of increasing their sensitivity when forced to deal with a problematic preterm infant [36]. Secure mothers, in comparison with insecure ones, are significantly more sensitive to their infants. Coppola and her colleagues found that sensitivity of secure mothers increases from full-term to premature birth conditions. Sensitivity is important but not sufficient to explain the quality of attachment. Responsiveness and parent-infant synchrony can also explain attachment quality.

7.2.1.1 Maternal Sensitivity

Maternal sensitivity is the ability of the mother to recognize, interpret, and respond promptly and appropriately to the needs and demands of the child [82]. Sensitive mothers also know how to respond to the gradual reciprocity in social interaction and to the infant's growing initiative [62]. Sensitive mothers are mothers who provide appropriate feedback to the infant, though it does not always mean giving what the child seems to want [82]. The mother can offer an acceptable alternative. The adequacy of the response thus depends, among other factors, on the age of the child. Hence, a sensitive behavior is one that adapts to the resources and age of the child [67]. Sensitive caregiving is a significant buffer to hyperreactivity of the stress response, whereas an insensitive caregiver can be a significant source of stress [8]. When mothers are quick to respond to their children with smiles, there is an increase in how quickly children are able to initiate interactions later on [83]. Moreover, mothers who are sensitive to their children's interests and needs and engage in rich language interactions are providing a learning environment for children to develop their language competency [84]. The same researchers found that consistent maternal sensitivity across time was particularly important for cognitive and social development in preterm-born infants. Children born very preterm, who are at high medical risk, may particularly benefit from parenting that is sensitive and non-intrusive in timing and nature [66]. Maternal sensitivity has also been associated with children's early regulatory abilities in preterm populations [85]. Maternal sensitivity in early dyadic interactions has been studied because of its potential long-lasting impact on child development [20]. It has been shown in the literature that maternal sensitivity, especially during the first year of life, is the most important predictor of attachment security [67].

7.2.1.2 Infant Responsiveness

Maternal involvement and infant responsiveness appear to be the best predictors of infant cognitive development, which underscores the importance of bi-directionality in infant development [86]. Responsiveness is the first form of infant sociability. Sociability is an important link mediating between maternal behavior and infant cognitive status. Infant sociability and responsiveness might be important factors mediating the link between early caregiving and cognitive outcome [86]. Parent's responsiveness is also important. Maternal responsiveness plays an important role in developing secure attachment and effective bonding patterns between mother and infant [87]. More than full-term infants, preterm infants seem to stimulate the kind of attentive and warm parenting often described as "responsive"[84]. Researchers hypothesize that the quality of parental responsiveness comes to effectively support preterm infants' difficulties with regulation and attention. That is, they bring about parenting skills that more stable newborns call upon less frequently.

7.2.1.3 Parent-Infant Synchrony

The synchrony of parent-infant interactions is related to the timeliness of infants' and parents' responses to each other. Synchrony refers to individuals' temporal coordination during social interactions. According to Delaherche et al. [88], synchrony is the dynamic and reciprocal adaptation of the temporal structure of behaviors between interactive partners. In a systematic review of synchrony during mother-child interactions, Leclère et al. [89] report the most common terms relating to synchrony as being mutuality, reciprocity, harmonious interaction, turn-taking, and shared affect. Synchrony may occur across different sensory modalities as it involves a coordination of multiple coupled behaviors. By definition, for each behavior produced by one partner, there is a limited window of time for the other partner to produce a coordinated behavior [88]. Parent-infant synchrony develops through early childhood, from biological rhythms during pregnancy to later symbolic exchanges involving language [90]. With immature infants, synchrony depends on the parent having a good understanding of how to effectively communicate with and respond to his or her child [13]. During face-to-face interactions, the mother assists the infant by adjusting her behavior to the infant's abilities, thus fostering similar inner psychological states between herself and the infant [8]. Synchronous interactions, in which both mothers and infants are mutually responsive, are both important for developing attachment and particularly challenging for preterm infants [83]. Premature birth interferes with the emergence of parent-infant synchrony [6]. The dyadic system between parents and preterm infants is less synchronous and mutually adaptive [47]. Premature infants are most dependent on mutual regulation for their social development. Yet, they have great difficulty eliciting synchronous parenting. Feldman and Eidelman [6] showed that the interactions of fathers and mothers with their premature 3-month-old child were less synchronous than in dyads with a full-term child. The authors associated theses less synchronous behaviors with an immaturity of the vagal system. Feldman [47] found that neonatal vagal tone predicts the degree of mother-infant synchrony at 3 months corrected age. She also points to the role of neonatal physiological regulation in the emergence of parent-infant synchrony. Feldman and Eidelman [6] observed infant-mother and infant-father synchrony, as well as maternal and paternal affectionate touch at 3 months corrected age for premature and full-term infants. At this age, lower levels of mother-infant and father-infant gaze synchrony were observed between parents and preterm infants, but no differences emerged in the mothers' or the fathers' affectionate touch. Preterm infants were alert for only a small percentage of the interaction's duration (only 10%); however, mothers responded to infant alertness only one-third of that time. Mothers of preterm infants were less able to grasp the rare opportunities of social readiness in their child and to respond with synchronized behavior. Moreover, these researchers showed that the coordination of maternal behavior with infant alertness is longitudinally related to the formation of a mutually regulated parent-infant dialogue at 3 months of age.

To conclude on parent-infant synchrony, during these coordinated exchanges with their parents, premature infants are sensitized to micro-levels of changes in facial signals, including direction of gaze, tone of voice, and changes in muscle tone. These cues constitute opportunities for infants to read and respond in synchrony to their parents during social exchanges. Parent-child synchrony has a strong positive influence on cognitive development and social-emotional competence at 24 months of age [13]. If parents are able to respond in sync with their preterm infant's behaviors, they may feel more confident about their role as the central figures in their child's cognitive, social, and emotional development.

7.2.2 Intrusiveness/Insecure Attachment

Some researchers have described mothers of premature infants as less sensitive when interacting with their infant [33, 71]. Fuertes, Faria, Soares, and Crittenden [91] found that only 33% of premature infants were securely attached. The authors observed that this result was due to the significant lack of maternal sensitivity in mothers of premature infants. Maternal unresponsiveness is related to later problems in mother-child interactions with the mother expecting the child to initiate interactions [92]. Moreover, mothers who are not responsive can also have low expectations of their children, which may limit their language-based interactions with them, and ignore their children's' expressions of important needs. These types of interactions can in turn impact the development of competence and skill for these children [84]. Parents of children born extremely preterm appear less sensitive to their children's cues and more intrusive during problem solving or play interactions than parents of full-term children [11, 85]. Mothers of infants born very preterm showed more intrusiveness and difficulty scaffolding as well as less sensitivity than mothers of term infants. The interactive behavior of these mothers is often characterized by excessive stimulation and intrusiveness, hence, inadequate and insensitive, because it induces more gaze avoidance and less attention on the part of the preterm infant [71]. Nevertheless the results of Wijnroks's study [86] suggested there is no indication that the pattern of increased maternal activity (and thus intrusiveness) impedes the development of cognitive competence and attention in preterm infants. It is only maternal involvement at 6 months (e.g., active encouragement and amount of verbal stimulation) that contributes to cognitive outcome at age two. These authors concluded that the 6 first months of life might be of special importance for the infant's later cognitive development, in particular for the acquisition of language.

Insecure attachment is observed when inadequate responses are provided to the child's expression of needs despite a general protective stance. The child then develops adaptation strategies that will either be avoidance or resistance. The proportion of insecure attachment was found to be higher in a premature infant population than in full-term infant population: 47 percent of preterm infants show an insecure pattern at 12 months, whereas the proportion is around 33% in full-term samples [20]. Results showed a significant correlation between the severity of perinatal problems and the risk of insecure attachment measured at 12 months. More specifically, Laganiére et al. [62] showed high-risk preterm infants have more insecure attachment than full-term infants. Low-risk premature infants have an intermediate level of insecure attachment, between full-term and high-risk preterm infants' levels. Severity of neonatal complications increases the likelihood of developing insecure attachment. These results underline the importance of medical-biological factors. The researchers suggest that children develop a low sense of control over their environment and are less likely to experience active safety-seeking behaviors in anxiety-provoking situations. In their first year of life, preterm infants live in a context that is less conducive to secure attachment relationship than children born at term [62]. These consequences may be mediated by other factors such as infant temperament, coping behavior, and maternal sensitivity [93]. In a systematic review of the literature on early mother-infant relationships in preterm populations, Korja et al. [2] indicated that the prevalence of insecure attachment patterns is not higher in preterm than in full-term infants assessed at 1 year. Thus preterm birth does not have a negative impact on the quality of attachment representations [94].

7.2.3 Disorganized Attachment

The disorganized attachment style was identified by Main [95] in addition to secure and insecure attachment styles. Children with disorganized attachment demonstrate contradictory behavioral sequences, which gives the impression of disorganized strategies or behaviors. The attachment figure is both a source of security and a source of fear. It does not protect or seem to protect, and it arouses fear in the child. Disorganized attachment can be described as the breakdown of an otherwise consistent and organized strategy of emotion regulation [48]. Disorganized infant attachment is not just the consequence of parental insentivity. Wolke, Eryigit-Madzwamuse, and Gutbrod [96] investigated the prevalence and etiology of attachment insecurity and disorganization in very preterm infants. The authors found that very preterm infants were not more insecurely attached than their full-term counterparts. However, very preterm infants were found to have disorganized attachment more often than full-term infants. Neurological impairment is indicated by distress crying at 3 months and developmental delay at 18 months, which are predictors of disorganized attachment. The risk of disorganized attachment appears to be one of a range of adverse outcomes associated with preterm birth and neurodevelopmental problems despite sensitive parenting [96].

7.3 NICU Interventions Aimed at Supporting or Restoring Optimal Parent-Preterm Infant Relationships

The physical and social characteristics of the NICU environment have a critical influence on neurodevelopmental outcomes in premature infants [8]. The effects of the characteristic NICU environment on the quality of parent-infant interaction may be an important factor in infant development. There is a growing consensus that supporting early parent-infant relationship in the NICU is crucial [97]. The effects of the NICU environment are linked to epigenetic factors that influence neural development [1, 98]. The importance of parental involvement in neonatal services, and especially in NICUs, is now well established. All staff agree that providing support for the developing infant-parent attachment relationship in the NICU is important [60]. Nowadays, NICU environments have undergone some major changes (e.g., architectural structure and organizational culture), and parents are now more actively involved in the daily care for their infant than ever before. Accordingly, the degree of proximity between parents and premature infants has improved [94]. Parents are increasingly acknowledged as primary caregivers for their preterm infant [98]. Most NICUs try to facilitate early parent-infant attachment and encourage parents to stay with their infants as much as possible [99]. NICU proposals may be varied but aim at supporting early parent-preterm infant closeness during hospital care, through dispositions such as architectural structure, organizational care involving parents (NIDCAP), direct contact (skin-to-skin, kangaroo care), breastfeeding, vocal exchange, massage, observation and interpretation of the behavior of preterm infants.

7.3.1 Architectural Structure

In order to encourage parents to visit their preterm infants, the single-family room model is growing in popularity with the provision of comfortable armchairs and beds. Many NICUs enable the whole family to be together round-the-clock, as much as possible. Parents who can stay in parent rooms at the units spend more time close to their infant and are more involved in their infant's care than parents who stay at family hotels, at home, or in a separate maternity ward [100]. Baylis et al. [10] observed parental bonding with preterm babies in two different NICU contexts, one which included an adult bed and privacy screens to allow parents to stay with their infants round-the-clock and the other which included only an armchair at every care space, making it uncomfortable for a parent to be present round-the-clock. The authors concluded that parents who had the opportunity to sleep in the NICU and to participate in their infants' care without unjustified limitations were more present and involved in their infant's care. Parents' round-the-clock presence in the NICU promotes parent-infant closeness, which helps parents to become more sensitive and to respond in synchrony to the infant's behavioral signals (see Sects. 7.1.6 and 7.2.1.3).

Open-bay units with three preterm infants are often present in NICUs. Environmental adaptations have been undertaken in order to decrease ambient noise (silent alarms, sound absorbing materials, modified equipment, increased staff awareness) and generate cyclical lighting. As mentioned earlier (Sect. 7.1.3), the incubator walls isolate the infant from human speech sounds. NICU architecture should encourage parents to actively engage with talk to, read to, or sing to their infants during visitation time (see Sect. 7.3.6).

7.3.2 Organizational Culture of the NICU

NICU practices try to moderate the effect of the environment, minimizing painful and stressful procedures, reducing parent-infant separation, and facilitating parent-infant closeness and interaction [77]. The authors compared 25 NICUs as a function of 2 indices: one which measured parent involvement in the care of their infant and in developmentally oriented care interventions and another which measured the procedures used for reducing infant pain. In a NICU with a high level of developmental care practice, parents were allowed to spend the night in the unit whenever they chose to, even when the infant's condition was critical. They were encouraged to hold their infant and to practice kangaroo care, both of which they did more of the time than in a NICU with a low level of developmental care practice. Infants from units with a high level of developmental care practice had better attention and self-regulation skills, were less excitable, were less hypotonic, and less stressed, suggesting that they had greater physiologic and behavioral stability than infants from units with a low level of developmental care practice. Thus, environmental factors such as developmental care and pain control have beneficial effects on infant neurodevelopment [77]. Epigenetic variations might be used to document the biological correlates of the beneficial effects of developmental care practices [1].

7.3.3 NIDCAP

The Newborn Individualized Developmental Care Assessment Program (NIDCAP) is an individualized program of integrated, early developmental care centered on the child and his/her family [101]. NIDCAP is based on four assumptions: (1) Detailed observations of infant behavior during daily interactive care (before, during, and after). (2) Healthy parents are the best people to help the child develop as harmoniously as possible. (3) The healthcare team is trained to integrate behavioral signals into the overall organization of medical and nursing care and to change its vision of care through regular reflective practice. (4) Comprehensive care will lead to the improvement of long-term child outcome, parent well-being and competencies, and to positive orientation in staff and personal development. NIDCAP promotes preterm infant interaction with parents, prevents infant stress, pain, over-stimulation and isolation while supporting goal orientation, competence and self-regulation [102]. The dialogue with the infant and individualization of care is equally relevant and vital, if the infant is supported by mechanical technology and/or simultaneously held by the parent in kangaroo position (see section just below).

The beneficial effects of NIDCAP have been shown in terms of shorter intensive care and overall hospital stay, greater weight gain, and improved behavioral outcomes that persist beyond infancy [103]. Studies have also documented that the NIDCAP approach enhances neurodevelopment, functional competence, and life quality for preterm infants at 1-week and 9-month CA [104]. NIDCAP intervention also has lasting beneficial effects on brain function at 8 years of age [105].

7.3.4 Skin-to-Skin/Kangaroo Care

Kangaroo mother care (KMC) consists of early, prolonged skin-to-skin care (SSC), for as long and as often as circumstances permit. Facilitating early skin-to-skin contact is one way to promote closeness and early parent-infant attachment. The core component is skin-to-skin contact. There is a potential for extended use of skin-to-skin care to reduce separation between infant and parents. Physical closeness with the baby is a major strategy though which the mother gains intimate knowledge about her infant and is able to demonstrate parental confidence to the NICU [106]. Being able to see, hold, and interact with her infant in the NICU contributes to the development of a mother's sense of herself as mother [10]. KMC is often associated with the promotion of breastfeeding (see next section). NICU staff have a crucial role to play in promoting and assisting parents in setting up SSC with their infant as soon as possible (e.g., early after birth) even in environments with high-tech incubator care [107]. The authors describe initiation and extent of parents' application of skin-to-skin care with their preterm infant at two Swedish neonatal intensive care units. The authors observed that the earlier the SSC was initiated after birth, the more skin-to-skin contact the infant received each day of its hospital stay. Moreover, infants whose first experience of SSC was with their father had a longer total duration of SSC during their hospital stay than infants who started SSC with their mother, due to the fact that the mother's medical care prevented her from doing SSC right after birth. This confirms that, during sensitive periods in the maturation of certain skills, even small inputs can have a major effect [39]. At discharge, mothers who provided kangaroo care believed that they had helped the baby while in the hospital more so than their counterparts who did not provide kangaroo care [64]. Facilitation of early skin-to-skin contact in the first hours after birth could contribute to a more gentle adjustment to extrauterine life with improved physiological stability, i.e., less invasive ways in surfactant administration, avoidance of early mechanical ventilation, and maintenance of adequate body temperature [98]. These effects persist in the long term. By 10 years of age, premature infants who received SSC immediately after birth showed more mature autonomic functioning, organized sleep, attenuated stress response, better cognitive control, and more reciprocal mother-child relationship [39]. Skin-to-skin contact has been shown to reduce maternal depression while increasing maternal sensitivity [108]. During traditional skin-to-skin contact, face-to-face gaze is impossible due to vertical infant positioning. Recently, Buil et al. [109] proposed a kangaroo "supported diagonal flexion" (SDF) positioning in order to enhance early communication (e.g., eye-to-eye contact as well as maternal vocalization, smiles, and gentle stroking) during mother-infant skin-to-skin contact.

In summary, research has demonstrated that skin-to-skin contact applied during this sensitive period is safe and should be viewed as a means of humanizing the process of giving birth in a context of prematurity.

7.3.5 Breastfeeding

Mother-infant interaction has been described as an important component during breastfeeding [12]. Breastfeeding promotes biological caregiving predispositions [9]. It also stimulates the secretion of oxytocin, which is very important for the formation of the attachment bonds. Moreover, breastfeeding is known for its nutritional, immunological, and cognitive benefits. Maternal sensitivity during infant feeding experience was positively related to mutual parent-child enjoyment [83]. These authors found that early risk factors, such as days spent on a ventilator, were positively related to maternal perception of worry and less maternal sensitivity during feeding. Moreover, mothers of very low birth weight preterm infants respond with less sensitivity than mothers with older gestational age infants during breastfeeding. Many mothers are focused on the feeding task and may miss infant communicative behaviors for engagement. Reyna et al. [110] studied maternal-infant synchrony during feeding interaction between a mother and her preterm infant and the change in these communicative behaviors over time. At the beginning, the mother considered breastfeeding as a way of being close to the infant with reciprocal pleasure, comfort, and attachment. Then, breastfeeding became a complex process, with great concern, for example, for whether the infant consumed enough milk. Thereafter breastfeeding became a privileged form of interaction where both the mother and the infant were active. When the mother succeeded in making the infant breastfeed exclusively, she felt secure and was proud of being such a good mother [110]. To conclude, it is important to support parents as interpreters of their premature infants' communicative behavior during feeding. It could help parents to be sensitive and feel more comfortable communicating with their infants during feeding.

7.3.6 Vocal Exchanges

Compared to the fetus of the same gestational age, there is a dearth of language experience for preterm infants in incubators during a critical time in their early development (see Sect. 7.1.3). Caskey et al. [54] have shown that the more the preterm is exposed to adult language in the NICU, the greater the number of reciprocal vocalizations that occur between parents and infants. These findings support the powerful effects of parent visiting in the NICU on the emergence of early vocalizations among preterm infants. Exposure to human speech during NICU stay, especially the mother's voice, is crucial for initial wiring of the brain for language acquisition [52]. These authors showed that recorded maternal sounds, as a supplement to parental visits, provide expanding opportunities for maternal speech exposure even when the mother is not physically present. Live vocal intervention seemed to be less studied than recorded interventions [56]. Yet recorded speech or songs are not contingent on the infant's responses and solicitations. Moreover, infants who benefit from contingent singing, based on such infant-inclusive singing style as lullaby and playsong, are better able to maintain self-regulation during social interaction with an adult: they are less irritable, cry less, and are more positive in their response to adult handling [111]. Music Therapy (MT) is highly appropriate and may promote the social and neurological development of preterm infants. Moreover, in a systematical review and meta-analysis on the effect of MT on preterm infants and their parents during NICU hospitalization, Bieleninik, Ghetti, and Gold [112] observed an important favorable effect of music therapy on infant respiratory rate and maternal anxiety. The effects are always better when it's a kin song sung by parents: there is a decrease in parental stress between before and after the lullaby. Similarly, there is an increase in the amount of active sleep, an increase in nutritional sucking, and an increase in calories intake between before and after the lullaby. There is also a decrease in heart rate during the lullaby, supporting the soothing influence of the voice, especially when the lullaby is sung by a parent. Encouraging parents to sing for their preterm infants and offering them an environment supportive of what they want to sing is another proposal for NICUs to promote a closer parent-infant relationship.

7.3.7 Massage

Preterm infants are prematurely deprived of the cutaneous stimulation provided during intrauterine development and of the continuous postnatal contact with their parents [113]. At the Touch Research Institute in Miami (Florida), T. Field and her colleagues have developed a preterm infant massage program. Although preterm infants may seem to be particularly fragile, some pressure is needed for the massage to be effective. In most of Field's studies, massage periods were 15 min long with moderate pressure (moving over skin) and occurred three times per day until hospital discharge [114]. Studies on massage therapy in many parts of the word [115] document greater weight gain in preterm newborns compared to standard care. Data also show increased vagal activity and gastric activity, which could lead to more efficient food absorption and increased weight gain [116]. During behavioral observations that followed the massage, preterm infants showed significantly less active sleep, fussing, crying, movement, and stress behavior (hiccupping) [117]. The authors instructed first-child parents how to massage. VLBW premature infants who received maternal massage had higher probability of earlier hospital discharge than those who did not receive the intervention. The maternal tactile-kinesthetic stimulation might have enabled an early positive mother-infant interaction [118].

Massage with Auditory, Tactile, Visual, and Vestibular stimulation (ATVV) is a form of massage that involves moderate stroking, eye contact with, talking to, and rocking the infant [119]. Mothers taught to provide the ATVV intervention for their infants exhibited more positive interactive behaviors than control mothers [120]. Mothers using the ATVV intervention reported significantly higher ratings for learning new ways to stimulate and teach their babies [64]. The ATVV intervention provided a method by which mothers could explore and become familiar with their infants. Álvarez et al. [113] performed a systematic review on therapeutic massage to preterm neonates during their stay in the NICU. It suggests that a clear benefit is obtained from the administration of massage therapy in hospitalized preterm infants, a finding that should encourage the more generalized use of massage in NICUs.

7.3.8 Parents Coaching to Observe and Interpret the Behavior of Their Preterm Infant

Early interventions focusing on the premature baby and its specific needs are useful. Careful observation of the baby during the hospital stay makes it possible for parents to better understand and adapt to the characteristics of their child, thus leading to a more flexible and affective parental response as the child develops [27].

Creating Opportunities for Parent Empowerment (COPE) is an educational-behavioral intervention program. Parents receive information and behavioral activities about the appearance and behavioral characteristics of preterm infants and how best to parent them. Intervention with parents of premature infants that starts early during the NICU stay results in less maternal stress, more positive parent-infant interactions during the hospital stay, leading to earlier hospital discharge, and less maternal anxiety and depressive symptoms after hospitalization [121]. Mothers and fathers who participated in the COPE program reported stronger beliefs in their ability to understand their preterm infants' behaviors and cues. Parents interacted with their preterm infants in a more sensitive manner than those in the comparison group (without Cope intervention).

Other special training programs have been developed to enable parents to recognize, understand, and respond to their infant's signs as early as possible [3]. Mothers who participated in the training program were more likely to keep the appropriate distance to their child and to use an adjusted tone of voice with them than mothers who had not participated in the training program. Benzies, Magill-Evans, Hayden, and Ballantyne [122] proposed an educational program that includes information about infant growth and development, demonstrations of infant behavior and active involvement of the parent in interaction with the infant, and then discussion with feedback from a professional. Parents learned to increase their recognition of the infant's subtle signs. They were also receptive to the infant's limited capacity to respond to stress. Parental educational intervention may increase parental knowledge and skill in caring for preterm infants and subsequently increase parenting self-efficacy and decrease stress.

These diverse programs have in common that they are implemented just after preterm birth and very early on during the NICU stay and that they are centered on the parent-child dyad.

7.4 Conclusion

Preterm birth is a high-risk situation for parent-child interaction. Any setup that supports positive and well-adapted interactions as often as possible should be promoted by healthcare professionals, institutions, and politicians. This entails providing help with decoding and progressive day-to-day tailoring of care including infant-specific characteristics and parental emotional responses. Therapeutic "education" of the needs of high-risk infants and their often emotionally stressed parents should be made highly and easily accessible.

References

1. Montirosso R, Provenzi L (2015) Implications of epigenetics and stress regulation on research and developmental care of preterm infants. J Obstet Gynecol Neonatal Nurs 44(2):174–182. https://doi.org/10.1111/1552-6909.12559
2. Korja R, Latva R, Lehtonen L (2012) The effects of preterm birth on mother-infant interaction and attachment during the infant's first two years. Acta Obstet Gynecol Scand 91(2):164–173. https://doi.org/10.1111/j.1600-0412.2011.01304.x
3. Steinhardt A, Hinner P, Kühn T, Roehr CC, Rüdiger M, Reichert J (2015) Influences of a dedicated parental training program on parent-child interaction in preterm infants. Early Hum Dev 91(3):205–210. https://doi.org/10.1016/j.earlhumdev.2015.01.012
4. Bekhechi-Mistycki V, Guedeney N (2008) Evaluation des représentations maternelles de la protection dans la grande prématurité. Dev Dent 20(1):5–33. https://doi.org/10.3917/dev.081.0005
5. Alvarez-Garcia A, Fornieles-Deu A, Costas-Moragas C, Botet-Mussons F (2014) Maturational changes associated with neonatal stress in preterm infants hospitalised in the NICU. J Reprod Infant Psychol 32(4):412–422. https://doi.org/10.1080/02646838.2014.937411
6. Feldman R, Eidelman A (2007) Maternal postpartum behavior and the emergence of infant–mother and infant–father synchrony in preterm and full-term infants: the role of neonatal vagal tone. Dev Psychobiol 49:290–302. https://doi.org/10.1002/dev
7. Vigod SN, Villegas L, Dennis C-L, Ross LE (2010) Prevalence and risk factors for postpartum depression among women with preterm and low-birth-weight infants: a systematic review. BJOG 117(5):540–550. https://doi.org/10.1111/j.1471-0528.2009.02493.x
8. Weber AM, Harrison TM, Steward DK (2012) Schore's regulation theory: maternal–infant interaction in the NICU as a mechanism for reducing the effects of allostatic load on neurodevelopment in premature infants. Biol Res Nurs 14(4):375–386. https://doi.org/10.1177/1099800412453760
9. Guédeney N, Beckechi V, Mintz A-S, Saive AL (2012) L'implication des parents en néonatologie et le processus de caregiving. Dev Dent 24(1):9–34. https://doi.org/10.3917/dev.121.0009
10. Baylis R, Ewald U, Gradin M, Hedberg Nyqvist K, Rubertsson C, Thernström Blomqvist Y (2014) First-time events between parents and preterm infants are affected by the designs and routines of neonatal intensive care units. Acta Paediatr:1045–1052. https://doi.org/10.1111/apa.12719
11. Borghini A, Pierrehumert B, Miljkovitch R, Muller-Nix C, Forcada-Guex M, Ansermet F (2006) Mother's attachement representations of their premature infant at 6 and 18 months after birth. Infant Ment Health J 27(5):494–508. https://doi.org/10.1002/imhj

12. Flacking R, Ewald U, Nyqvist KH, Starrin B (2006) Trustful bonds: a key to "becoming a mother" and to reciprocal breastfeeding. Stories of mothers of very preterm infants at a neonatal unit. Soc Sci Med 62(1):70–80. https://doi.org/10.1016/j.socscimed.2005.05.026
13. Treyvaud K, Anderson VA, Howard K, Bear M, Hunt RW, Doyle LW, Anderson, J P (2009) Parenting behavior is associated with the early neurobehavioral development of very preterm children. Pediatrics 123(2):555–561. https://doi.org/10.1542/peds.2008-0477
14. Holditch-Davis D, Santos H, Levy J, White-Traut R, O'Shea TM, Geraldo V, David R (2015) Patterns of psychological distress in mothers of preterm infants. Infant Behav Dev 41:154–163. https://doi.org/10.1016/j.infbeh.2015.10.004
15. Mellier D (2017) L'enfant prématuré: développement et soins psychologiques. In: Miljkovitch R, Morange-Majoux F, Sander E (eds) Traité de psychologie du développement. Masson, Paris, pp 1–36
16. Obeidat H, Bond E, Callister LC (2009) The parental experience of having an infant in the newborn intensive care unit. J Perinat Educ 18(3):23–29. https://doi.org/10.1624/105812409X461199
17. Miles MS, Burchinal P, Holditch-Davis D, Brunssen S, Wilson SM (2002) Perceptions of stress, worry, and support in black and white mothers of hospitalized, medically fragile infants. J Pediatr Nurs 17(2):82–88. https://doi.org/10.1053/jpdn.2002.124125
18. Schappin R, Wijnroks L, Uniken Venema MMAT, Jongmans MJ (2013) Rethinking stress in parents of preterm infants: a meta-analysis. PLoS One 8(2):1–19. https://doi.org/10.1371/journal.pone.0054992
19. Singer LT, Salvator A, Shenyang G, Collin M, Lilien L, Baley J (1999) Maternal psychological distress and parenting stress after the birth of a very low-birth-weight infant. J Am Med Assoc 281(9):799–805
20. Udry-Jorgensen L, Pierrehumbert B, Borghini A, Ansermet F, Muller-Nix C (2011) Quality of attachment, perinatal risk, and mother-infant interaction in high-risk premature sample. Infant Ment Health J 32(3):305–318. https://doi.org/10.1002/imhj
21. Ionio C, Colombo C, Brazzoduro V, Mascheroni E, Confalonieri E, Castoldi F, Lista G (2016) Mothers and fathers in nicu: the impact of preterm birth on parental distress. Eur J Psychol 12(4):604–621. https://doi.org/10.5964/ejop.v12i4.1093
22. Chertok IRA, McCrone S, Parker D, Leslie N (2014) Review of interventions to reduce stress among mothers of infants in the NICU. Adv Neonatal Care 14(1):30–37. https://doi.org/10.1097/ANC.0000000000000044
23. Zelkowitz P, Bardin C, Papageorgiou A (2007) Anxiety affects the relationship between parents and their very low birth weight infants. Infant Ment Health J 28(3):296–313. https://doi.org/10.1002/imhj
24. Meijssen D, Wolf MJ, van Bakel H, Koldewijn K, Kok J, van Baar A (2011) Maternal attachment representations after very preterm birth and the effect of early intervention. Infant Behav Dev 34(1):72–80. https://doi.org/10.1016/j.infbeh.2010.09.009
25. Parker L (2011) Mothers' experience of receiving counselling/psychotherapy on a neonatal intensive care unit (NICU). J Neonatal Nurs 17(5):182–189. https://doi.org/10.1016/j.jnn.2010.12.001
26. Gerstein ED, Poehlmann-Tynan J (2015) Transactional processes in children born preterm: influences of mother-child interactions and parenting stress. J Fam Psychol 29(5):777–787. https://doi.org/10.1037/fam0000119
27. Borghini A, Müller-Nix C (2015) Traumatisme parental et conséquences lors d'une naissance prématurée. Contraste 41(1):65. https://doi.org/10.3917/cont.041.0065
28. Holditch-Davis D (2003) Posttraumatic stress symptoms in mothers of premature infants. J Obstet Gynecol Neonatal Nurs 32(2):161–171. https://doi.org/10.1177/0884217503252035
29. Kersting A, Dorsch M, Wesselmann U, Lüdorff K, Witthaut J, Ohrmann P et al (2004) Maternal posttraumatic stress response after the birth of a very low-birth-weight infant. J Psychosom Res 57(5):473–476. https://doi.org/10.1016/j.jpsychores.2004.03.011
30. Deater-deckard K (1998) Parenting stress and child adjustment: some old hypotheses and new questions. Clin Psychol Sci Pract 5:314–332

31. Muller-Nix C, Forcada-Guex M, Borghini A, Pierrehumbert B, Ansermet F (2009) Prématurité, vécu parental et relations parents/enfant: éléments cliniques et données de recherche. Psychiatr Enfant 52(2):423. https://doi.org/10.3917/psye.522.0423
32. Gerstein ED, Poehlmann-Tynan J, Clark R (2015) Mother-child interactions in the NICU: relevance and implications for later parenting. J Pediatr Psychol 40(1):33–44. https://doi.org/10.1093/jpepsy/jsu064
33. Muller-Nix C, Forcada-Guex M, Pierrehumbert B, Jaunin L, Borghini A, Ansermet F (2004) Prematurity, maternal stress and mother-child interactions. Early Hum Dev 79(2):145–158. https://doi.org/10.1016/j.earlhumdev.2004.05.002
34. Korja R, Savonlahti E, Ahlqvist-Björkroth S, Stolt S, Haataja L, Lapinleimu H et al (2008) Maternal depression is associated with mother-infant interaction in preterm infants. Acta Paediatr (6):97, 724–730. https://doi.org/10.1111/j.1651-2227.2008.00733.x
35. Lacombe M, Bell L (2006) L ' attachement parent (s) -enfant: un défi pour la pratique infirmière lors de la visite postnatale. L'infirmière Clinicienne 3(1):11–18
36. Coppola G, Cassibba R, Costantini A (2007) What can make the difference?. Premature birth and maternal sensitivity at 3 months of age: the role of attachment organization, traumatic reaction and baby's medical risk. Infant Behav Dev 30(4):679–684. https://doi.org/10.1016/j.infbeh.2007.03.004
37. Als H, Butler S, Kosta S, McAnulty G (2005) The assessment of preterm infants' behavior (APIB): furthering the understanding and measurement of neurodevelopmental competence in preterm and full-term infants. Ment Retard Dev Disabil Res Rev 11(1):94–102. https://doi.org/10.1002/mrdd.20053
38. Als H (1983) Infant individuality: assessing patterns of very early development. In: Call JD, Galenson E, Tyson RL (eds) Frontiers in infant psychiatry. Basic Books, New York, pp 363–378
39. Feldman R, Rosenthal Z, Eidelman AI (2014) Maternal-preterm skin-to-skin contact enhances child physiologic organization and cognitive control across the first 10 years of life. Biol Psychiatry 75(1):56–64. https://doi.org/10.1016/j.biopsych.2013.08.012
40. Buil A (2011) Impacts des expériences sensorielles discontinues sur le développement des prématurés. Evolut Psychomotr 23(92):72–82
41. Bullinger A, Goubet N (1999) Le bébé prématuré, acteur de son développement. Enfance 52(1):27–32. https://doi.org/10.3406/enfan.1999.3127
42. Stevens B, Grunau RE (2002) Pain in vulnerable infants. Clin Perinatol 29:4–6. https://doi.org/10.1016/S0095-5108(02)00023-4
43. Haley DW, Weinberg J, Grunau RE (2006) Cortisol, contingency learning, and memory in preterm and full-term infants. Psychoneuroendocrinology 31(1):108–117. https://doi.org/10.1016/j.psyneuen.2005.06.007
44. Bagner DM, Sheinkopf SJ, Vohr BR, Lester BM (2010) A preliminary study of cortisol reactivity and behavior problems in young children born premature. Dev Psychobiol 52:574–582. https://doi.org/10.1002/dev.20464
45. Doussard-Roosevelt J, Porges S, McClenny BD (1996) Behavioral sleep states in very low birth weight preterm neonates: relation to neonatal health and vaga maturation. J Pediatr Psychol 21(6):785–802
46. Porges W (1995) Porges, 1995, cardiac vagal tone: a physiological index of stress. Neurosci Biobehav Rev 19(2):225–233
47. Feldman R (2006) From biological rhythms to social rhythms: physiological precursors of mother-infant synchrony. Dev Psychol 42(1):175–188. https://doi.org/10.1037/0012-1649.42.1.175
48. Moe V, Braarud HC, Wentzel-Larsen T, Slinning K, Vannebo UT, Guedeney A et al (2016) Precursors of social emotional functioning among full-term and preterm infants at 12 months: early infant withdrawal behavior and symptoms of maternal depression. Infant Behav Dev 44:159–168. https://doi.org/10.1016/j.infbeh.2016.06.012
49. Olafsen KS, Ronning JA, Handegärd BH, Ulvund SE, Dahl LB, Kaaresen PI (2012) Regulatory competence and social communication in term and preterm infants at 12 months corrected age. Results from a randomized controlled trial. Infant Behav Dev 35(1):140–149. https://doi.org/10.1016/j.infbeh.2011.08.001

50. Eckerman CO, Oehler JM, Hannan TE, Molitor A (1995) The development prior to term age of very prematurely born newborns' responsiveness in en face exchanges. Infant Behav Dev 18(3):283–297. https://doi.org/10.1016/0163-6383(95)90017-9
51. Tremblay-leveau H, Lemaitre-Boquer L, Megan A, Renard S, Delauney H (1999) Les actions de communication chez les bébés prématurés à haut risques. Enfance 1:33–42
52. Rand K, Lahav A (2014) Maternal sounds elicit lower heart rate in preterm newborns in the first month of life. Early Hum Dev 90(10):679–683. https://doi.org/10.1016/j.earlhumdev.2014.07.016
53. Rand K, Lahav A (2014) Impact of the NICU environment on language deprivation in preterm infants. Acta Paediatr 103(3):243–248. https://doi.org/10.1111/apa.12481
54. Caskey M, Stephens B, Tucker R, Vohr B (2011) Importance of parent talk on the development of preterm infant vocalizations. Pediatrics 128(5):1–7. https://doi.org/10.1542/peds.2011-0609
55. Caskey M, Vohr B (2013) Assessing language and language environment of high-risk infants and children: a new approach. Acta Paediatr 102(5):451–461. https://doi.org/10.1111/apa.12195
56. Filippa M, Panza C, Ferrari F, Frassoldati R, Kuhn P, Balduzzi S, D'Amico R (2017) Systematic review of maternal voice interventions demonstrates increased stability in preterm infants. Acta Paediatr:1–10. https://doi.org/10.1111/apa.13832
57. Filippa M, Devouche E, Arioni C, Imberty M, Gratier M (2013) Live maternal speech and singing have beneficial effects on hospitalized preterm infants. Acta Paediatr 102(10):1017–1020. https://doi.org/10.1111/apa.12356
58. Mahmoudzadeh M, Dehaene-Lambertz G, Fournier M, Kongolo G, Goudjil S, Dubois J et al (2013) Syllabic discrimination in premature human infants prior to complete formation of cortical layers. Proc Natl Acad Sci U S A 110(12):4846–4851. https://doi.org/10.1073/pnas.1212220110
59. Provasi J, Anderson DI, Barbu-Roth M (2014) Rhythm perception, production, and synchronization during the perinatal period. Front Psychol 5:1048. https://doi.org/10.3389/fpsyg.2014.01048
60. Twohig A, Reulbach U, Figuerdo R, McCarthy A, McNicholas F, Molloy EJ (2016) Supporting preterm infant attachment and socioemotional development in the neonatal intensive care unit: staff perceptions. Infant Ment Health J 37(2):160–171. https://doi.org/10.1002/imhj
61. Landsem IP, Handegård BH, Tunby J, Ulvund SE, Rønning JA (2014) Early intervention program reduces stress in parents of preterms during childhood, a randomized controlled trial. Trials 15:1–13. https://doi.org/10.1186/1745-6215-15-387
62. Laganiére J, Tessier R, Nadeau L (2003) Attachement dans le cas de prématurité: un lien médiatisé par les perceptions maternelles. Enfance 55(2):101–117. https://doi.org/10.3917/enf.552.0101
63. Agostini F, Neri E, Dellabartola S, Biasini A, Monti F (2014) Early interactive behaviours in preterm infants and their mothers: influences of maternal depressive symptomatology and neonatal birth weight. Infant Behav Dev 37(1):86–93. https://doi.org/10.1016/j.infbeh.2013.12.003
64. Holditch-Davis D, White-Traut R, Levy J, Williams KL, Ryan D, Vonderheid S (2013) Maternal satisfaction with administrering infant interventions in the NICU. J Obstet Gynecol Neonatal Nurs 42(6):641–654. https://doi.org/10.1037/emo0000122.Do
65. Feldman R (2007) Parent–infant synchrony: biological foundations and developmental outcomes. Curr Dir Psychol Sci 16(6):340–345. https://doi.org/10.1111/j.1467-8721.2007.00532.x
66. Forcada-Guex M, Borghini A, Pierrehumbert B, Ansermet F, Muller-Nix C (2011) Prematurity, maternal posttraumatic stress and consequences on the mother-infant relationship. Early Hum Dev 87(1):21–26. https://doi.org/10.1016/j.earlhumdev.2010.09.006
67. Matos I, Tereno S, Wendland J, Guedeney N, Dugravier R, Greacen T et al (2014) Sensibilité maternelle et sécurité de l'attachement de l'enfant au sein d'une population à haut risque psychosocial. Dev Dent 26(1):5. https://doi.org/10.3917/dev.141.0005
68. Bozzette M (2007) A Review of Research on Premature Infant-Mother Interaction. Newborn Infant Nurs Rev 7(1):49–55. https://doi.org/10.1053/j.nainr.2006.12.002
69. Crawford JW (1982) Mother infant interaction in premature and full-term infants. Child Dev 53(4):957–962

70. Greene JG, Fox NA, Lewis M (1983) The relationship between neonatal characteristics and three-month mother-infant interaction in high-risk infants. Child Dev 54(5):1286–1296
71. Field TM (1977) Effects of early separation, interactive deficits, and experimental manipulations on infant-mother face-to-face interaction effects of early separation, interactive deficits, and experimental manipulations on infant- mother face-to-face interaction. Child Dev 48(3):763–771. https://doi.org/10.2307/1128325
72. Goldberg S, Perrotta M, Minde K (1986) Maternal behavior and attachment in low-birth-weight twins and singletons. Child Dev 57(1):34–46
73. Kennell JH, Trause MA, Klaus MH (1975) Evidence for a sensitive period in the human mother. Ciba Found Symp (33):87–101
74. Mehler K, Wendrich D, Kissgen R, Roth B, Oberthuer A, Pillekamp F, Kribs A (2011) Mothers seeing their VLBW infants within 3 h after birth are more likely to establish a secure attachment behavior: evidence of a sensitive period with preterm infants. J Perinatol (6):31. 404–410. doi: 10.1038/jp.2010.139
75. Roué J-M, Kuhn P, Lopez Maestro M, Maastrup RA, Mitanchez D, Westrup B, Sizun J (2017) Eight principles for patient-centred and family-centred care for newborns in the neonatal intensive care unit. Arch Dis Child Fetal Neonatal Ed 102(4):F364–F368. https://doi.org/10.1136/archdischild-2016-312180
76. Gray L, Watt L, Blass EM (2000) Skin-to-skin contact is analgesic in healthy newborns. Pediatrics 105(1):e14. https://doi.org/10.1542/peds.105.1.e14
77. Montirosso R, Del Prete A, Bellù R, Tronick E, Borgatti R (2012) Level of NICU quality of developmental care and neurobehavioral performance in very preterm infants. Pediatrics 129(June):1–9. https://doi.org/10.1542/peds.2011-0813
78. Reynolds LC, Duncan MM, Smith GC, Mathur A, Neil J, Inder T et al (2013) Parental presence and holding in the neonatal intensive care unit and associations with early neurobehavior HHS public access. J Perinatol 33(8):636–641. https://doi.org/10.1038/jp.2013.4
79. Boukydis CFZ, Bigsby R, Lester BM (2004) Clinical use of the neonatal intensive care unit network. Pediatrics 113(3):679–689. https://doi.org/10.1542/peds.113.3.S1.679
80. Latva R, Lehtonen L, Salmelin RK, Tamminen T (2004) Visiting less than every day. Arch Ped Adolesc Med 158:1153–1157
81. Tissier J, Bouchouchi A, Glaude C, Legge A, Désir S, Greacen T, Dugravier R (2011) Une intervention préventive communautaire en pé rinatalité. Prat Psychol 17(2):107–117. https://doi.org/10.1016/j.prps.2010.11.006
82. Ainsworth MDS, Blehar MC, Waters E, Wall S (1978) Patterns of attachment: A psychological study of the strange situation, vol xviii. Lawrence Erlbaum, Oxford, 392p
83. Boyce LK, Cook GA, Simonsmeier V, Hendershot SM (2015) Academic outcomes of very low birth weight infants: the influence of mother-child relationships. Infant Ment Health J 36(2):156–166. https://doi.org/10.1002/imhj
84. Smith KE, Landry SH, Swank PR (2005) The influence of decreased parental resources on the efficacy of a responsive parenting intervention. J Consult Clin Psychol 73(4):711–720. https://doi.org/10.1037/0022-006X.73.4.711
85. Clark CAC, Woodward LJ, Horwood LJ, Moor S (2008) Development of emotional and behavioral regulation in children born extremely preterm and very preterm: biological and social influences. Child Dev 79(5):1444–1462. https://doi.org/10.1016/j.infbeh.2012.11.002
86. Wijnroks L (1998) Early maternal stimulation and the development of cognitive competence and attention of preterm infants. Early Dev Parenting 7(1):19–30. https://doi.org/10.1002/(SICI)1099-0917(199803)7:1<19::AID-EDP160>3.0.CO;2-R
87. Lai MM, D'Acunto G, Guzzetta A, Boyd RN, Rose SE, Fripp J et al (2016) PREMM: preterm early massage by the mother: protocol of a randomised controlled trial of massage therapy in very preterm infants. BMC Pediatr 16(1):146. https://doi.org/10.1186/s12887-016-0678-7
88. Delaherche E, Chetouani M, Mahdhaoui A, Saint-Georges C, Viaux S, Cohen D (2012) Interpersonal synchrony: a survey of evaluation methods across disciplines. IEEE Trans Affect Comput 3(3):349–365

89. Leclère C, Viaux S, Avril M, Achard C, Chetouani M, Missonnier S, Cohen D (2014) Why synchrony matters during mother-child interactions: a systematic review. PLoS One 9(12):e113571. https://doi.org/10.1371/journal.pone.0113571
90. Guedeney A, Guedeney N, Tereno S, Dugravier R, Greacen T, Welniarz B, Saias T, Tubach F (2011) Infant rhythms versus parental time: promoting parent-infant synchrony. J Physiol Paris 105(4–6):195–200. https://doi.org/10.1016/j.jphysparis.2011.07.005
91. Fuertes M, Faria A, Soares H, Crittenden P (2009) Developmental and evolutionary assumptions in a study about the impact of premature birth and low income on mother-infant interaction. Acta Ethologica 12(1):1–11. https://doi.org/10.1007/s10211-008-0051-4
92. Dix T, Cheng N, Day WH (2009) Connecting with parents: mothers' depressive symptoms and responsive behaviors in the regulation of social contact by one- and young two-year-olds. Soc Dev 18(1):24–50. https://doi.org/10.1111/j.1467-9507.2008.00488.x
93. Fuertes M, Dos Santos PL, Beeghly M, Tronick E (2006) More than maternal sensitivity shapes attachment: infant coping and temperament. Ann N Y Acad Sci 1094:292–296. https://doi.org/10.1196/annals.1376.037
94. Tooten A, Hall RAS, Hoffenkamp HN, Braeken J, Vingerhoets AJJM, van Bakel HJA (2014) Maternal and paternal infant representations: a comparison between parents of term and preterm infants. Infant Behav Dev 37(3):366–379. https://doi.org/10.1016/j.infbeh.2014.05.004
95. Main M, Solomon J (1986) Discovery of an insecure-disorganised/disoriented attachment pattern. In: Brazelton TB, Yogman M (eds) Affective development in infancy. Abex, Norwood, NJ, pp 95–124
96. Wolke D, Eryigit-Madzwamuse S, Gutbrod T (2014) Very preterm/very low birthweight infants' attachment: infant and maternal characteristics. Arch Dis Child Fetal Neonatal Ed 99(1):F70–F75. https://doi.org/10.1136/archdischild-2013-303788
97. Flacking R, Lehtonen L, Thomson G, Axelin A, Ahlqvist S, Moran VH, Ewald U, Dykes F (2012) Closeness and separation in neonatal intensive care. Acta Paediatr 101(10):1032–1037. https://doi.org/10.1111/j.1651-2227.2012.02787.x
98. Kristoffersen L, Støen R, Rygh H, Sognnæs M, Follestad T, Mohn HS et al (2016) Early skin-to-skin contact or incubator for very preterm infants: study protocol for a randomized controlled trial. Trials 17(1):593. https://doi.org/10.1186/s13063-016-1730-5
99. Nuss T, Kelly KM, Campbell KR, Pierce C, Entzminger JK, Blair BK et al (2014) The impact of opening visitation access on patient and family experience. J Nurs Adm 44(7/8):403–410. https://doi.org/10.1097/NNA.0000000000000090
100. Wigert H, Berg M, Hellström AL (2010) Parental presence when their child is in neonatal intensive care. Scand J Caring Sci 24(1):139–146. https://doi.org/10.1111/j.1471-6712.2009.00697.x
101. Als H (1986) rev 2008, ©. MA: NIDCAP Federation International Boston; Program Guide – Newborn Individualized Developmental Care and Assessment Program (NIDCAP): an Education and Training Program for Health Care Professionals. http://nidcap.org
102. Als H, McAnulty GB (2011) The newborn individualized developmental care and assessment program (NIDCAP) with kangaroo mother care (KMC): comprehensive care for preterm infants. Curr Womens Health Rev 7(3):288–301. https://doi.org/10.2174/157340411796355216.The
103. Als H (2015) Program guide newborn individualized developmental care and assessment program (NIDCAP) an education and training program for health care professionals NIDCAP education and training for professionals consultation and guidance in NIDCAP care implementation. NIDCAP Federatio International
104. McAnulty G, Duffy FH, Butler S, Parad R, Ringer S, Zurakowski D, Als H (2009) Individualized developmental care for a large sample of very preterm infants: health, neurobehaviour and neurophysiology. Acta Paediatr 98(12):1920–1926. https://doi.org/10.1111/j.1651-2227.2009.01492.x
105. McAnulty GB, Duffy FH, Butler SC, Bernstein JH, Zurakowski D, Als H (2010) Effects of the newborn individualized developmental care and assessment program (NIDCAP) at age 8 years: preliminary data. Clin Pediatr 49(3):258–270. https://doi.org/10.1177/0009922809335668

106. Fenwick J, Barclay L, Schmied V (2008) Craving closeness: a grounded theory analysis of women's experiences of mothering in the special care nursery. Women Birth 21(2):71–85. https://doi.org/10.1016/j.wombi.2008.03.006
107. Blomqvist YT, Ewald U, Gradin M, Nyqvist KH, Rubertsson C (2013) Initiation and extent of skin-to-skin care at two Swedish neonatal intensive care units. Acta Paediatr 102(1):22–28. https://doi.org/10.1111/apa.12056
108. Tessier R, Cristo M, Velez S, Giron M, de Calume Z, Ruiz-Palaez J et al (1998) Kangaroo mother care and the bonding hypothesis. Pediatrics 102(2):e17. https://doi.org/10.1542/peds.2005-1877
109. Buil A, Carchon I, Apter G, Laborne FX, Granier M, Devouche E (2016) Kangaroo supported diagonal flexion positioning: new insights into skin-to-skin contact for communication between mothers and very preterm infants. Arch Pediatr 23(9):913–920. https://doi.org/10.1016/j.arcped.2016.04.023
110. Reyna BA, Brown LF, Pickler RH, Myers BJ, Younger JB (2012) Mother-infant synchrony during infant feeding. Infant Behav Dev 35(4):669–677. https://doi.org/10.1016/j.infbeh.2012.06.003
111. Malloch S, Shoemark H, Crncec R, Newnham C, Paul C, Prior M et al (2012) Music therapy with hospitalized infants - the art and science od fommunicative musicality. Infant Ment Health J 33(4):386–399. https://doi.org/10.1002/imhj
112. Bieleninik L, Ghetti C, Gold C (2016) Music therapy for preterm infants and their parents: a meta-analysis. Pediatrics 138(3):e20160971. https://doi.org/10.1542/peds.2016-0971
113. Álvarez MJ, Fernández D, Gómez-Salgado J, Rodríguez-González D, Rosón M, Lapeña S (2017) The effects of massage therapy in hospitalized preterm neonates: a systematic review. Int J Nurs Stud 69:119–136. https://doi.org/10.1016/j.ijnurstu.2017.02.009
114. Field T (2001) Massage therapy facilitates weight gain in preterm infants. Curr Dir Psychol Sci 10(1999):51–54. https://doi.org/10.1111/1467-8721.00113
115. Field T, Diego M, Hernandez-Reif M (2010) Preterm infant massage therapy research: a review. Infant Behav Dev 33(2):115–124. https://doi.org/10.1016/j.infbeh.2009.12.004
116. Field T (2014) Massage therapy research review. Complement Ther Clin Pract 20(4):224–229. https://doi.org/10.1016/j.ctcp.2014.07.002
117. Mendes EW, Procianoy RS (2008) Massage therapy reduces hospital stay and occurrence of late-onset sepsis in very preterm neonates. J Perinatol 28(12). 815–820. doi: 10.1038/jp.2008.108
118. Field T (2002) Preterm infant massage therapy studies: an American approach. Semin Neonatol 7(6):487–494. https://doi.org/10.1053/siny.2002.0153
119. White-Traut R (2004) Providing a nurturing environment for infants in adverse situations: multisensory strategies for newborn care. J Midwifery Womens Health 49(4 Suppl 1):36–41. https://doi.org/10.1016/j.jmwh.2004.05.004
120. White-Traut RC, Nelson MN (1988) Maternally administered tactile, auditory, visual, and vestibular stimulation: relationship to later interactions between mothers and premature infants. Res Nurs Health 11(1):31–39
121. Melnyk BM, Feinstein NF, Alpert-Gillis L, Fairbanks E, Crean HF, Sinkin R a et al (2006) Reducing premature infants' length of stay and improving parents' mental health outcomes with the creating opportunities for parent empowerment (COPE) neonatal intensive care unit program: a randomized, controlled trial. Pediatrics 118(5):e1414–e1427. https://doi.org/10.1542/peds.2005-2580
122. Benzies KM, Magill-Evans JE, Hayden KA, Ballantyne M (2013) Key components of early intervention programs for preterm infants and their parents: a systematic review and meta-analysis. BMC Pregnancy Childbirth 13(Suppl 1):S10. https://doi.org/10.1186/1471-2393-13-S1-S10

Depression Is Not Gender-Biased: Maternal and Paternal Depression and Early Parent-Infant Interactions

8

Isabelle Mueller, Marjorie Beeghly, and Ed Tronick

Experiencing the *baby blues*—feeling increased levels of stress, sadness, loneliness, and anxiety—is common for many new parents during the immediate days or weeks after giving birth. But for approximately 14% of new mothers and 4% of fathers [1], the *blues* fails to resolve and turns into a severe and lasting form of postpartum depression, affecting parents' daily lives, personal relationships, and their infant's development. Infants of depressed parents are at increased risk for developmental problems, including mental health problems, such as affective disorders or behavioral conduct problems later in life [2]. This increased child vulnerability is often attributed to differences in early caregiving and parenting practices, linked to parents' postpartum condition. To explore potential mechanisms underlying these associations, we will discuss several factors linked to parental depression and adverse infant developmental outcomes. First, we will review the characteristics and the importance of the early parent-infant interaction based on the mutual regulation model [3–5]. Second, we will discuss how interactional processes may be altered by parental gender differences in parenting style and psychopathology, as well as research indicating that infant boys are at higher risk for adverse effects of parental depression than girls. Finally, we will consider environmental and biological factors that may contribute to individual differences in infant risk or resilience beyond parent-infant interactional processes in the context of parental depression.

I. Mueller
University of Massachusetts Boston, Boston, MA, USA

M. Beeghly
Wayne State University, Detroit, MI, USA

E. Tronick (✉)
University of Massachusetts Boston, Boston, MA, USA

Harvard Medical School, Boston, MA, USA
e-mail: ed.tronick@umb.edu

© Springer Nature Switzerland AG 2019

G. Apter et al. (eds.), *Early Interaction and Developmental Psychopathology*,
https://doi.org/10.1007/978-3-030-04769-6_8

8.1 Mutual Regulation Model

An infant's ability to cope with everyday stressors becomes more robust during the first year of life and is an important achievement during infancy. Throughout this period, interactions with primary caregivers are an important learning environment, a primary developmental context, and source of external regulation for the child [3, 6, 7]. The infant's ability to regulate its emotions, attention, and behavior is powerfully shaped by the interactive emotional exchange during face-to-face interactions and other social-emotional engagements with caregivers [4, 8]. By attending to the emotional expressions and underlying needs of the infant, a caregiver's actions can scaffold the infant to organize and shape its own responses, facilitating desired emotions and helping the infant overcome unwanted ones.

Successful parent-infant interactions, however, are not just simply the result of adult social skills but rather are highly reciprocal. By actively responding to each other's emotional and behavioral affective displays and communicative signals, the infant and the parent form a dyadic unit—a dyadic open system—in which both partners co-regulate the other's affective and attentional states. This regulatory process is characterized by a dynamic flow of matching states of parent-infant expressions and intentions, followed by the occurrence of mismatching states of non-corresponding intentions and subsequent repairs of the mismatches to matching states. Each participant, parent and infant, aims to regulate mismatches or interactive disorganization in a bidirectional process communicating cues and receiving information from the other [3, 9]. Successful mutual regulation is thus highly dependent on each partner's ability to read their partner's affective and behavioral cues and respond appropriately. Though not lacking impressive communicative and regulatory capacity, the immature infant's capacities are limited, and sensitive scaffolding by the parent is crucial for successful mutual regulation [4].

The mutual regulation model [3, 5] describes a theoretical framework for how infant regulatory abilities develop in a bidirectional parent-infant system, through moment-by-moment infant-parent affective communicative exchanges. For instance, when an infant is hungry or needs a diaper change, it has the capacity to communicate this need through fussing or crying. In turn, the parent reads those cues and responds in the best way possible to alleviate the problem and comfort the infant. On the other hand, a coy smile of the infant may elicit gentle positive stimulation by the parent. A well-attuned response is one in which the parent focuses on the meaning of the infant's emotional display, rather than on the behavior per se, and aims to meet the need or intention underlying the infant's affective signals, in a clear and consistent way. Through successful and unsuccessful encounters in this bidirectional relationship, there emerges an increased understanding of the infants' emotional displays on the part of the typical parent, as well as an increase in their effectiveness in adjusting the level of stimulation to match that of the infant and modulation the infants' level of arousal. Over time with reiterated dyadic experiences, the infant also develops an implicit or procedural knowing of how *we*—infant and parent—are together [3, 4], and a feeling of safety and trust with the parent emerges, gradually leading to the formation of a secure attachment.

On the other hand, the parent may misread the infant's cues or the parent's response may lack sensitivity and attunement. When this mismatching is prolonged and happens on a regular basis, the needs of the infant are repeatedly not met. The dyad fails to establish successful co-regulation. Those persistent interactive disruptions may leave the caregiver helpless or frustrated, and the infant dysregulated. Over time, the infant fails to develop an implicit sense of trust and closeness in the relationship, and chronic dysregulation impairs the infant's ability to engage positively with the world of people and objects.

But brief mismatches and ruptures in the typical parent-infant interaction are more common than often thought; on average merely 30% of the mother-infant interaction takes place in coordinated matching states [9]. That is, dyadic mismatches are "normal" as is the stress which travels with them, and successful repairs of mismatches back to matches are a vital part of the infant's experience and foundational to its development [10]. If the parent-infant dyad is well attuned and can reliably repair ruptures in engagement, the experience of reparation enables the child to develop an implicit or procedural sense that even when conflicts, misunderstandings, and miscommunications happen, can be transformed into positive states again. Repeated reparatory experience helps support the infant's capacity to engage in age-possible self-regulatory skills and, over time, leads to greater self-efficacy, a sense that negative events can be transformed into positive states by one's own efforts, which in turn generates a resilience [11]. Thus, the quality and quantity of reparatory events, as compared to synchronous events, are a prime process driving developmental change for good or for ill.

8.2 Characteristics of Mother- and Father-Infant Interaction

The development of a mutually regulated parent-infant relationship is a "natural" but demanding task, especially for first-time parents. Although we know that this transition involves dynamic transactions among complex biological, mental, and social factors, until recently, only a limited literature has evaluated the caregiver's subjective experience of the emerging relationship with the infant. In a longitudinal study of first-time Canadian middle-class parents, Tronick and Bell found that the family unit dynamically evolves during the postpartum period [12, 13]. The dominant themes reported by new parents during the first weeks after delivery include finding a rhythm with their newborn and exploring their new relationship. While mothers focus more on meeting the infant's physical needs and fathers are more fascinated by the infant's early capacities, the overriding aims for both parents are developing a connection with the infant and "getting to know" the infant.

Throughout the next months, the initially homogeneous parental system differentiates and gender/parental-specific roles emerge. First-time fathers focus on overcoming their own insecurities with the infant, whereas mothers begin to initiate complementary interactions to deepen their relationship with the child [13]. The mother's greater focus on developing a relationship with their infant may reflect her sense that she already "knows" what her infant is like from the time of pregnancy.

Over time, the couple evolves past their somewhat unbounded triadic relationship in which the father often plays a peripheral role supporting the mother. Now each parent shows distinct, gender-specific characteristics in their interactions with the infant. Notably, as distinctive patterns of mother-infant and father-infant interaction emerge and each parent focuses increasingly on his/her own relationship with the infant, both parents begin to report a greater distancing in their marital relationship during the early months of the postpartum period [12]. This early differentiation appears to have a significant reorganizing impact on the emerging family system. It enables the parents to establish a new triadic *family* unit by 4 months postpartum, with emerging complementary roles for the parents in relation to the infant and to each other [12, 13].

The complementary roles of mothers and fathers are observed in several aspects of parenting. For instance, it is often reported that the amount of time a mother and a father spends with their infant is inversely related [14, 15]. But whether this observation is related to maternal gatekeeping and paternal compensatory behavior, or whether it is linked to the quality of the interaction, has yet to be addressed. Additionally, mothers and fathers show differences in their interaction style with their child. Play activities may be more characteristic for father-infant interactions, whereas mothers engage in more basic caregiving and affective behaviors. Mothers are found to be more sensitive with their infants during a natural play interaction than fathers, and, consistent with this observation, infants are more likely to cooperate with their mothers than with their fathers [16]. In addition since mothers often spend more time with the infant than fathers, they may have more opportunity to increase sensitive attunement with the infant.

However, families are not insular systems. Rather, they are dynamic systems that are influenced by multiple transacting contextual factors such as parental level of education, adequacy of financial resources, parental mental health, amount of social support, and cultural beliefs and values. Bell and colleagues' [12, 13] account of the transitions in family and couple relations may aptly characterize the experience of middle-class Canadian families, but may not necessarily generalize to other families in other settings. Further research on the transition to parenthood in larger, more diverse samples is needed.

8.3 Parental Mental Health

That said, it is likely the case for all families everywhere that parental psychological factors such as mental health play a fundamental role in the emerging parent-infant relationship. Maternal and paternal depression, along with exposure to other stressors such as poverty or trauma, may diminish a parent's capacity to be emotionally available for their infant and to repair interactive ruptures that occur during routine caregiving exchanges. Tronick [17] has argued that parental resources utilized to cope with these factors deplete parental resources that otherwise could more effectively be used for regulating the interaction with the infant. Consequently, this diminished capacity undermines the quality of the emerging parent-infant interaction and the organization of the family system [12, 13].

8.4 Maternal Depression

Maternal depression is a relatively common condition that affects maternal parenting behavior and is associated with withdrawal or increased negative emotions, irritability, and a loss of interest in activities. Maternal depression not only compromises a mother's ability to read her infant's cues accurately, it also continuously exposes the infant to an environment that is characterized by negative emotions and disconnection [4]. A depressed adverse emotional parenting climate disrupts the dynamic interaction of the parent-infant dyad and limits joint positive experiences of matching states and, more importantly, successful reparations. Cohn and Tronick [18] were among the first to demonstrate that 3-month-old infants already have a distinct behavioral reaction to maternal withdrawal. In a face-to-face setting, mothers were asked to simulate depression by speaking in a flat voice, keeping their face expressionless, and limiting touch and movement toward the infant. Infants in this simulated depression condition showed more negative affect compared to infants whose mothers engaged in normal interactive behavior. In addition, the infants in the depressed experimental condition displayed a higher proportion of behaviors denoting protest, wariness, and gaze aversion from their mothers. In contrast, when these same mothers resumed their typical natural interaction, their infant exhibited a coherent cycle of positive affect, social monitoring, and play. Overall, the infants showed distinct patterns of behavior that were specific to their mother's emotional displays [18]. These findings suggest that even a 3-min episode of simulated depression has a strong impact on the infant's emotional experience and communicative response in the moment.

The findings from the simulation study suggest that if exposure to depressed maternal behavior and affect were to become "real" and chronic, it would have a far-reaching significant impact on the infants' behavior and eventual outcomes. With a depressed parent, the infant chronically faces an environment dominated by withdrawal and negative affect [19]. This limits the infant's experience of engaging in joint positive affect matching, coordination, and reparation with the mother [20]. The mother's ability for scaffolding her infant's regulation of attention and negative emotion is also compromised, resulting in an increased disconnection of the dyad. Lacking effective external support, the infant has to self-regulate, a demanding task that can only succeed briefly, given the infant's limited regulatory abilities. The chronic experience of being in mismatched dyadic states and failing to experience reparation, as well as not receiving the scaffolding needed to self-regulate, leads to increased infant dysregulation and disengagement from people and the inanimate world. As a result, infants of chronically depressed mothers exhibit increased negative affect, passivity, and self-comforting behaviors, compared to infants of non-depressed mothers [21].

The chronic maternal withdrawal and negative affect associated with postpartum depression, and the failure of the dyad to experience reparation, may have cumulative toxic effects and place the infant at heightened risk for emotion regulation problems, relationship, and attachment insecurity, which in turn are linked to social emotional problems in later childhood [4]. The quality of mother-infant interaction is also linked to the infant's cognitive development. For example, in a large study of 570 mother-infant dyads from low-income backgrounds, Sheinkopf and colleagues report that maternal positive engagement with the infant at 4 months of age predicts the child's later verbal and performance IQ at 4 and 7 years [22]. Indeed, these effects may be amplified as the child's early development is compromised by chronic maternal depression, and in turn the child's altered behavior further compromises the mother's capacity for regulating the mother-infant interaction effectively, a potentially vicious and developmentally compromising cascade.

8.5 Sex Differences in Infant Vulnerability

Inasmuch as the mother-infant interaction is co-regulated by each partner and is bidirectional in nature, it is important to consider whether sex differences in infant regulatory capacities contribute to mother-infant interactive processes. For instance, Weinberg and colleagues report that infant girls show greater self-regulatory skills than infant boys, whereas infant boys display higher affective reactivity and need more maternal scaffolding than infant girls [23]. These gender-specific self-regulatory patterns can also be observed in distinct differences in the dyadic organization of mother-son and mother-daughter interactions [20]. For instance, several researchers demonstrate that mother-son and mother-daughter dyads exhibit a different pattern of affect attunement. Mother-son dyads exhibit more matching affective states (both positive and negative) and higher synchrony than mother-daughter dyads [9, 23]. Weinberg et al. [23] further show that infant girls engage significantly more in object play than infant boys and mother-daughter dyads engage in less positive affect matching aside from object engagement [24].

A growing literature additionally suggests that the withdrawn and disengaged behavioral patterns observed in depressed mothers may have a greater impact on infant boys than girls, perhaps because boys may need more regulatory support from their caregivers. This gender-specific vulnerability is well documented in the scientific literature [20, 24, 25].

Weinberg et al. [26] investigated the impact of maternal depression on several features of the mother-infant interaction at 3 months postpartum in a challenging social context, the Face-to-Face Still-Face (FFSF) paradigm. Male infants of depressed mothers showed an overall increase in negative emotion compared to female infants of depressed mothers or to infants of non-depressed mothers. Boys of depressed mothers displayed significantly more negative affect and disengagement during the reunion episode of the FFSF paradigm. In turn, depressed mothers had more negative interactive patterns if they had an infant boy than if they had an infant girl. The negative emotional display of depressed mothers and the infant boys of depressed mothers increased from an initial play episode and peaked after exposure to a social stressor (FFSF reunion episode). A similar increase in negative affect among the male infants of depressed mothers during the FFSF paradigm has also been observed in several other studies [24, 27, 28]. These findings not only suggest that the exposure to maternal depression may pose an increased challenge for dyads' ability to repair mismatches and successfully co-regulate social interactions, but the derailment is greater when a mother is interacting with a son. Moreover, the findings on the interactive problems of depressed infant-mother dyads after the still-face indicate that such dyads are more vulnerable to stress than non-depressed dyads.

Other research has focused specifically on the effect of maternal depression on dyadic matching and mismatching states during mother-infant interaction. This literature as expected suggests that the critical interactive event is not the frequency of mismatches but rather the form and quality of the repair of mismatches. One such measure is the dyad's latency to repair mismatches [29]. Mothers with diagnosed clinical depression compared to healthy mothers without depression have less capability to match their infant's positive affect. For instance, depressed mothers need more time to initiate a first positive coordination with the infant during a natural play situation, which may undermine the dyad's ability to repair mismatching states [29]. Moreover, the increased disruptions in mother-infant interactions associated with maternal depression are more challenging for infant boys, again perhaps due to their increased need for more maternal scaffolding and support to regulate negative affect.

In a longitudinal study by Beeghly and colleagues [30], mothers with high versus normative levels of depressive symptoms were followed over the first year postpartum. Mothers' level of depressive symptomatology remained relatively stable over time. Mothers meeting high symptom criteria at 2 months postpartum were more likely to continue to experience a high level of depressive symptoms at subsequent time points during the first postpartum year. Moreover, depressed mothers of infant sons were more likely to continue to experience a high level of depressive symptoms at 3 months postpartum than depressed mothers of infant girls [30]. Though more research is needed, the increased disengagement and lack of coordination between depressed mothers and their infant sons may be what is contributing to these dyads' difficulties in adjustment. Furthermore, the increased need of male infants for maternal scaffolding and support may add an additional demand for resources when mothers have clinically significant levels of postpartum depression.

In other research, Beeghly et al. [31] evaluated the dynamics of maternal postpartum depression in a large sample of African American mother-infant dyads over the first 18 months postpartum. Findings indicate that risk factors such as lower socioeconomic status and young maternal age at delivery increase the risk for a higher level of maternal depressive symptoms over time, whereas social support has a positive influence on maternal mental health status. Most importantly, results show that maternal depressive symptom trajectories have a differential impact on boys' and girls' attachment outcomes by 18 months. If maternal symptoms of depression increase over the postpartum period, boys are less likely to show attachment security at 18 months. In contrast, mother-daughter dyads display no significant relation between security of attachment and maternal postpartum depressive trajectories.

Sex differences are also reported for infants' vulnerability to other types of maternal psychopathology. In a longitudinal study that followed 69 mothers with an anxiety disorder over the first 8 months postpartum, Müller et al. [27] found significant effects of infant sex and age. Unlike many studies that focus solely on infant negative affect, this study focused on infants' self-comforting behavior, which is usually characterized as internalizing behaviors indicative of distress in the infant [32]. In the maternal anxiety group, boys under the age of 3 months displayed increased self-comforting behaviors during the FFSF paradigm compared to girls, whereas girls over the age of 5.5 months showed significantly decreased regulation by self-comfort compared to the boys and to infants of mothers in the healthy control group. These gender-specific findings for maternal anxiety are similar to those reported for maternal depression. That is, younger boys of anxious mothers seem to experience significantly more stress during a challenging social situation than girls of anxious mothers. In addition, the observation that older girls display less self-comforting behavior or distress during the FFSF procedure suggests that female infants have more mature regulatory skills and are less affected by maternal psychopathology even in experimental situations that elicit social stress.

8.6 Paternal Depression

Given that mothers are traditionally the primary caregiver of infants and depression is a relatively common condition among postpartum women, a majority of research is based on the impact of depression on the mother-infant interaction. Although fathers nowadays are increasingly involved in child care, there is still a paucity of research on paternal depression and its influence on parent-infant interaction and early child development.

A meta-analysis looking at the effects of parental depression on infants and young children shows that the effects of paternal depression are comparable to those of maternal depression [33]. Depressed fathers exhibit increased negative behavior, increased withdrawal, and decreased positive affect during interactions with their infants. These findings are stronger for younger fathers compared to older fathers. The greater impact of depression on younger fathers may reflect the fact that younger fathers have less experience with infants, leading to a lack of confidence during father-infant interaction. This insecurity may represent an additional challenge for young fathers during father-infant interaction, compounding the other behavioral characteristics of depression such as withdrawal and negative affect. These factors may minimize the capacity of depressed fathers to engage in co-regulated interactions with the infant.

In addition to paternal age, other factors also moderate these associations. Ethnicity is one such factor. Wilson and Durbin [33] report a stronger correlation between paternal depression symptoms and adverse parenting among non-Caucasian fathers than for Caucasian fathers [33]. Paternal perceptions of their infant's temperament may also play a role. A study looking at 3-month-old infants shows that fathers with clinical symptoms of depression describe their children as more distressed than healthy fathers, indicating a relationship between paternal psychopathology and negative perceptions of their infant's temperament [34]. Longitudinal research also indicates that paternal depression during the postpartum period may have a differential impact on boys than girls. For instance, preschool boys are more likely to display conduct problems when their fathers had reported high levels of depressive symptoms during their child's early infancy [35]. This, again, implies that boys may be more sensitive than girls to the characteristic lack of attunement and scaffolding that is often associated with parent-infant interaction in the context of parental depression. Conduct problems describe a child's persistent inability to successfully regulate mood and behavior, leading to increased aggression and antisocial behaviors in the context of distress. A direct connection between a lack of father-infant co-regulation during infancy through paternal depression and boys' later self-regulatory problems emphasizes this observed increased vulnerability of male infants, as well as perhaps the greater developmental importance of fathers to their sons.

The observations on paternal depression, as well as maternal depression, can be easily framed within the tenets of the mutual regulation model. This model proposes that successful co-regulation and repairs in the dyad during infancy enable the child to develop self-regulation strategies, leading to increased resilience and a better ability to cope with stressors later in life. More longitudinal research focusing on boys' and girls' developmental outcomes in the context of maternal and paternal depression is needed to gain insight in the underlying mechanisms leading to this gender-specific vulnerability to later child psychopathology.

But paternal mental health problems do not only affect the infant; couples also report increased conflict and disharmony in their own relationship when fathers have high depressive symptoms [34]. Evaluating the family as a triadic unit and assessing the degree of paternal involvement in childrearing are also important and are receiving increased attention during the past years. As described in Bell et al. [12], mothers and fathers of a young infant build a highly differentiated unit with triadic interdependencies and complementary behaviors. Maternal depression affects not only the infant but also most likely the father, and in turn, the mental health problems of the father most likely affect the entire triadic or multimember family system [34]. For instance, although parental depression is relatively common during the postpartum period and can be found in 14% of new mothers and 4% of fathers [1], maternal and paternal depressive symptoms are often correlated. In a recent review, the amount that fathers self-report depressive symptoms increases to 24–50%, when their partner is also affected by postpartum depression [36, 37]. This finding implies that paternal and maternal mental health is not just an isolated occurrence but both present a dynamic interaction that may impact the well-being of the entire family, including the infant. More insidiously, from a systemic viewpoint, parental depression, or for that matter any mental health problem that affects family members' capacity for engaging in positive interactions with other family members, is likely to affect others in a negative manner, which in turn further amplifies the problems of all the individuals in the family unit.

Notably, greater paternal involvement in childcare is often described as a potential protective factor buffering the infant from the effects of maternal postpartum depression. For instance, paternal involvement may reduce some of the adverse aspects for the infant via its effects in supporting the mother in her condition. Furthermore, engaging in more positive interactions with the infant when the father is an equally involved caregiver may alleviate some of the depriving effects of maternal withdrawal. But given the possible association between maternal and paternal mental health, greater paternal involvement may have the opposite effect as well. When both parents experience high levels of symptoms of depression, the infant's exposure to a climate of negative affect is increased [38].

There is also evidence that paternal depression is associated with compromised patterns of father-infant interaction (Tronick, personal communication 2017). Specifically, maternal and paternal depressive symptoms are negatively correlated with mother-infant and father-infant mutual engagement evaluated during a natural play interaction. In addition, paternal depression is negatively associated with social engagement during father-child interaction, whereas maternal depressive symptoms are negatively associated with mutual engagement.

Methodological differences among studies of paternal depression make this literature difficult to interpret. One problem is that different studies use different methods for assessing depression and the quality of paternal parenting [33]. The quality of parenting can be assessed by evaluating interactive behaviors such as sensitivity, warmth, matching, synchrony, positive, and negative emotional displays. But not all of those parenting measurements may be equally affected by paternal depression. Additionally, the methods used to assess paternal parenting have typically been drawn from work with mothers, but fathers are reported to differ from mothers in several dimensions of interactive behavior with their children [16]. It may not be appropriate to use the same measures to capture the quality of paternal and maternal interactions. More research is needed, not just for how postpartum depression in fathers affects their parenting but especially for how the effects of paternal depression manifest in the family as a complex unit and the possible adverse or alleviating influence of gender, parental age, as well as cultural and ethnic differences on paternal parenting behavior and child outcomes.

8.7 Buffering and Transduction Model

The buffer-transducer model [17, 39] aims to expand the mutual regulation model by including sociocultural and underlying biological mechanisms that may impact the infant's development beyond the "cocoon" of the parent-infant dyadic interaction itself. The buffer-transducer model starts by emphasizing the importance of dyadic engagement as a central component or common pathway for the mediation effects of many different factors. Infants are immature and have limited capacity to self-regulate, so parental scaffolding is essential to help the child regulate and organize attentional and emotional states. In addition, this model aims to highlight underlying factors and mechanisms that influence the dyad, either buffering or transducing those effects on infant development. For instance, what are commonly referred to as risk factors are conceptualized in the model as either resource-depleting or resource-enhancing factors. These resources include physiological, psychological, and regulatory factors that influence the functioning of the dyad. One example is parental education. Lower levels of parental education are often associated with poorer parental self-regulatory skills, and a lower capacity to self-regulate may impact the parent's ability to provide necessary or well-attuned scaffolding for the infant during parent-infant interaction [39]. Thus the inability of the parent to self-regulate is transduced to the infant via poorer mutual regulation during parent-infant interaction. As such, resources that could be put to better use such as enhancing the child's engagement with people and things are depleted in the service of infant self-regulation [40]. Several other enhancing or depleting factors such as socioeconomic status, social support, exposure to violence, and, of course, parental depression have a significant impact on the quality of the dyadic interaction between parent and infant.

The buffer-transducer model goes on to consider biological influences on developmental outcomes and the dyads itself. For instance, genetic predispositions, as well as epigenetic factors, may influence the likelihood for developing disorders such as depressive symptoms, therefore enhancing or depleting resources that may affect the quality of the parent-infant interaction and the infant's development. In turn, the quality of the interaction will have reciprocal effects on epigenetic mechanisms. Similarly, other members of the immediate family and the infant's social ecology can function as a buffering factor for the infant when a parent is affected by postpartum depression but only when those family members/individuals are in good mental health themselves. By contrast, if close relatives suffer from depression or other mental health problems themselves, or the infant's social ecology is stressful and resource depleting, they may increase the adverse effects of parental depression on the parent-infant relationship and the infant's long-term outcomes [38].

8.8 Conclusion

What is typically referred to as "normal" development and what we refer to as psychopathology are phenomena that emerge early out of chronically reiterated parent-infant social-emotional engagements, such that the infant's ways of being in the world become increasingly self-organized and more tightly organized over the long course of ontogeny. Exposure to parental postpartum depression has distorting effects on the quality of the infant's and child's interactions with parents, with associated reductions of the reparation of dyadic mismatches and positive affect, and increases in shared negative affect, such as sadness and anger. These compromising effects make us aware of how these dynamic parent-infant mutual regulatory processes sculpt development. Research on parental postpartum depression emphasizes how depression's effects systemically include both the father and mother and clearly suggest the role of other caregivers if they are a regular part of the child's interactive world. Moreover, the effects of postpartum depression on infants have to be understood in terms of a dynamic system in which different components—different individuals with different characteristics—affect the functioning of other components, the other individuals, over time, leading either to amplification of the dyadic system or to its dissipation. Fathers may ameliorate the negative effects of maternal postpartum depression by their greater involvement in child care or may actually amplify it. Over time, both parents and the child co-create a family system that becomes increasingly stable, that is, increasing internally organized and increasingly resistant to change. Pointedly, the process by which postpartum depression alters the parent-infant relationship is no different than the process generating normal development, and further examination is needed about how postpartum depression operates to undermine negative dyadic reparation processes. Moreover, as presented in the buffer-transducer model, the interplay of multiple other factors, both external and internal, has to be considered as inherently and dynamically part of the dynamics of the process. Furthermore, these considerations should not be limited to the parents but must include the buffering or transducing effect of others, as well as the broader social organizations in the child's social ecology. Perhaps most importantly, research that is based on the buffer-transducer model could build a greater awareness of how resources that could—can we say "should"—be used for supporting children's positive growth and development are diverted to overcoming the depleting effects of postpartum depression. Such research would highlight fragility and sturdiness, as well as the centrality of the parent-infant/child system in an individual's mental health.

Acknowledgment A version of this paper was presented for the *Reiss-Greenberg Chair, an endowed chair of the Reiss-Davis Child Study Center and Institute*, January 2017, by Dr. Tronick. The research in this paper was supported by Grants from the National Institute of Child Development and the National Science Foundation, E. Tronick PI.

References

1. Davé S, Petersen I, Sherr L, Nazareth I (2010) Incidence of maternal and paternal depression in primary care: a cohort study using a primary care database. Arch Pediatr Adolesc Med 164(11):1038–1044
2. Lovejoy MC, Graczyk PA, O'Hare E, Neuman G (2000) Maternal depression and parenting behavior: a meta-analytic review. Clin Psychol Rev 20(5):561–592
3. Tronick EZ (1989) Emotions and emotional communication in infants. Am Psychol 44(2):112–119
4. Tronick E, Beeghly M (2011) Infants' meaning-making and the development of mental health problems. Am Psychol 66(2):107–119
5. Weinberg MK, Tronick EZ (1997) Depressed mothers and infants: failure to form dyadic states of consciousness. In: Murray L, Cooper PJ (eds) Postpartum depression and child development. The Guildford Press, New York/London, pp 54–81
6. Gunnar MR, Donzella B (2002) Social regulation of the cortisol levels in early human development. Psychoneuroendocrinology 27(1):199–220
7. Mesman J, van IJzendoorn MH, Bakermans-Kranenburg MJ (2009) The many faces of the still-face paradigm: a review and meta-analysis. Dev Rev 29(2):120–162

8. Tronick E, Als H, Adamson L, Wise S, Brazelton TB (1978) The infant's response to entrapment between contradictory messages in face-to-face interaction. J Am Acad Child Psychiatry 17(1):1–13
9. Tronick EZ, Cohn JF (1989) Infant-mother face-to-face interaction: age and gender differences in coordination and the occurrence of miscoordination. Child Dev 60(1):85–92
10. Tronick E (2007) The neurobehavioral and social-emotional development of infants and children. In: New York. WW Norton & Company, London
11. Beeghly M, Tronick E (2011) Early resilience in the context of parent-infant relationships: a social development perspective. Curr Probl Pediatr Adolesc Health Care 41(7):197–201
12. Bell L, Goulet C, Tribble DSC, Paul D, Boisclair A, Tronick EZ (2007) Mothers' and fathers' views of the interdependence of their relationships with their infant a systems perspective on early family relationships. J Fam Nurs 13(2):179–200
13. Bell L, Tribble DSC, Goulet C, Paul D, Tronick EZ (2007) Mothers' and fathers' early relationship with their infant: similar yet temporally discordant themes. Can J Midwifery Res Pract 6(3):30–41
14. Horn WF (2000) Fathering infants. In: Osofsky JD, Fitzgerald HE (eds) WAIMH handbook of infant mental health: parenting and child care. Wiley, New York, NY, pp 270–297
15. Lamb ME, Lewis C (2004) The development and significance of father–child relationships in two-parent families. In: Lamb ME (ed) The role of the father in child development, 4th edn. Wiley, New York, NY, pp 272–306
16. Fuertes M, Faria A, Beeghly M, Lopes-dos-Santos P (2016) The effects of parental sensitivity and involvement in caregiving on mother–infant and father–infant attachment in a Portuguese sample. J Fam Psychol 30(1):147–156
17. Tronick E (2018) The caregiver-infant dyad as a buffer or transducer of resource enhancing or depleting factors that shape psychobiological. Dev J 38(4):561–572. https://doi.org/10.1002/anzf.1274
18. Cohn JF, Tronick EZ (1983) Three-month-old infants' reaction to simulated maternal depression. Child Dev 54(1):185–193
19. Tronick EZ (2002) Infant moods and the chronicity of depressive symptoms: the co-creation of unique ways of being together for good or ill. Paper 1: the normal process of development and the formation of moods. Z Psychosom Med Psychother 49(4):408–424
20. Tronick E, Reck C (2009) Infants of depressed mothers. Harv Rev Psychiatry 17(2):147–156
21. Reck C, Hunt A, Fuchs T, Weiss R, Noon A, Moehler E, Downing G, Tronick EZ, Mundt C (2004) Interactive regulation of affect in postpartum depressed mothers and their infants: an overview. Psychopathology 37(6):272–280
22. Sheinkopf SJ, Tenenbaum EJ, Messinger DS, Miller-Loncar CL, Tronick E, Lagasse LL et al (2016) Maternal and infant affect at 4 months predicts performance and verbal IQ at 4 and 7 years in a diverse population. Dev Sci:1–11
23. Weinberg MK, Tronick EZ, Cohn JF, Olson KL (1999) Gender differences in emotional expressivity and self-regulation during early infancy. Dev Psychol 35(1):175–188
24. Weinberg MK, Beeghly M, Olson KL, Tronick E (2008) Effects of maternal depression and panic disorder on mother–infant interactive behavior in the face-to-face still-face paradigm. Infant Ment Health J 29(5):472–491
25. Schore AN (2016) All our sons: the developmental neurobiology and neuroendocrinology of boys at risk. Infant Ment Health J 38(1):15–52
26. Weinberg KM, Olson KL, Beeghly M, Tronick EZ (2006) Making up is hard to do, especially for mothers with high levels of depressive symptoms and their infant sons. J Child Psychol Psychiatry 47(7):670–683
27. Müller M, Tronick E, Zietlow AL, Nonnenmacher N, Verschoor S, Traeuble B (2016) Effects of maternal anxiety disorders on infant self-comforting behaviors: the role of maternal bonding, infant gender and age. Psychopathology 49(4):295–304

28. Sravish AV, Tronick E, Hollenstein T, Beeghly M (2013) Dyadic flexibility during the face-to-face still-face paradigm: a dynamic systems analysis of its temporal organization. Infant Behav Dev 36(3):432–437
29. Reck C, Noe D, Stefenelli U, Fuchs T, Cenciotti F, Stehle E et al (2011) Interactive coordination of currently depressed inpatient mothers and their infants during the postpartum period. Infant Ment Health J 32(5):542–562
30. Beeghly M, Weinberg MK, Olson KL, Kernan H, Riley J, Tronick EZ (2002) Stability and change in level of maternal depressive symptomatology during the first postpartum year. J Affect Disord 71(1):169–180
31. Beeghly M, Partridge TR, Tronick E, Muzik M, Rahimian Mashhadi M, Boeve JL, Irwin JL (2017) Associations between early maternal depressive symptom trajectories and toddlers' felt security at 18 months: are boys and girls at differential risk? Infant Ment Health J 38(1):53–67
32. Müller M, Zietlow AL, Tronick E, Reck C (2015) What dyadic reparation Is meant to do: an association with infant cortisol reactivity. Psychopathology 48(6):386–399
33. Wilson S, Durbin CE (2010) Effects of paternal depression on fathers' parenting behaviors: a meta-analytic review. Clin Psychol Rev 30(2):167–180
34. Ramchandani PG, Psychogiou L, Vlachos H, Iles J, Sethna V, Netsi E, Lodder A (2011) Paternal depression: an examination of its links with father, child and family functioning in the postnatal period. Depress Anxiety 28(6):471–477
35. Ramchandani P, Stein A, Evans J, O'Connor TG, ALSPAC Study Team (2005) Paternal depression in the postnatal period and child development: a prospective population study. Lancet 365(9478):2201–2205
36. Goodman JH (2004) Paternal postpartum depression, its relationship to maternal postpartum depression, and implications for family health. J Adv Nurs 45(1):26–35
37. Paulson JF, Bazemore SD (2010) Prenatal and postpartum depression in fathers and its association with maternal depression: a meta-analysis. JAMA 303(19):1961–1969
38. Mezulis AH, Hyde JS, Clark R (2004) Father involvement moderates the effect of maternal depression during a child's infancy on child behavior problems in kindergarten. J Fam Psychol 18(4):575–588
39. Liu C, Tronick E (2016) Neurobehavioural development in infancy: the buffering and transducing role of the mother/caretaker-infant dyad. Child Psychol Psychiatr:17–23
40. DiCorcia JA, Tronick E (2011) Quotidian resilience: exploring mechanisms that drive resilience from a perspective of everyday stress and coping. Neurosci Biobehav Rev 35(7):1593–1602

Part III

Early Interactive Assessment and Therapeutic Management

Assessment Tools for Parent-Infant Interaction and Their Contribution to Perinatal Clinical Care

9

Emmanuel Devouche, Sara Dominguez, and Gisèle Apter

Early face-to-face communication is seen as the cradle of all subsequent social abilities such as joint engagement or coordinated attention and as supporting interpersonal engagement, sharing of meaning and processes of intentional communication [1–4]. Infant development is itself an interactive process, involving both interactions with social partners and with aspects of the physical environment. The developmental continuity between early processes supporting face-to-face communication and the cognitive basis for crucial abilities such as joint attention is no longer a question of debate [4–6]. Because the young infant interacts mainly with parents, a constant co-regulation is needed to maintain a balance between two asymmetrical partners ([6–9], see Chaps. 2 and 3, Part I). Importantly, communication also involves interactive dysregulation and rewarding repairs are an essential part of typical healthy interactions [10].

When parent-infant interaction presents a high risk of distortion, there is a need to develop specialized care dedicated to support the emergence or restoration of healthy parent-child relationships [11]. Indeed, when one or both partners are affected by psychopathology, interactive "errors" are less readily accounted for and spontaneously "repaired". Patterns of response and initiative are indeed modified by psychopathological factors, generating more distorted behaviour from both partners [12–14]. The interactive system that develops is the result of failed attempts on the part of both partners to find or regain a more satisfying connection together [15].

E. Devouche (✉)
Laboratoire de Psychopathologie et Processus de Santé, Paris Descartes University, Paris, France

Groupe Hospitalier du Havre, Université de Rouen Normandie, Mont-Saint-Aignan, France

S. Dominguez
Psychologist at Early Years Psychology, The Hague, The Netherlands

G. Apter
Groupe Hospitalier du Havre, Université de Rouen Normandie, Mont-Saint-Aignan, France

© Springer Nature Switzerland AG 2019

G. Apter et al. (eds.), *Early Interaction and Developmental Psychopathology*,
https://doi.org/10.1007/978-3-030-04769-6_9

And because the infant is an astonishingly rapidly developing being, the distorted interactive patterns come to form the basis of the infant's interaction "expectancies" [16]. What's more, the infant considers these patterns as the *usual* way of interacting with its closest partners [17]. The distorted patterns become a normalized way in which the infant engages with the world and consequently with the future partners he or she will encounter [18].

Although the tools presented in this chapter were initially elaborated within a clinical setting for the detection of vulnerabilities and interactive risks in infants, they can also be used as training tools for clinicians and as research tools to study the development of infant-parent interaction, both in typical and in atypical contexts. The tools provide a structured observation of the early parent-infant interaction system. Some of these tools require a structured setting, whereas others are based on observation during free play. All these tools use detailed observation grids that guide description and interpretation of the interaction.

9.1 Selection of Tools

In this section, we will focus on the following scales: The Brazelton Neonatal Behavioral Assessment Scale (NBAS; Brazelton [19]), the CARE-Index [20], the guide-book for assessing the dialogue between the adult and the child (GEDAN; Roten and Fivaz-Depeursinge [21]), the Global Ratings Scales for Mothers-Infant Interactions (GRS; Fiori-Cowley and Murray [22]), The Coding Interactive Behaviour (CIB; Feldman [23]) and the Parent-Child Early Relational Assessment (PCERA; Clark [24]). These different tools differ in their underlying theoretical approaches, in the aspects of the interaction they evaluate, in the duration and complexity of conducting the assessment, and in the age of infants they can be used with. They have been selected because of their specific focus on social interaction and are not exclusively centred on one or the other partner involved in the infant's care (for an extensive review of scales and tools, see [25]). Because the focus of the present book is on social interaction during the first year of life, tools assessing only infant attachment were excluded. Moreover, the mutual regulation model [26, 27] is not included in this chapter as it is addressed in previous sections of this book (see Chap. 3, Part I).

9.1.1 The Brazelton Neonatal Behavioural Assessment Scale (NBAS) (Brazelton [19]; See Part III, Chap. 10)

T.B. Brazelton's evaluation scale [28] aims to objectify the infant's skills from birth. Yet, this scale relies on the subjective experience of the examiner and thus represents an unparalleled newborn assessment tool that explores the full complexity of neonatal behaviour. In order to be assessed with this tool, the newborn must have a gestational age of at least 37 weeks, but the optimal period for examination is between the 3rd and the 10th day of postnatal life.

With infants born prior to this age, it is necessary to use an equivalent scale tailored to premature infants, the APIB (Assessment of Preterm Infant Behaviour [29]). The NBAS must be conducted by a trained observer who has acquired the ability to adapt to the particularities of the newborn baby's expression. This is what Brazelton calls the "flexibility of the examiner". Indeed, identification with the newborn results in acceptance of physical sometimes regressive movements that must be taken into account by the examiner. Whatever the circumstances, the items of the scale should not be applied to the child in a prescriptive manner but rather according to particular rhythm and manifestations of the newborn during the evaluation. Thus, the baby's strategies for adapting to exchanges with the examiner must be carefully observed precisely because they are part of the assessment. Specialists are also careful not to subject the newborn to the solicitations beyond its abilities. Signs of stress but also crying or unexpected drowsiness are examples of strategies used by newborns to counter maladapted solicitations.

In the last version of the scale [30], neonatal skills are grouped into six sets or "clusters": habituation, orientation, motor system, state regulation, state organization and autonomous system.

The NBAS has also been used as a therapeutic intervention tool intended to support the establishment of the first bonds between a newborn and its mother by arousing processes of co-attention between parents and their babies, similar to those it implied with the newborn and the examiner during the assessment. Parents are indeed thought as participants in the assessment process. This offers parents a useful grid for reading and interpreting the social and emotional signals of their newborn during the first month, which is a period of intense adjustment for all members of the family and of relative vulnerability for infants. In this perspective, the use of this tool, when it is well controlled, constitutes a therapeutic support for the establishment of the first emotional bonds between parents and babies (see Chap. 10, Part III).

9.1.2 The CARE-Index [31]

The CARE-Index is a screening tool developed by P. Crittenden [20, 31] that identifies risk for distorted early relations by evaluating the quality of adult-infant interaction. This tool is based on the Dynamic-Maturational Model (DMM) of attachment theory [32]. The assessment provided by the CARE-Index focuses on adult sensitivity in a dyadic context. Through this assessment format, Crittenden highlights the idea that sensitivity is not an individual characteristic of the parents but rather a characteristic of a specific relationship, suggesting thus that an adult could display different degrees of sensitivity with different children. In this sense, it is truly a dyadic assessment tool, evaluating the "goodness of fit" between adult and infant. It focuses on the interpersonal quality and meaning of behaviours of both adult and infant. Indeed, it describes the attitude of each partner towards the other and thus enables the identification of possible maternal dysfunctions at the origin of future maltreatment or negligence towards the child.

This tool can also serve as a guide for an intervention plan and as a tool for the process of intervention itself. The CARE-Index provides insight into the nature of child-centred adult behaviour and of the child ability to participate. These insights can help focus intervention [32]. Moreover, within the process of intervention, video-recorded interactions are viewed during replay sessions with the adults. Video feedback constitutes an invaluable framework within which families can think about their interactions with their child, analysing them with supportive guidance in order to develop their own observational skills and adaptive behavioural repertoires. Video interaction guidance is now well recognized by practitioners the world over [33].

This assessment tool can be used with children from birth to 15 months of age, and, in an adapted format, with toddlers up until 2.5 years of age. The parent (or other adult caregiver) is asked to play freely with the infant for at least 3 min, though the play session can be longer as long as it respects the natural length of interactions for the age of the infant's age-appropriate needs and abilities. Videotaping can be done in different contexts such as in the home environment, in a clinical setting or at a research laboratory. Coding is done in real time and thus does not involve microanalysis of behaviour.

The CARE-Index has been applied to the general population and to at-risk populations such as adolescent mothers [34], substance-abusing mothers [35] and mothers with other psychiatric disorders [36].

The CARE-Index focuses on seven aspects of adult and infant behaviour: facial expression, vocal expression, position and body contact, expression of affection, pacing of turns, control and choice of activity. Scores are given separately to adult and infant, but by definition the rating of the behaviour of one partner is performed in the context of the other partner's behaviour. The different scores are combined to generate 7 subscale scores, namely, sensitivity, control and unresponsiveness for the adult; cooperation, compulsivity, difficulty and passivity for infants from birth to 15 months; and cooperativeness, compulsiveness, threatening coerciveness and disarming coerciveness from 15 to 30 months of age [37]. For each scale, the scores range from 0 to 14. A 0 sensitivity score refers to perilous insensitivity, a score of 7 refers to a sensitivity norm, and 14 suggests remarkable sensitivity. It is important to note that extensive training, with practice and reliability tests, is needed in order to use the CARE-Index in both clinical and research settings.

9.1.3 The Parent-Child Early Relational Assessment (PCERA; Clark [24])

The PCERA is designed to assess the quality and tone of parent-infant interactions. This scale was included in the present non-exhaustive review because of its specific theoretical basis. Indeed, the postulate underlying the PCERA is inspired by both Vygotsky's work and his well-known concept of the zone of proximal development [38], and Mary

Ainsworth's attachment theory [39]. It assesses the behavioural style and affective quality of an interaction [40]. In this perspective, parents are considered as having a regulatory role in infant development, and attention is paid to the parents' experience of the child, to the child's experience of the parents, to the affective and behavioural characteristics that they each bring to the interaction and to the tone or quality of the interaction.

The PCERA was initially developed to assess the quality of mother-child interaction with mothers presenting psychiatric disorders [41]. The tool has been further modified, and the present version can be used with infants and children from 2 to 60 months of age in interaction with the mother or the father. It can be used with both high-risk children populations (premature infants, children with developmental delays) and high-risk parent populations (adolescent parents, parents with substance abuse problems), as well as with a normative sample [24, 40, 42].

The quality of the interaction is assessed from four videotaped situations lasting 5 min each: feeding, structured task, free play and separation/reunion. These situations provide four windows enabling exploration of how parent and child communicate. Indeed, each situation is likely to be experienced differently, with some eliciting feelings of competence in the parenting role and others eliciting conflictual feelings. The first situation is the feeding one during which the parent is told to behave as he/she usually does with the child. After this feeding or snack time, parent and child are invited to participate in a structured task which varies according to the child's age: under 7 months the parent is asked to change a diaper and capture the baby's attention with a rattle; between 8 and 12 months, the parent is asked to hide a toy under a cup; and from 13 months onwards the parent is asked to build a tower with wooden blocks. For the free play situation that comes after, the parent is asked to choose toys among a set of toys and to play freely with the child. In the last situation, the separation/reunion, the parent leaves the child alone for a few minutes and then returns. The PCERA includes scales that evaluate the child (30 domains), the parent (29 domains) and the dyad (8 domains). The child domains included in this assessment are mood/affect, behaviour/adaptive abilities, activity level, regulatory capacities, communication and motoric competences. Parent domains are expressed affect and mood, expressed attitude towards child, affective and behavioural involvement with child and parenting style. Dyadic domains are affective quality of interaction, mutuality and sense of security in relationship with the parent. Ratings are made on a five-point Likert scale for each domain, with prior training to rating being recommended.

This assessment highlights both areas of strength and concern in the parent, the child and the dyad, and it can be used as part of an initial diagnostic evaluation to define relationship issues and to focus intervention as well as to follow the dyad at different moments during clinical care. Moreover, the videotapes are viewed with the parent during a video replay session in order to assess the parents' perceptions, attitudes and goals during each situation.

9.1.4 A Guide-Book for Assessing the Dialogue Between the Adult and the Child (GEDAN; Roten and Fivaz-Depeursinge [21])

Created in 1992 by Roten and Fivaz-Depeursinge, the GEDAN is a guide for assessing the quality of adult-infant interaction. It is inspired by microanalytic observations of adult-infant interactions through a systems approach. According to this approach, an interaction can be analysed from two complimentary perspectives; on the one hand, the interaction is seen as a unitary system, and on the other hand its internal organization is taken into account by paying attention to the respective contributions of each individual composing the system.

This tool can be used with infants in their first semester of life, from 5 to 6 weeks up to 6 months of age. The adult (mother, father or stranger) and infant are placed in a face-to-face situation, and the adult is asked to play freely with the infant, while they are video recorded. The dyad can also be recorded in a feeding or diaper change context, with minor modifications to the procedure. This tool has been widely used with both healthy dyads and at-risk populations [21]. The assessment is made in real time from the video recordings that can last up to 6 min, and it consists of multiple choice questions that describe the behaviours of each partner.

As stated above, the GEDAN considers both the dyadic unit and the contributions of the individuals composing it. In order to do so, the observer focuses attention on the degree of engagement of both partners. This leads to an evaluation of the dyad's interactional mode, from three main interactive dimensions, namely, position, posture and visuofacial features.

The coding and analysis of these dimensions in space and time make it possible to classify the dyad on a scale of dyadic engagement. The categories of the scale are located on a continuum ranging from sufficiently predictable engagement and adjusted to dialogue to rigidly unadjusted disengagement. Adult-infant interactions are characterized according to three modes: consensual, conflictual and paradoxical.

Within the consensual mode, the partners are engaged at all levels (position, posture, visuofacial features); dialogue appears possible and is observed. In the conflictual mode, the adult organizes the bodily and visuofacial context specific to the dialogue so that the child has the possibility of engaging or not, the child being able to avert attention to the partner. Dialogue is feasible but does not take place. In the paradoxical mode, dialogue is not possible due to lack of a clear interactive framework that does not allow the predictability of adult behaviours. Indeed, the adult proposes an ambiguous context that does not permit the infant to understand what is expected, fostering disengagement.

It is important to note that prior training in observation is needed to use this tool. Moreover, the authors propose that GEDAN can be useful for both researchers and clinicians, in particular it can serve as a tool for training in the skill of observation [21].

The nature of the information collected with this tool (objective and subjective information, temporal and spatial information, dyadic and individual information) provides a global portrait of the adult-infant interaction.

9.1.5 The Global Rating Scales for Mother-Infant Interactions (GRS; Fiori-Cowley and Murray [22])

The GRS were developed by Fiori-Cowley and Murray [22] to identify interactive specificities of dyads in which the mother had experienced postnatal depression. The GRS are a video-based assessment of the quality of mother-infant interaction and can be applied to infants aged from 2 to 5 months, at home or in a laboratory setting. Mothers are asked to play freely with their infants (as they usually do) but without any toys, during 5 min. This duration of face-to-face exchange is presented by authors as sufficient to rate behaviours of both partners and their interaction.

The GRS evaluate maternal behaviour, infant behaviour and the quality of the overall mother-infant interaction. Maternal behaviour is assessed on four dimensions that describe the degree to which a mother's behaviour is appropriately adjusted to her infant: (1) sensitivity, (2) intrusiveness, (3) remoteness and (4) overt behaviour relevant to clinical levels of depression (such as happiness, energy level, self-absorption and tension). Infant behaviour is coded on three dimensions, describing (1) the infant's positive engagement in the interaction, (2) behaviour on a lively-inert scale and (3) behaviour on a fretful-contented scale. A final dimension assesses the quality of the overall interaction between mother and infant. Each item in each dimension is coded on a Likert scale ranging from 1 to 5, where 5 is the best coding and 1 the least positive one.

The GRS are an easy-to-use and objective tool that allows the detection of specificities of early depressed mother-well infant interactions. It is also adapted to a clinical setting. The ecological dimension of the tool is specifically adjusted to the observation of mother-infant interaction in a familiar context for the dyad. It is well tailored to infants as young as 2 months and offers a quick overview of potential interactive distortions [43].

Although originally developed to assess the differences in mother-infant interaction between groups of women with or without postnatal depression, the scales have also been used with different clinical groups such as mothers with schizophrenia [44] or borderline personality disorder [45].

9.1.6 The Coding Interactive Behaviour (CIB; Feldman [23])

The CIB is the most recent tool of the selection reviewed in this chapter. Developed by Feldman and her colleagues [23], the scale is designed to assess mother-infant, father-infant and caregiver-infant interactions from birth to 36 months of age. The scale focuses on the appreciation of the sequence of interactive behaviours, on the way each partner engages in the exchange and on their respective individual styles. The rationale of the scale is embedded in different theoretical approaches such as Ainsworth's attachment theory [39], Winnicott's concept of "holding" [46], Brazelton's work on neonatal behavioural states [19] and Stern's concept of intermodal affective attunement [47].

The scale includes 43 items evaluating parental or caregiver behaviours, infant behaviours and the dyad as a whole. During the first year of life, six dimensions are assessed: parental sensitivity and intrusiveness, infant's social engagement and withdrawal, dyadic reciprocity and negative states. Two other dimensions are added for infants 2 years and older: parental limit setting and infant's compliance. We will focus here on the first year. The dimension of parental sensitivity measures the way parental behaviours show evidence of responsiveness to infant's needs and behavioural manifestations and includes items such as imitation, visual attention and infant-directed speech. Parental intrusiveness represents the opposite unadjusted behaviours and includes items such as physical manipulation-forcing, intrusion, negative affect/anger and hostility. Infant's social engagement includes observable behaviours such as visual attention, emotions, vocalizations and assessment of tiredness, emotional lability and avoidance. Dyadic reciprocity refers to reciprocity and mutual adjustment and regulation, and the dimension of negative states refers to restriction and stress inside the dyad.

Rating is made on a five-point Likert scale for each item on the basis of a video recording of a parent-infant free play interaction situation. A rating of one represents a weak occurrence of a behaviour or emotion. And a rating of five translates a high level of appearance of that behaviour or emotion in the interaction. Complementary scales were added to take into account other contexts for assessment such as feeding context, family context or premature birth [48, 49]. Moreover, an intensive training to ratings is compulsory, and double-blind rating is recommended. The CIB has been validated in multiple studies and fruitfully applied to different at-risk populations such as premature babies or parents with psychiatric disorders [50–52]. Because the scale can be used throughout infancy, it permits follow-up of dyadic interaction at successive points in time, including the opportunity to assess the impact of clinical care.

9.1.7 Rethinking Clinical Care Through Research on the Development of Interactions: A Comprehensive Approach

As stated above, these tools are indicative of the parent-infant interactive system and its possible risks through the developmental process. Because these tools rely on observation grids with well-defined behaviours, they support structured observation of specific moments of interaction between parents and infants. These observation frameworks can provide information and useful evaluation in a clinical setting: they enable objective assessment of the intersubjective processes that unfold during clinical parent and infant observations. They also offer deeper insight into the interactive regulation system and can serve as a guide for the clinician's interventions, providing means to promote and offer more adapted, non-judgemental clinical care.

Moreover, these tools, with the exception of the NBAS, require video recording and then coding of the interaction between the infant and the adult. Interestingly, video recording alone carries benefits for the clinician. It offers the possibility of watching the video of the interaction many times. Video recording can thus be used to support more comprehensive clinical assessments within professional teams, as a tool to train clinicians and, in some circumstances, as a means to scaffold parenting. And the coding and interpretation of the recorded interaction provided by the validated tools we have reviewed and which are all based on specific observation grids provide an important detailed and circumscribed level of analysis of interactive partners' behaviours.

Watching and coding video recordings might appear time-consuming and of little use at first sight. Indeed, the identification of predefined behaviours requires extensive training (compulsory for most of the tools), i.e. it is time-consuming from the start of the training phase. However, training in observation has long-term benefits in and of itself for both professionals and for caregivers [53]. It also helps to foster a common language based on common knowledge that is worthwhile when considering and evaluating human behaviour.

9.1.8 The Example of Joint Therapy

Proposals for caring interventions during the peripartum begin earlier and earlier and are characterized by a joint interest in the parent, the baby and the interactive "system". Several schools are at the origin of the development of joint parent-infant therapy. In the United States, Selma Fraiberg [54] went into the community to meet the "hard-to-reach" families whom she followed at home. She was a pioneer in introducing systematic short or long-term psychotherapeutic work with mothers and their babies. She stressed in particular how maternal fantasies can invade the functioning of the baby. In France, Serge Lebovici [55] worked on the phantasmagoric interactions and transgenerational mandates that bear on early parent-infant relations, and he developed innovative therapeutic consultation program. In Geneva, Cramer and Palacio-Espasa [56] focussed on the projective identifications of parents in order to identify parental conflicts, and they initiated new forms of short mother-baby therapy.

However, these various therapeutic approaches, although they were developed adaptively for the management of both the mother and the baby, have shown their limitations when a parent presents severe mental illness. Le Nestour et al. [57] have observed that a parent with borderline personality disorder tends to mobilize their therapist in a particular manner, often entailing a loss of focus towards the parent-infant dyad and in favour the parent alone. The team led by Le Nestour at L'Aubier in France decided to set up weekly co-therapy sessions in the presence of two therapists where one therapist focuses attention on observation and exchanges with the adult, centred on the behavioural and phantasmagorical aspects of parental interaction, and the other therapist is "dedicated" to careful observation of the baby. Based on Esther Bick's direct observation method, the second therapist focuses his/her attention on the baby's relationship to both the parent(s) and the therapists. This therapeutic framework allows each partner of the dyad to be taken into account without risk of being excluded from the relationship.

Yet, the co-therapy situation, although it is a step forward to understanding the early functioning of a parent-infant dyad, does not permit a full-scale appreciation of how parent-infant interaction functions in an everyday context. Not only because the clinical setting is not a natural one but also because of the presence of the therapists. The window opened on the parent-infant world by the co-therapy situation could be indeed further enlarged by observing the parent and infant together in a situation with no other identified partners. Given the complexity of the dynamics of interaction, it is hard to observe even with a highly trained view. How can the clinician's observations be enriched and broadened?

9.2 Conclusion

The tools described in this chapter have been elaborated to offer the opportunity to observe what is likely to occur in everyday life between the infant and the parent, that is, in situations that remain intimate and rarely accessible to outsiders. This constitutes another major advantage of their use by clinicians. Early detection of interactive distortion provides a window of opportunity for clinical intervention focused not only on parental or infant symptoms but on the dyad itself.

		Partner				Situation					Context			
	Age	Mother	Father	Caregiver	Stranger	Free play	Structured play	Feeding	Diaper change	Separation/ reunion	Maternity ward	Home	Clinical setting	Research lab
NBAS	Neonate (until 1 month). Premature neonate with APIB	✓	✓	✓	✓						✓	✓	✓	✓
Care Index	0–15 months and 15–30 months (toddler form)	✓	✓	✓		3 min						✓	✓	✓
CIB	Birth to 36 months	✓	✓	✓		✓	✓	✓	✓					
GEDAN	5–6 weeks to 6 months	✓	✓		✓	Up to 6 min		✓	✓					✓
GRMII	2–5 months	✓				5 min						✓	✓	✓
PCERA	2–60 months	✓	✓			5 min	✓	✓		✓				

References

1. Bruner JS (1990) Acts of meaning. Harvard University Press, Cambridge, MA
2. Gratier M, Devouche E (2011) Imitation and repetition of prosodic contour in vocal interaction at 3 months. Develop Psychol 47(1):67–76
3. Reddy V (2008) How infants know minds. Harvard University Press, Cambridge, MA
4. Trevarthen C (1998) The concept of foundations of infant intersubjectivity. In: Bråten S (ed) Intersubjective communication and emotion in early ontogeny. Cambridge University Press, Cambridge, UK, pp 15–47
5. Bakeman R, Adamson LB (1984) Coordinating attention to people and objects in mother-infant and peer-infant interaction. Child Develop 55(4):1278–1289
6. Tronick EZ (1989) Emotions and emotional communication in infants. Am Psychol 44(2):112–119
7. Beebe B, Jaffe J, Markese S, Buck K, Chen H, Cohen P, Feldstein S (2010) The origins of 12-month attachment: a microanalysis of 4-month mother–infant interaction. Attachm Human Develop 12(1–2):3–141
8. Tronick EZ, Cohn JF (1989) Infant-mother face-to-face interaction: age and gender differences in coordination and the occurrence of miscoordination. Child Develop 60(1):85–92
9. Fogel A, Nwokah E, Dedo JY, Messinger D, Dickson KL, Matusov E, Holt SA (1992) Social process theory of emotion: A dynamic systems approach. Soc Dev 1(2):122–142
10. Tronick E (2005) Why is connection with others so critical? The formation of dyadic states of consciousness and the expansion of individuals' states of consciousness: coherence governed selection and the co-creation of meaning out of messy meaning making. In: Nadel J, Muir D (eds) Emotional development. Oxford University Press, New York, pp 293–316
11. Apter G, Devouche E, Gratier M (2011) Perinatal mental health. J Nerv Mental Dis 199(8):575–577
12. Apter G, Devouche E, Garez V, Valente M, Genet MC, Gratier M et al (2016) The still-face: a greater challenge for infants of mothers with borderline personality disorder. J Personal Dis 31(2):156–169
13. Murray L, Fiori-Cowley A, Hooper R, Cooper P (1996) The impact of postnatal depression and associated adversity on early mother-infant interactions and later infant outcome. Child Develop 67(5):2512–2526
14. Reck C, Hunt A, Fuchs T, Weiss R, Noon A, Moehler E et al (2004) Interactive regulation of affect in postpartum depressed mothers and their infants: an overview. Psychopathology 37(6):272–280
15. Weinberg KM, Olson KL, Beeghly M, Tronick EZ (2006) Making up is hard to do, especially for mothers with high levels of depressive symptoms and their infant sons. J Child Psychol Psychiat 47(7):670–683
16. Sander L (1980) Investigation of the infant and its caregiving environment as a biological system. In: Greenspan SI, Pollock GH (eds) The course of life: psychoanalytic contributions toward understanding personality development, Vol. 1. Infancy and early childhood. Mental Health Study Center, Division of Mental Health Service Programs, National Institute of Mental Health, U.S. Dept. of Health and Human Services, Public Health Service, Alcohol, Drug Abuse, and Mental Health Administration, Adelphi, MD, pp 177–202
17. Tronick E, Beeghly M (2011) Infants' meaning-making and the development of mental health problems. Am Psychol 66(2):107–119
18. Field T, Healy B, Goldstein S, Perry S, Bendell D, Schanberg S et al (1988) Infants of depressed mothers show "depressed" behavior even with nondepressed adults. Child Develop 59(6):1569–1579
19. Brazelton TB (1973) Neonatal behavioral assessment scale. Lippincott, Philadelphia
20. Crittenden PM (1985) Maltreated infants: vulnerability and resilience. J Child Psychol Psych 26(1):85–96
21. Roten Y, Fivaz-Depeursinge E (1992) Un guide pour l'évaluation du dialogue adulte-nourrisson (GEDAN). La Psych L'enfant 35(1):157–195

22. Fiori-Cowley A, Murray L (1996) Global ratings for mothers-infant interactions at two and four months. Winnicott Research Unit, University of Reading, Department of Psychology, Reading, UK
23. Feldman, R. (1998). Coding interactive behavior manual. Unpublished manual.
24. Clark R (1985) The parent-child early relational assessment: instrument and manual. University of Wisconsin Medical School, Department of Psychiatry, Madison
25. Lotzin A, Lu X, Kriston L, Schiborr J, Musal T, Romer G, Ramsauer B (2015) Observational tools for measuring parent–infant interaction: a systematic review. Clin Child Family Psychol Rev 18(2):99–132
26. Weinberg MK, Tronick E (1994) Beyond the face: an empirical study of infant affective configuration of facial, vocal, gestural, and regulatory behaviors. Child Develop 65:1503–1515
27. Weinberg MK, Tronick E (1996) Infant affective reactions to the resumption of maternal interaction after the still face. Child Develop 67:905–914
28. Brazelton TB, Nugent JK, Bruschweiler-Stern N (2001) Echelle de Brazelton: évaluation du comportement néonatal. Médecine & hygiène
29. Als H, Lester BM, Tronick EZ, Brazelton TB (1982) Toward a research instrument for the assessment of preterm infants' behavior (APIB). In: Theory and research in behavioral pediatrics. Springer, Boston, pp 35–132
30. Brazelton TB, Nugent JK (1995) Neonatal behavioral assessment scale. Cambridge University Press, Cambridge, MA
31. Crittenden PM (1979–2004) CARE-index: coding manual. Unpublished manuscript, Miami, FL. Available from the author
32. Crittenden PM (2005) Teoria del l'attaccamento, psicopatologia e psicoterapia: l'approccio dinamico maturativo. Psicoterapia 30:171–182
33. McPheat G (2013) Video interaction guidance: a relationship-based intervention to promote attunement, empathy and Well-being. Practice 25(5):369–370
34. Pacquette D, Bigras M, Zoccolillo M, Tremblay R, Labelle M-È, Azar R (2001) Comparison de la sensibilité parentale entre des mères adolescentes et des mères adultes peu scolarisées. Revue de Psychoéducation et d'Orientation 30(2):283–298
35. Ciotti F, Lambruschi F, Pittino B, Crittenden P (1998) La valutazione della relazione precoce madre-bambino in una popolazione di madri con una storia di tossicodipendenza attraverso l'uso del CARE-Index. Psicoterapia Cognitiva e Comportamentale 4:53–59
36. Mullick M, Miller LJ, Jacobsen T (2001) Insight into mental illness and child maltreatment risk in mothers with major psychiatric disorders. Psych Services 52(4):488–492
37. Hautamäki, A., Mothers and infants. in Farnfield, S., & Holmes, P. (Eds.). (2014). The Routledge handbook of attachment: assessment. New York, NY, US: Routledge/Taylor & Francis Group
38. Vygotsky L (1978) Interaction between learning and development. In: Cole M, John-Steiner V, Scribner S, Souberman E (eds) Mind in society. Harvard University Press, Cambridge, MA, pp 79–91
39. Ainsworth M (1979) Infant-mother attachment. Am Psychol 34(10):932–937
40. Clark R (1999) The parent-child early relational assessment: a factorial validity study. Edu Psychol Measure 59(5):821–846
41. Musick JS, Clark R, Cohler BJ (1981) The mothers' project: a clinical research program for mentally ill mothers and their young children. In: Weissbourd B, Musick J (eds) The social and caregiving environments of infants. NAEYC, Washington, DC, pp 111–127
42. Clark R, Paulson A, Conlin S (1993) Assessment of developmental status and parent infant relationships: the therapeutic process of evaluation. In: Zeanah C (ed) The handbook of infant mental health. Guilford, New York, pp 191–209
43. Zarate-Guerrero G, Devouche E, Espinosa-Gómez C, Apter G (2013) Comment évaluer les difficultés interactives entre une mère déprimée et son bébé de 3 mois à partir d'un jeu libre? Neuropsych L'Enfance L'Adolesc 62(1):47–52
44. Riordan D, Appelby L, Faragher B (1999) Mother-infant interaction in post-partum women with schizophrenia and affective disorders. Psychol Med 29:991–995

45. Crandell LE, Patrick MP, Hobson RP (2003) Still-face'interactions between mothers with borderline personality disorder and their 2-month-old infants. Br J Psych 183(3):239–247
46. Winnicott DW (1960) The theory of the parent-infant relationship. Int J Psycho-Anal 41:585–595
47. Stern D (1985) The interpersonal world of the child. A view from psychoanalysis and developmental psychology. Basic Books, New York
48. Keren M, Feldman R (2002) Le rôle de l'évaluation des interactions lors du repas dans l'évaluation psychopathologie usuelle du jeune enfant. Devenir 14(1):5–16
49. Silberstein D, Feldman R, Gardner J, Karmel B, Kuint J, Geva R (2009) The mother-infant feeding relationship across the first year and the development of feeding difficulties in low-risk premature infants. Infancy 14(5):501–525
50. Feldman R, Eidelman AI (2003) Direct and indirect effects of maternal milk on the neurobehavioral and cognitive development of premature infants. Develop Psychobiol 43(2):109–119
51. Feldman R, Eidelman AI (2007) Maternal postpartum behavior and the emergence of infant-mother and infant-father synchrony in preterm and full-term infants: the role of neonatal vagal tone. Develop Psychobiol 49(3):290–302
52. Keren M, Feldman R, Tyano S (2001) Diagnoses and interactive patterns of infants referred to a community-based infant mental health clinic. J Am Acad Child Adoles Psych 40(1):27–35
53. Trowell J, Miles G (2012) Evaluation of the application of infant observation in the training of frontline professionals working with children and families. In: Urwin C, Sternberg J (eds) Infant observation and research: emotional processes in everyday lives. Routledge/Taylor & Francis Group, New York, NY, US, pp 33–43
54. Fraiberg S, Fraiberg L (1980) Clinical studies in infant mental health: The first year of life. Basic Books
55. Lebovici, S. (1989). L'évaluation des interactions précoces entre le bébé et ses partenaires. Eshel; Médecine et Hygiène
56. Cramer B, Palacio Espasa F (1993) La pratique des psychothérapies mères-bébés. Études cliniques et techniques (The practice of mother-infant psychotherapies. Clinical and technical studies). Presses Universitaires de France, Paris
57. Le Nestour A, Apter G, Heroux C, Mourgues B, Patouillot-Slatine I (2007) Parentalités limites et prises en charge thérapeutiques. La psychiatrie de l'enfant 50(1):125–177

The NBAS: Supporting the Newborn and Its Family at Birth

10

Drina Candilis-Huisman

Originally a pediatrician, but enlightened by his psychoanalytical training and his knowledge of empirical research on early interactions (very novel at that time), Brazelton wanted to encourage the medical world, especially neonatologists and pediatricians in maternity wards, to change their views about the newborn and therefore about its family and the way it would reorganize around the newborn after birth.

This, according to Brazelton, had two direct consequences: on the one hand, to consider the baby as an interactive partner from the start and, on the other hand, if the establishment of the first ties between a baby and its parents did not go as well as hoped for, not to stick to the dogma of exclusive parental responsibility and specifically not to stigmatize mothers. The demonstration of deep individual differences, whose effects are expressed as early as the first moments after birth, made him realize that infants may actively participate in fostering interactive dysfunctions. With this new and essential idea in mind, T. B. Brazelton became concerned with making parents more familiar with their infant's specific features, thus enhancing and supporting finer adaptation to their baby.

According to Brazelton, developed countries have completely entrusted the care of their child to health professionals. This has somehow undermined parents who have lost confidence in their child's inner competencies and resources and possibly also in their own. This actually highlights how Winnicott, in his BBC radio talks, used to remind parents and families in postwar Britain that babies are ready to interact from the start and that parents might intuitively know best, or at least *well enough*, how to communicate with and care for them [1].

This chapter draws on my experience as a Brazelton trainer, certified by the Brazelton Center at the Children's Hospital in Harvard, Boston, and my practice as a clinical psychologist in perinatal care. For a complete description in French, see a book entitled *Rencontre avec T. B. Brazelton, Que nous apprennent les nourrissons*? (Editions Eres, Toulouse, 2011) [2].

D. Candilis-Huisman (✉)
Université Paris Diderot, Paris, France

© Springer Nature Switzerland AG 2019

G. Apter et al. (eds.), *Early Interaction and Developmental Psychopathology*,
https://doi.org/10.1007/978-3-030-04769-6_10

Early observation of the newborn consists in relying on the child's ability to restore parental self-esteem based on their own intuitive knowledge, one that might have been partly "confiscated" by the technical medical world. This ambitious approach was based on Brazelton's considerable knowledge of the already complex organization of a neonate at birth and his will to share this knowledge during the examination carried out in the presence of and for the parents. The Brazelton examination (original name of the NBAS) requires a practioner who has expertise in newborn competencies and is able to share it with the parents. The practitioner must thus willingly agree to a partnership with the parents, supporting their observations and feelings during the examination and valuing and respecting their knowledge about the needs of their baby.

Observation of the baby fosters a form of alliance between parents and clinician, and the days following birth are a favorable period to form strong alliances. As captured in the fairy tale *Sleeping Beauty*, the acts and words of each person over the cradle take on a unique meaning and power.

Observation of the newborn child thus achieves two major goals. First, it increases interest in the baby inspiring better training of clinicians involved in the examination of newborns and upholding the opportunity for more scientific research and knowledge about the neonate. Second, it encourages early preventive intervention aimed at minimizing later developmental and emotional disorders which is harder to manage once solidly established.

By taking an interest in very early life, T.B. Brazelton unhesitatingly links the observation of the child to the clinician's way of interacting with the infant as a sort of personal commitment on the part of the clinician. It is necessary to go "in search of the baby" with all that one has got: one's body and one's emotions included, in order to "enter the dance" that the examination represents. Then, practitioners must be capable of accepting the baby's guidance, letting it play and lead. Being able to maintain renewed wonder and astonishment in the adult-child exchange with every new infant is essential. This allows the clinician to grasp the infinite diversity of individual differences. In fact, Brazelton insists on the necessity to endorse the child's own ability to find within himself/herself the resources necessary to fuel his/her developmental needs. He also emphasizes the emotional impact for the clinician and the parents of the specifics of every birth process and its consequences for the family and its internal relationships. To try to acknowledge and understand the child as he/she is per se and to accept him/her without preconception becomes the practitioner's guideline; and this is extremely useful in the case of vulnerable children (premature or disabled) or with infants born in cultural or social contexts unfamiliar to the practitioner.

10.1 The Construction of the Scale and Its Principles

The first scale was developed in 1973. Five main characteristics distinguished it from the other assessment approaches available at that time [3].

First and foremost, from the very beginning, the NBAS was underpinned by the idea that the newborn is a complex organism. It hypothesized that the newborn is capable of protecting itself from negative stimuli, that it has the capacity to control (some of) its motor responses in order to make them available for response to external stimuli, and, finally, that the neonate is able to solicit stimuli in the environment, this being a vital necessity to fuel development at all levels, motor, emotional, social, and cognitive.

Secondly, one of the main aims of the child's examination is to provide the optimal conditions to obtain the "best performance" possible. This implies that the examiner has undergone thorough training and will be able to repeatedly provide a reliable enhanced assessment, thus letting parents be aware of the infant's visible "best" capacities. This consequently links the quality of the examiner's training with the quality of the child's examination, i.e., the better the child performs, the better the examiner is rated. This completely distinguishes the scale from any objective approach to an infant's behavior. It is indeed the clinician's intersubjectivity that is at the forefront, one that is carefully and continually put to test by repeated use of the scale with a clinician who is also trained to teach.

Thirdly, the baby's behavioral responses guide the order of administration of the items on the scale. The entire examination aims to entice the infant from an active sleeping state to a calm awakened one, then to a less available state, such as a crying state, and finally to bring it back to a quiet awake state. The line of the examination thus follows a sort of ascending and descending pattern. This of course would seem to depend on the infant. However, it also means that the examiner's ability to follow the child's moves and adequately elicit state changes from stimulation to soothing is put to test.

Fourthly, the examiner must know how to use the infant's specific characteristics, insofar as they enable or prevent a certain quality of response. Actions and reactions of a child strongly depend on its state of alertness. The state of a baby reflects both its availability to the outside world and its response to what is perceived of it. T.B. Brazelton sometimes uses the metaphor of the interface to describe what goes on between the infant and himself. This interface is capable of both transmitting and receiving external or internal information depending on how infant alertness status can filter this material. Thus, for example, it is pointless to propose orientation items (gaze tracking of an object or moving toward a sound source) if the infant has not, even briefly, reached an awakened state.

And lastly, it becomes understandable that the aim of the examination is not to rate a performance positively or negatively. This would have a disastrous impact on parents. It is meant to be an analysis of the child's response strategies to what is being offered within its own particular context. A highly trained clinician is able to summarize and present a developmental profile, obtained thanks to answers grouped in general clusters, and thus give insight on how an infant might be on at risk trajectory rather than poised to follow a typical course of development. The assessment accurately describes each item on the scale with nine different scores per item. This has at least two advantages. One is that this enforces reliability between examiners, and the other is that infants are observed with minute detail instead of recorded average performances. The result is that it reduces the risk of flattening out individual differences, including specific strengths and potentials.

The guidelines, defined in the 1970s, have never varied since, although several reviews of the scale have updated it to comply with novel scientific knowledge and have thus adjusted the diagnostic and clinical scope of the examination. Changes were first undertaken in 1984 [4] and then in 1995 [5] in order to improve the scale in two directions:

1. To offer a clearer understanding of an infant's strengths and vulnerabilities.
2. To place greater importance on the qualitative part of the assessment by integrating the examiner's subjective experience and his/her empathic movements.

With the "eight additional items" in the last version, the examiner establishes the quality of the baby's attention, how durable it can be, the confidence it inspires, and specifically if the infant is able to elicit an adult's attention. This is a much more subjective approach to the infant as an individual. It attempts to summarize the level of the intersubjective exchanges that the newborn shows itself capable of. This is considered to reflect its level of maturity.

10.2 The Scale and Its Added Touchpoints: Environment as a Window to the Antenatal Period

In spite of the giant steps that research has accomplished thanks to ultrasound exploration, intrauterine life is captured only in the aftermath of its effects. It has been coined the "first chapter" of life, but full term gestation is still necessary to fully apprehend the givens of the human infant.

Some prerequisites are necessary to use the NBAS. It is essential to take gestational age into account in order to analyze the quality of the assessment. The minimum threshold for a baby to be examined using the scale is 37-week gestational age (i.e., definition of a full-term infant). For an infant under 37-week GA at birth, the items will be too demanding, and therefore the evaluation will lack validity and reliability. Information about health issues in pregnancy, such as maternal malnutrition, addictive behaviors (i.e., abuse of toxics, alcohol, drugs, tobacco, etc.), and existence of at-risk conditions during pregnancy whether due to maternal illness (pre-eclampsia, gestational diabetes) or infections directly affecting the fetus (toxoplasma, cytomegalovirus, etc.), needs to be included in order to adequately use the NBAS. And of course, information related to birth and delivery is equally crucial. All of these elements will impact neonatal behavior at birth. During pregnancy, the manner in which each fetus develops will be unique resulting at birth in a specific way of responding to the intersubjective world the infant encounters.

In utero development marks a vital period for the construction of the neonate as an already unique individual. The infant could be considered the product of an epigenetic evolution in which, from its conception, embryonic biological development interacts with the uterine environment, including the placenta and its multiple characteristics. Therefore, far from seeing the baby as a tabula rasa or as a brand new being, one could consider that it is the result of complex interactions that are difficult to examine before birth. Metaphorically, this means that, well before birth, the infant has been endowed with genetic and epigenetic material, a family, and a cultural background and therefore that it is already engaged in a personal trajectory.

Careful consideration should therefore be given to pregnancy. It is a window of opportunity to start working with parents on their representations of their future child. T.B. Brazelton considers such opportunities offered to future parents as the first step of his touchpoint program (for detail of touchpoints program, see Brazelton [6]). According to Brazelton and Sparrow, touchpoints are periods during the first years of life when children's development reaches a transformational acceleration that can disrupt the family as a system, due to the necessity to quickly adapt to the infant's developmental acceleration and transformation [6, 7].

Pregnancy is thus considered the first of the 13 touchpoints they have identified, highlighting the importance of preparation and support of upcoming parenthood before the infant's birth. This first meeting between parents and clinician, which occurs in the last weeks of pregnancy, offers a unique opportunity to recognize parental misgivings, potential fears, and the ambivalence they may feel about the arrival of the baby and to support them and to promote reflection around the fetus, and future newborn, and its skills. These consultations are unfortunately rarely implemented during pregnancy. They could provide a very interesting opportunity for prevention. In this manner, parents could be better prepared to acknowledge infants' needs and to cope with them. It might also add more resources to what is often felt as helplessness on the part of parents and lower their sense of unpreparedness or of lurching into the unknown when their child is born.

10.2.1 The Scale: A Witness to the Upheaval of Birth

More than ever, we have to remember that "a baby does not exist alone," not only because of its "absolute dependence" but also because, at all levels of its personal organization, the baby is programmed to find external support, in order to discover and be able to make use of its own internal motives and abilities. In other words, an infant depends on other people, not so much to act on his/her behalf or to do things for him/her, but rather to provide crucial opportunities that will enable him/her to rely on his/her own internal resources. Missing this point means that infants can become overwhelmed and silenced by overly knowledgeable partners who do not acknowledge and accept his or her role in fostering and building intersubjective relations.

Thus, contrary to what one usually thinks, newborn assessment is not so much a matter of evaluating the "skills" of a newborn baby; but rather a matter of giving oneself a tool to identify the strengths and vulnerabilities of a child confronted with an adult who seeks to provide him/her with the most suitable support for his/her capabilities during examination.

The observation of the newborn is based on a dynamic and hierarchical organization according to the following levels:

- **The neurovegetative system**, i.e., the identification of changes in the color of the skin, in involuntary movements such as jerks, and tremulations, in other words in what constitutes a very primitive form of protective shield. For this, one needs to also look for signs of stress: increased respiratory frequency, hiccups, regurgitations, yawning; all these autonomic behaviors require that the examiner take a pause and adapts to the baby, in order to respect the infant's rhythm and capacity to maintain attention, or to retreat and to take into account each infant specifically.
- **The tonic-motor system**, which assesses the tone as well as the quality of motor behavior, is obviously at the forefront of the evaluation of a child's maturity. Soft, controlled, and harmonious movements contribute to give parents an image of the infant as an individual in control and thus a sense of confidence in their infant. On the contrary, a baby with jerky movements or whose gestures seem to "go beyond his goal" (e.g., if the infant's hand seems to be released into nowhere) can confuse his/her parents who will find him/her "nervous" or who will somehow sense his/her fragility. The tonic system is also involved in the manner in which infants relate. So much so, that Ajuriaguerra spoke of the "tonic-emotional dialogue" to characterize the deep feelings shared by the mother and baby when being held [8].
- **The state of alertness regulation and organization of the system**. In newborn babies, six different states of alertness can be observed: two states of sleep that are cyclic, an intermediate state between wake and sleep (drowsiness), and finally three awake states (quiet awake, active awake, crying). How a baby reacts is assessed as the test moves forward. Will he/she wake up gradually or suddenly? Will he/she start crying? How will he/she self-comfort? Finally, does this child show a certain stability in his/her behavior, or does he/she have difficulty channeling his/her excitement in order to reach a quiet awake state appropriate for interaction? He/she will then develop strategies to regulate either by falling asleep in an untimely manner or by taking refuge in crying that is difficult to control, which are two different styles of breaking off from the outside world that reveal his/her vulnerability. However, tears are also an expression of the vitality of a baby especially if they are not the only recourse it has. The examiner is also concerned with the robustness of crying and the quality of sleep. It is not uncommon that during a 20-min examination, a baby crosses the six states on several occasions. The assessment of the organization and regulation of the states of alertness take into account both the qualitative aspect of each state and their quantitative manifestations.
- **The orientation and interaction system**. Auditory and visual capacities are a form of presence in the world that brings the newborn child closer to the adult communication system. A baby follows a moving face or object and tracks it when it moves along a vertical axis. He/she turns his/her head in the direction of a sound or a voice as if to search for it and fixes his/her gaze on the sound source

when he/she locates it. This visual activity mobilizes a motor and tonic resources, which for a short period help focus the baby's activity on the external mode. He/she can even send his/her arm toward the visual or sound source, as if to reach for it. The newborn also mobilizes all its other sensory channels (olfaction, touch) in a way more or less identifiable by the adult, in search of anchoring and thus of primitive recognition by the partner.

Orientation capacities can be deployed only on condition that the three preceding subsystems are in balance with one another, not in a homeostatic way as assumed by the Freudian hypothesis of primary narcissism but permanently in two minds: This makes the environment or the other person a support for the expression of the personal abilities of the baby.

The work of the examiner is to **"simplify" the world for the baby** by "questioning" him/her in a simple and rigorous way about his/her abilities. Paradoxically, this means the examiner tries to be in a position that is essentially receptive to the movements of the baby. This emphasizes the importance of the environment for the baby at the beginning of life and the fact that this interactive dance with a partner must leave the baby free to play his/her own game. The adult partner must exercise continuous empathy toward all the infant's sensory dimensions during the interaction. This positioning on the part of the examiner is very different from a purely experimental or simply medical evaluation approach. Above all, it is based on the state the baby is in during the assessment and the visible modifications as the examination sequence unravels. Acting on the environment to bring the world within reach of the more vulnerable infants is one of the major lessons that the Brazelton assessment scale teaches us for everyday practice.

10.2.2 The Scale Seen Through a Clinical Illustration

After the invisible intimacy of what goes on during pregnancy, between the body of the mother (to-be) and her fetus/baby (to-be), birth can be seen as a disruption: the mother will need to rapidly discover the new little human being that she has dreamed of and perhaps imagined, with or without the support of the ultrasound image; recognizing the real infant in front of her with its innate capacity to entice the outside world, grip and retain its proximity in order to survive. This is the first major asymmetry, after the separation of physical birth, that early relationship aims to rectify. Being together, but separately, is the challenge that the dyad is faced with. They will build life as a pair, replacing the intimacy of pregnancy by a proximity made of smell, touch, gaze, and nourishment. Winnicott, in his theory of parent-infant relationships, emphasized the part played by the child and the part played by the parents in the construction of intersubjective relationships [9]. The Brazelton NBAS scale serves as a guideline to try to understand what is happening from the point of view of the threesome involved, the newborn, its parents, and the clinician.

The following clinical consultation will illustrate the complexity of these various interactions:

We have an appointment with Benjamin's family because his mother has already phoned the PMI (Maternal and Child Protection Service) several times during her pregnancy and since the baby was born. She needs to share her various difficulties and asks for advice. The nurse, even though she has never met the mother, suggests that she comes to assess the baby with the Brazelton scale, in a framework that is generally offered for first appointments.

During these first meetings with the parents, consultations last an hour on average, often longer. A sufficient amount of time necessary for a complete examination of the baby and touchpoint/supportive dialogue with the family needs to be planned. It is not uncommon afterward to offer a follow-up, regardless of how far away the families' homes are. This first, apparently very ordinary, consultation will show how the observation of the baby's behavior gives insight about the infant's state and how it interacts with his/her mother and family. It also allows us to respond to and discuss the parents' questions.

Benjamin is 3 weeks old. His parents are both in their thirties and very proud of their first baby. The father seems to be extremely sensitive to his son and observes him carefully. The parents present very differently. The father is wearing a suit; he seems to have taken time off work to come to the consultation. The mother is in jeans and seems quite casual. She looks younger than her age. She says she does not really know what awaits her (she appears unclear about what to expect from the consultation).

The baby is in a crib, nicely dressed in soft woolens. At 3 weeks, he has already had several consultations for colic, and the pediatrician has advised medication. These small concerns do not undermine the pride of the father, who mentions the measurements of his boy and the speed of his growth. The mother stands somewhat behind him. I lean over the cradle to introduce myself to the baby, and I see his nostrils expand as if he wants to discriminate by smell who this new person is rather than gaze at the face I am offering him at that moment. The father also notices this and is astonished but smiling. The father puts the infant on the examination table and moves slightly away. With the help of the mother, I delicately undress the child, who is a big, sturdy baby. I notice that his chin and legs tremble, no sooner is he undressed. He has a uniformly colored complexion even though a bit jaundiced; the assessments made at the maternity ward on several occasions have not confirmed this diagnosis. The discussion rapidly moves to the subject of the Caesarean section (that was the infant's mode of delivery) and then to the question of breastfeeding. The father informs me that the baby was put in an incubator just after birth to be warmed and that he had a bottle as his first meal 1 h after birth. I am surprised at this but do not express it, thinking that immediate breastfeeding is a relatively frequent practice but making a note of this unusual behavior. I wonder if, perhaps at that very moment, the staff did not grasp the mother's desire to breastfeed.

The baby is awake. The first interactions are very engaging: the baby shows good grasping reflexes and looks at me intensely. The mother comments on the fact that her baby does not see yet. It is a little more difficult to assess the infant's tone; when I release his arms and legs, he gazes intently at the mobile above his head, completely immobilizing himself. The father then suggests: "It's the mobile that he's looking at." The mother is skeptical due to her past belief. I bring the infant back into a sitting position in front of me, and, there again, he demonstrates great participation by firmly holding his head in a vertical position, wrinkling his forehead with the effort, as if to better mark his concentration on what I'm asking him to do. The mother is very surprised at the intensity of the active presence of the baby. I then try to put him in an upright position. He is at first very straight on his legs, but, contrary to what I had hoped and anticipated, he sat a little when I try to obtain automatic walking. He rests his entire bodyweight on my hands, which support him under his arms, and remains static. Replacing him then on his back in resting position, as gently as possible, triggers Moro bursts, as if he had the unpleasant sensation of being dropped. Then face to face, he looks at me, his gaze follows me with ease, and he seems less interested in sounds or voices. The mother then talks about her fear that the baby be blind; she has a young cousin who was blinded at birth as a result of an infection. She fears that the same thing will happen to her son. I ask her to quietly call her son so that he can turn to the sound of her voice, which is a part of the examination that is usually done during the assessment. She follows my suggestion while saying that he does not recognize her voice, and, to my surprise, she does not call him at any time by his first name or even by calling him baby. She continues to talk to me while waiting for the baby to reorient. I feel caught in a strange paradoxical communication. She finally tells me that she had told me so: the baby cannot do it. And she moves away a little, while the baby begins a clear movement of orientation toward her.

From then on, it is as if I also feel cast of, and when the baby, placed again on the examination table, starts to whine, I feel briefly a little distraught as to how to comfort him. I observe, first of all, that he again attempts and manages new and intense visual encounters, which calm him for a short while without any other intervention on my part. However, this undoubtedly requires too great an effort for him, and he starts thrusting and projecting his arms, which end up finally disorganizing him completely. He then starts to cry. I tell the parents that we will be able to understand together what can be done to comfort him. But here again, the task is more difficult than I had anticipated: neither my voice nor my close contact is sufficient; I must take him in my arms and walk while rocking him. I realize that he pulls away strongly from my shoulder to try to find my eyes and obtain visual contact. He visually clings to the contrasting tiles of the floor and to the toys in the consultation room while searching. The mother, seeing him in pursuit of a visual target that could hold back his tears, associates this with what happens in the evening with her at home, when he is hardly consolable and his gaze is fixed on a red cooking utensil swinging over the fridge, which he watches over her shoulder.

The searching gaze provides only a short-lived consolation, and the mother then offers to breastfeed him, thinking (rightly) that this is the best way to appease him. He quickly finds the nipple, and I observe how he suckles forcefully, his eyes closed, and he is rolled up into a ball in his mother's blouse; his hands are close to his mouth, almost clinging to her breast. There is no eye contact between them but a very close bodily adjustment. Benjamin relaxes and falls asleep, after three brief episodes of suckling.

The discussion with the parents continues for a while. The parents mention how they feel very affectionately surrounded but also stifled by their reciprocal families over two generations. The mother says, halfway through, that her own mother advises her not to give in to the baby even though she notices that her grandmother did exactly the opposite. A form of paradoxical communication played out at a transgenerational level can be noted here and is underlined by the mother herself.

The consultation that was initially requested for breastfeeding and nursing barely addressed these issues. Yet, I would like to defend the idea that the most complete and accurate observation possible of the baby, in the framework I have described, allows us to better approach the unique situation of each child and its family, here Benjamin.

Concerning breastfeeding, which was the original focus here, it must be acknowledged that it constitutes a difficult transition for the mother. It can take place between the second and fourth day after delivery, but obviously it is influenced by what happened during pregnancy and birth, by what happens here and now, and by everything that the baby contributes to it. It is a period of total reorganization for the mother, an acutely chaotic moment that cannot be avoided. Nine women out of ten go through a feeling of wanting to stop breastfeeding because of discomfort, breast pain, or their own anxiety. The role of care providers is to respect this course of action and postpone the start of breastfeeding if this proves to be too difficult. Breastfeeding is not a medical prescription; it is cultural in the broad sense, i.e., a process of humanization. Finally, the fact that Benjamin was not immediately breastfed after birth is easier to understand retrospectively, when one considers the dynamics of this examination and consultation. On several occasions, I connected (empathized, identified with) what the baby felt and with what his mother felt with her relatives, as she was able to describe it at the end of the consultation. That is to say, I acknowledged a mixture of presence and absence on the part of the parent, which I have called here paradoxical communication.

10.3 Comments and Analysis of the Clinical Vignette Through the NBAS and More

In her lessons on the psychoanalytic observation of babies, Esther Bick's ideas offer a valuable insight into the place of breastfeeding in the beginning of children's psychological life. She wrote in 1967 [10]:

My thesis is that, in their primitive state, the parts of the personality are felt to have no binding force between them and therefore must be held together passively through the skin functioning as a border (…). This internal function of containing the parts of self depends on the introjection of an external object experienced as capable of fulfilling this function. It seems fairly obvious that the experience of suckling as a prototype of the introjection of the object plays a central role in this experience of an object capable of performing this function.

Thus, shivers, sneezing, and disorganized movements in the baby (which can also be included under the heading "stress signs" in Brazelton's terminology) are moments of non-integration (disorganized/reorganizing states) in a baby, and efforts should be made to observe how he/she experiences them and tries to readjust and adapt. For Esther Bick, they decrease when the mother tolerates closer contact with the baby at times when the baby has no immediate needs.

I find this idea very interesting when considering Benjamin and his parents and how worried the mother is that the baby in front of her will not look at her nor hear her, thus failing to reassure her. She can bury him in the warmth of her body and feel that he is always able to suckle even if she is in doubt concerning other sensory interactions. I pointed out to the parents that Benjamin is a baby who has put on more than a kilo in 3 weeks, which made his father very proud and also demonstrates the mother's investment and competence in the activity of feeding. She started talking to me while showing herself capable of this very close intimate bodily contact during feeding. Similarly, she spoke to me while waiting for the baby to turn to her during the orientation tests. Perhaps this could help us hypothesize some of the aspects linked to the baby being "colicky" and how he has difficulty falling asleep at night. There are moments when he experiences an increase in his states of non-integration, and the mother ails to provide him with an answer other than through breastfeeding. The more he is fed, the more he becomes at risk of increasing the colic linked to larger quantities of food that are the sole way found to respond to Benjamin's stress.

A little later in her article, Esther Bick talks about a baby who strongly re-minds us of Benjamin. She writes about a child who seems to grip at his mother though every sensory canal available. She comments that he seems to hold himself or self-contain through gaze, listening, self-touch, and tone, as if all of his sensory energy was concentrated on holding on [10]. At this very early stage, there seems to be no differentiation between sensory responses: they all serve as suction cups for adhesiveness, or in NBAS terms, they are all used for regulating purposes. Esther Bick goes on to point out that the same proximity needs to exist for the mother. She uses the metaphor of the mother being like an astronaut who has lost her space suit during this peripartum period, exploring unknown territories without the proper equipment. This gives importance to the fact that the mother also needs to be nurtured, soothed, and recognized by those around her.

So what does Benjamin tell us when he seeks visual stimulus with such constancy? Probably his need to use visual communication channels as a way to cling to a form of Winnicottian holding, a "containment function" that is insufficient for him at this moment. The mother unravels the same need to be held and to hold onto him. She has difficulty explaining how the appropriate distance and closeness are too complex to establish, oscillating between extreme proximity and body closeness and too much distancing (for Benjamin anyhow) on the other sensory canals such as gaze or voice. It is as if both of them, mother and infant, agree to tell us, "we are doing very well together when we touch and hold but physically separated from one another we are lost." This search for proximity cannot be more natural during this period, so soon after birth. However, the need for closeness can only be satisfied by breastfeeding, both for the infant and its mother; thus rendering any form of physical separation increasingly difficult. We often hear mothers say they are unable to “frustrate the child” and restrain from feeding. Nevertheless, this is in fact quite paradoxical, since this is frustration that is impossible by default, that is to say due to the inability to offer another type of closeness.

But then what about the father? Benjamin’s father is, as can be seen here, extremely available and positively oriented toward the child. He actively observes him and is amused by him; he marvels at his infant and does not doubt what is in front of his eyes. Yet, beyond appearances, even if quite a reassuring figure for the baby, he partly fails to offer a sufficiently reliable environment for the mother. He follows her in her difficult quest to find a soothing link with the baby but cannot guide and steer her toward a larger variation of regulated sensory interactions. I can surmise the father’s delicate position as an external observer when my own demonstrations are objects of interest or of rejection for the mother and for the baby but do not trigger any response on her part.

Psychoanalytic thinking has opened our eyes to the shocking side of the pleasure of suckling for the child and the mother, because of the twofold nature of the breast for both of them, breast for baby and breast for partner, physical virtue of breastfeeding or sexually exciting breast, bosom of tenderness, and breast of passion. Acknowledging what a baby makes us experience during an evaluation supports this point of view. Through the NBAS setting, the extreme strength and consistency of the baby’s behavior in its quest for interactive mutuality and regulation are visible. As is the paradoxical energy that it takes for a woman to become a mother while being more or less prepared for this developmental change.

At a time, when the feeling of failure is anticipated by the mother and often by both parents, the individual characteristics of the baby are readily interpreted by them as a confirmation of their incapacity to offer the infant what it needs. An irritable baby can thus easily reinforce this feeling of failure and have a depressive impact on parents. On the contrary, a baby unencumbered by these preexisting representations can contribute to caring for its parents and underlining its capacities will then enhance parental attitudes. “He looks at me, he recognizes me,” the mother tells herself, gratified.

As we see in the case of Benjamin and his parents, the examination has offered a much more complex picture than one would have had just by observing the manifest behaviors of infant and parent. The examiner’s feelings and the manner in which he or she is able to translate them avoids simply acknowledging the stereotypical “perfect” family image completed by the arrival of a beautiful healthy baby. The parent’s interrogations and their stressful experiences can be shared from the inside, whether they be linked to misunderstandings of themselves and their desires or to those of their representations of their infant’s problems. The baby, on the other hand, uses the unfulfilled parts of his/her vital manifestations to inform the parents of his/her needs and insistently imposes his/her demands. Finally, the assessment using the NBAS becomes a genuine consultation, and this is what we have endeavored to show in this observation.

10.4 To Continue on with the NBAS

The underlying theme of our work is based on the conviction that effective action to support families must be based on the early alliance and long-term support that can be established with them, relying on a network of actors that share common objectives. In our community-based clinic, much of our activity with parents and their children in the first month of life is inspired by the principles developed by the Boston team. Brazelton examinations are offered to primiparous families as a preventive intervention for mothers who are in at-risk situations (risk of maternal depression, single mothers, teenage or very young mothers, couples in low socioeconomic and with low levels of education and integration in the community). Loneliness and helplessness, absence of social support, and isolation have increased in highly dense urban areas, thus heightening the challenges of parenthood and infant daily care. The NBAS scale seems to us a particularly appropriate tool in this endeavor. It can not only can help early identification of potential developmental issues or subtler interactive dysregulation but also support parents in recognizing and acknowledging their early experiences with the infant. Moreover, it allows for shared interventions by professionals and the family and by professionals between themselves (pediatric nurses, doctors, pediatricians, and psychologists). We surmise that good physical development of the child will improve parental self-esteem, dignity, and respect thus providing a better future for all.

References

1. Winnicott DW (1987) Child, the family, and the outside world. Addison-Wesley, Reading, MA
2. Candilis-Hisman D (2011) Rencontre avec T. B. Brazelton. Que nous apprennent les bébés? Éditions Érès, Toulouse
3. Als H, Tronick E, Lester B, Brazelton TB (1977) The brazelton neonatal behavioral assessment scale. J Abnorm Psychol 5(3):215–231
4. Brazelton TB (1984) Neonatal behavioral assessment scale, Clinics in Developmental Medicine, vol 88, 2nd edn. Spastic International Medical Publications, London
5. Brazelton TB, Nugent JK (1995) Neonatal behavioral assessment scale, Clinics in Developmental Medicine, vol 137, 3rd edn. Spastic International Medical Publications. Translated into French by Nadia Bruchsweiler-Stern and Drina Candilis-Huisman/Médecine et Hygiène, London/Geneva
6. Brazelton TB (1992) Touchpoints: emotional and behavioral development. Addison-Wesley, Reading, MA
7. Brazelton TB, Sparrow JD (2001) Touchpoints. Perseus, Cambridge, MA, pp 3–6
8. de Ajuriaguerra J (1985) Organisation neuropsychologique de certains fonctionnements: des mouvements spontanés au dialogue tonico-postural et aux modes précoces de communication. Enfance 2(3):265–277
9. Winnicott DW (1971) La théorie des relations parents-nourrissons. In: Pédiatrie à la psychanalyse. Payot, Paris
10. Bick E (1998) L'expérience de la peau dans les relations d'objet précoces. In: Harris Williams M (ed) Les Ecrits de Martha Harris et Esther Bick. Editions du Hublot, Larmor-Plage, pp 141–152

Early Psychomotor Therapy: Support for Vulnerable Babies and Their Families

11

Aude Buil

Psychomotor care is the youngest paramedical profession in France (the State Diploma was created in 1974). Its exercise is under medical prescription and under the dual supervision of the French Ministry of Health and the French Ministry of Higher Education and Research. This professional discipline stems from the synergistic integration of various developing functions including muscle tone in relation to body movement, sensory perception, emotion, interpersonal relations, and cognition. Synergy here reflects a phenomenon whereby several factors acting together create a greater effect than the sum of the expected effects if they operated independently. This disciplinary approach finds its roots in the work of Wallon [1] and Ajuriaguerra de and Angelergues [2] by placing motor development within a social relational framework and considering it a precursor to language. Throughout life, individuals structure themselves, constructing and modifying their representations on the basis of this functional synergy and of developing relationships and interactions with the environment. In early childhood, psychomotricity evaluates and treats the development and integration of the aforementioned functions in synergy. There are a number of modes of intervention adapted to the particular characteristics of the baby and of the mother-baby relationship, from perinatal hospitalization to the parental home, in an institutional context or in private practice. Treatment in the practice of psychomotricity is concerned with the development of motor functions, language, and interpersonal relationships. It is part of the clinical triad of "evaluating, alerting, and providing support."

A. Buil (✉)
Laboratoire de Psychopathologie et Processus de Santé (LPPS), EA 4057, Neonatal Medicine and Toddler Developmental Center, Descartes University, Paris, France

© Springer Nature Switzerland AG 2019

G. Apter et al. (eds.), *Early Interaction and Developmental Psychopathology*, https://doi.org/10.1007/978-3-030-04769-6_11

11.1 Early Psychomotor Care

The early support provided by the psychomotor therapist is based on the acknowledgment of the synergy of the aforementioned psychomotor functions. A first meeting between psychomotor therapist, baby, and parents often works as a "consultation guidance" aimed at reassuring parents about their skills and responding to their concerns about developmental issues. The psychomotor therapist, together with the parents and through joint observation, determines the level of development reached by the baby. If the need for a therapeutic intervention proves necessary, regular, often weekly, sessions can be set up. Psychomotor monitoring can be carried out separately but is often integrated into a multidisciplinary care framework.

The specificity of psychomotor treatment is its focus on body tonus as a fundamental means by which the infant experiences the world and expresses itself. It is an interface between the internal and external environment. The psychomotor therapist uses body relaxation to improve the attention and concentration capacities of children from the youngest age. In clinical practice, the psychomotor therapist often deals with vulnerable infants who have been hospitalized in the perinatal period following either premature birth or a medical problem (anoxia, cerebrovascular accident, convulsions, etc.) with the risk of brain damage. Most of the time, they present regulation disorders with permanent motor agitation and impulsivity, operating in ON/OFF, all-or-nothing modes. They are constantly agitated and collapse into sleep consisting of micro-naps during the day or only in the evening for the night sleep. In such situations, various strategies can be used to provide support, such as help with sucking, rocking, vibrations (singing, stroller, car, etc.), and body proximity (in the arms).

The parent-child interactional style is intrinsically linked to sensorimotor functions. Children with sensorimotor ON/OFF functioning often have a "compulsive-compliant" pattern associated with mothers with a "controlling" style during the first months. When we meet these mothers during the first years, they also often reveal depressive symptoms. They are physically and psychologically exhausted by a child they fail to understand and who disrupts them in their capacity to be a mother.

This sensorimotor ON/OFF functioning takes root very early in the child's life. In fact, the vulnerable infant struggles to develop its regulatory competence. This is initially a tonic-emotional regulation through the transitions between the different states of alertness. This regulation presupposes a physical control toward an active awake state or, on the contrary, a letting go toward a progressive relaxation when falling asleep. Understanding this function in the light of the syntactic theory of development [3] makes it possible to assess what it entails for the young child and thus provides therapeutic options that cover the following domains: self-regulation, attention/interaction, motricity, states of consciousness, and physiology. Support provided by the psychomotor therapist helps children to reduce their (hyper) vigilance to the environment, to let go of their body weight and to reduce their speed of movement, to fall into drowsiness and then sleep, and finally to slow down their heart and respiratory rhythm.

Early tonic disorders, even transient ones, can permanently hinder interactions and relationships, development of the body pattern, and self-confidence (children's control of their bodies undermined by poorly controlled motor skills).

11.2 Psychomotor Care of Vulnerable Infants

Knowledge about the early competences of babies has grown significantly since the 1980s. Neuroscience and medical imagery have shed light on fetal life from its earliest stages. At the same time, advances in medicine make it possible to keep newborn babies alive from ever-younger ages. These premature newborns, different from fetuses and term-babies, show a particular psychomotor development, which needs to be tracked from hospitalization onward. Inpatient term newborns have different characteristics from healthy term neonates. During their hospitalization, they generally have a decreased basic tone, due to their initial medical problem and/or sedation drug used. Motor discharges appear to be the main bodily reactions to their environment. Thus, these vulnerable newborns will very soon present tonus regulation difficulties.

In fact, perinatal hospitalization immediately places the child and its parents in a dystimulating environment, for which none of them is prepared. The child develops by relying on sensory and motor systems that are still immature, partially functional, and exposed to atypical stimulations that break with the normal biological continuum [4]. As soon as the patient is hospitalized, the psychomotor therapist intervenes directly with the child and its family as well as indirectly with healthcare teams. The psychomotor therapist often works as a guide for the implementation of developmental care, with or without using the NIDCAP (Neonatal Individualized Developmental Care and Assessment Program) [3]. The sensory environment in which premature infants are placed (noise, light, odor, etc.) and the organization of the care provided must be adapted to the sensorimotor competences of the premature infants and encourage intuitive parenting, more focused on the relational aspects and less on the medical aspects of their child.

11.3 Early Neurodevelopmental Follow-Up

The psychomotor development of vulnerable children is currently scrutinized from an epigenetic perspective. Very early on, genetic, cerebral, environmental, and relational factors orient the tonic, motor, and relational organization of each child. After hospitalization and on the child's return home, neurodevelopmental follow-up involves organizing regular consultations, enabling the identification of warning signs and appropriate support for the family. It also allows a multidisciplinary follow-up to be set up with professionals specifically trained in the care of vulnerable newborns and their families.

Regular psychomotor assessment, at key ages during development, uses standardized tools accessible to all psychomotor therapists, such as the Revised Brunet Lezine [5], the Functional Motor Development from 0 to 48 months [6], the Assessment of Early Social Communication [7], the Dubowitz Neurological Assessment of the Newborn Infant [8], and the Neurological Assessment from 0 to 6 years [9]. Other tools requiring special training in their use are commonly employed, such as, at the neurobehavioral level, the Neonatal Behavioral Assessment Scale [10]) and the Assessment of Preterm Infant's Behavior [11]; at the motor level, the General Movement Assessment [12]; and at the sensorimotor level, the Bayley Scales of Infant and Toddler Development [13].

These tools are used in the context of follow-up consultations organized by networks dedicated to newborns at risk during their first 7 years. They are used by the psychomotor therapist alone and in multidisciplinary consultation with a pediatrician, a psychologist, a physiotherapist, a speech therapist, etc. according to the needs of the child and the institutional organizations in each geographical area. This developmental monitoring must continue during the first years of life in order to identify the difficulties that children and their families might face before they become lasting.

11.4 Sensory Development

A preterm infant has been a fetus living in an aqueous environment for at least 5 months. Its sensory capacities have developed according to a fixed temporal sequence, a phylogenetic inheritance, which staggers the sensory inputs to the developing brain. In this developmental sequence, the somatosensory structures appear anatomically first and then functionally at the beginning of the second trimester, prior to the oral chemosensory (taste) and nasal (olfaction) structures. It is only in the third trimester that the vestibular and then auditory and finally visual structures become functional.

The first months of fetal life are particularly rich in tactile experiences. It is the most mature sense, and is particularly called upon by the aqueous environment. The amniotic fluid exerts a homogeneous and therefore contained pressure on the body of the fetus. The fetus is in weightlessness, where gravity is contained by the body of the mother and the amniotic fluid, which promotes a liberated motor function. The frequency of movements is particularly intense in the second trimester before declining in the third [14]. The fetus experiences sliding on its skin created by its own movements within the uterine cavity and by the movements of the mother. These very early experiences support the development of reassuring body envelopes [15]. In this context, premature birth greatly alters the quality and type of sensations, which influence cerebral development in the constitution of its cortical architecture. Als et al. [16] and Mewes et al. [17] have shown that a longer incubator stay for a child who is born early impedes the expression of sensory skills and disrupts the development of perinatal discrimination, recognition, and location.

11.5 Development of Neuromotor Pathways

The development of neuromotor pathways within the central nervous system provides a fundamental theoretical basis for understanding the motor skills of children born prematurely. The subcortical and cortical systems diverge in phylogenesis and at the neurophysiological level [18]. The archaic subcortical system comes from the brainstem which is myelinated before cortical structures are[1]. It matures in an upward direction (from the feet to the head) between 24 and 34 weeks of gestation. It maintains posture by the antigravity extensor muscles, especially the lower limbs and the axis. It manages the quadriflexion of the limbs and controls the primary reflexes. The more recent cortical system is derived from the hemispherical cortex. Its myelination occurs later, between 32 weeks of gestation and 2 years. It matures downward and participates in the control of postural tone by its excitatory or inhibitory action on the motor neurons. It manages the tone of the flexor muscles of the shaft, the relaxation of limbs, and voluntary fine motor skills (independent finger movements, precision, and speed of manipulation) [18]. In utero, these two systems mature one after the other, without constraint in their expression, since weightlessness is present. Thus, in the second trimester, the fetus has subcortical-dependent extensional motor function in the lower limbs and the axis, which find support against the uterine wall, the placenta, and the bone and organic structure of the mother's body. The uterine enclosure contracts while supporting the fetus on it, which promotes the return to flexion of the lower limbs. Moreover, during the second trimester and the beginning of the third trimester, the child continues to grow and has less and less space within the uterine cavity. It adopts a posture by curving the axis of the body and grouping the upper and lower limbs.

It is also noted that when the mother perceives the movements of her baby, she naturally places her hands on her belly, with more or less pressure on the identified area. This action also supports the flexion of the lower limbs after an extension. It is the beginning of a dialogue between the fetus and its mother, initiated by the movements of the fetus. Feldman [19] describes this tuning in through the concept of synchrony, as a continuous "dance" between the two partners. Beginning during pregnancy, this is a rhythmic tuning based on biological elements (heart rhythm, hormonal regulation, etc.) in order to prepare newborns to enter into coordinated interactions immediately after birth. Haptonomy is based on this type of multisensory interaction, which can also be initiated by both parents through touching the mother's abdomen [20].

Thus, in utero, alongside the maturation of the cortical pathways, the flexion of the body axis and the limbs is physically favored by the uterine enclosure and actively by uterine reflex contractions and by the mother.

11.6 Hypertonia of the Posterior Plane of the Body

During premature birth, the fetus goes from an aqueous environment, with homogeneous pressure, to an aerial environment where the atmospheric polarized pressure is intense. This pressure is overwhelming. The premature infant has very limited

[1] An essential process to increase the conduction velocity of the nervous influx. It is a practical indicator of the maturation of a cerebral system: the myelination of the motor systems defines the type of motor function during the development of the child.

possibilities for moving. Before 32 weeks of gestation, it only has the subcortical system to fight gravity with, and maintain postural tone. Postural tone is the minimal muscle tone required to maintain a posture without moving and to restore postural attitudes against the action of weightlessness. Moreover, the premature baby has lost the uterine envelope, which actively contained its motor traction in extension and passively maintained its posture in a flexed position (see Fig. 11.1).

The input of the cortical system is observed between 34 weeks gestation and 2 years. This process allows the gradual equalization of the extensor muscles of the posterior plane and the flexors of the anterior plane of the body. In fact, the premature child must recreate a sensoritonic equilibrium to maintain a background tone and mobilize an action tone, enabling the gradual initiation of a rectification against gravity during active motor activity (raising an arm or the head from the plane of the bed, for instance).

The neurological immaturity at the origin of the overall hypotonia of the vulnerable child and the motor traction in extension, managed by the muscles of the posterior plane, lead to the development of pathogenic postures: cervical hyperextension, shoulder retraction elevation, decreased posterior pelvic tilt, and hip abduction and external rotation. These are sometimes reinforced by inadequate positioning [21–24]. With hypertrophy of the posterior plane, the child loses the opportunity to develop self-regulation strategies, such as putting his/her hands on the face and mouth and centering his/her hands and feet. He/she must be calmed from the outside, from the human environment to which the premature baby grips physically and psychologically.

The risk of developing hypertonia of the posterior plane is correlated with gestational age at birth. Premature births (before 28 weeks) are most at risk. A child born at 26 weeks presents an overall hypotonia for approximately 2 months and can only appeal to the subcortical system to maintain its postural tone and to start to move.

This muscle imbalance can have relational implications. For example, it is surprising for parents and caregivers to find that a child arriving after 30 weeks can turn

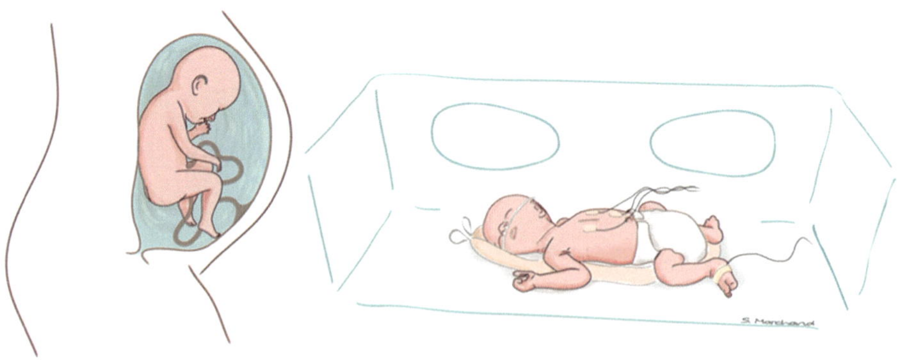

Fig. 11.1 From the uterine envelope to the incubator: when premature birth brings the fetus from free of moving and supported (on the left) to a pathogenic posture under an atmospheric polarized pressure (on the right)

his/her head when positioned on his/her stomach, when such a movement is too difficult when he/she is placed on the back. This is because, on the stomach, the baby mobilizes the extensor muscles of the neck instead of the flexor muscles of the neck when on the back. Without support, or with a non-adapted support, on the back, premature babies have their heads turned to the side with a parietal support. The head rests passively on the mattress. Because the cortical system begins myelination from 32 weeks, it is still very difficult for the child to maintain the head in the axis of the body (with an occipital support). This can lead to muscle shortening if good positioning practices are not followed for premature infants, with a regular alternation of positions. This alternation must take into account the cranial and corporeal supports of the child [24, 25]. The hypertonia of the posterior plane leads to greater ease in thoracic respiration (high and superficial) achieved by a movement of extension of the chest and a short exhalation phase. The latter requires relaxing muscles of the posterior plane of the body axis and of the upper limbs and slightly curving the body axis. Their respiratory rhythm is therefore rather rapid. The slowing of the respiratory, and therefore cardiac, rhythm requires a long and deep exhalation phase. This same difficulty is observed in children with genetic syndromes or with long-lasting axial and peripheral hypotonia. They recruit the tone of their posterior plane to breathe, move, and communicate, which durably affects their relational and motor patterns. Once engrammed at the brain level, these patterns will be used daily and will serve as a basis for further development and are likely to negatively impact the following steps like turning, sitting, babbling, spooning, etc. Supporting the axial flexion/extension balance during hospitalization and afterward at home would allow children to develop abdominal breathing at a normal rhythm for their age. The psychomotor therapist works at providing tools to support a less pathogenic posture, thus offering opportunities for the baby to enter into a relation with his/her social environment enhancing his/her ability to communicate.

However, there are also risks in the relationship between the parents and their child. In the example described above, parents regularly see their child turn his/her head. They therefore assume that this gesture is possible and pay little attention to the postural prerequisites that it supposes. Parents have lateral access to their child through the incubator windows. How will they react when their child (on his/her back at the moment in question) will not turn his/her head toward them when they speak to him/her? They may think that their child refuses to look at them, to make contact with them, and may believe that he/she does not want to, when in fact he/she is unable to. What are the implications of these everyday situations?

11.7 Providing Support to Parents through Psychomotor Care

During the consultation, parents may express a narcissistic wound in their parenthood related to the disabilities of their child. They often see him/her as courageous but very fragile, especially from the physical point of view. Smallness contributes a great deal to this feeling. When we mention touch and manipulation, they say they are afraid to “break” the child, like a small porcelain doll. It is up to us, as professionals, to support children bodily so that they can reveal and develop their motor and interactive skills. Work on incubator and cradle positioning is a prerequisite.

In parallel, providing parents with psychomotor care sessions will create a space, outside primary medical care, where attention is focused on the baby’s body. Its early preventive intervention is effective in enhancing parental sensitivity and infant attachment security. The parents discover it and communicate with their baby by following their own tonic, emotional, and rhythmic responses and those of their baby. The anxiety associated with perinatal risk and separation, the smallness of the baby, and the medical environment make it difficult for parents to develop their skills such as in holding and handling their baby. Their intuitive parenting is undermined [26]. The psychomotor therapist scaffolds the parents to encourage the holding of their baby with his/her flexion motor patterns. Parents will be able to understand their infant and his/her evolution better apart from the vital aspects. Inside this dedicated time frame, parents focus on another aspect of their child that is unknown to them. Interactions are often far from optimal, and parents experience difficulties in recognizing and adjusting to their infant’s signals, leading to a decrease in touch, vocalizations, and gaze [27]. This scaffolding helps parents to discover their place and their parenting skills with an infant who is kept alive and fed by others.

The psychomotor therapist provides support to the parents by helping them to observe and discover the sensori-tonico-motor and relational skills of their baby and their evolution over time. The psychomotor therapist provides a triple support: to the baby, to the parents, and to their mutual attunement. For example, in a situation of nursing or holding, a concrete stabilization of the baby’s body allows him/her to experience his/her exploratory skills toward him/herself, his environment, and the relationship with his/her parents. The psychomotor therapist also supports parents in their own posture and tonic-emotional regulation. The psychomotor therapist proposes body readjustements to the parents and the baby throughout the consultation, in order to facilitate their tonico-emotional atunement. Dialogue with the human environment is the preferred means of regulation. Tonus is a relational and communicational vector. It is the first means of expression of the baby who has to translate and transcribe to the world his/her emotional experience. Emotions take shape in tonus changes. This tone plays an important role in the postural function that supports or prepares the execution of a movement. Dialogue with the human environment is the preferred means of regulation. At this age, regulation is external and refers to the child’s interactions with his/her environment, according to Wallon’s [1] assertion that the baby belongs to his environment before belonging to himself.

Shared observation supports the budding relationship. The first experiences provide a basis for those that follow between a parent and his infant. This baby who seems strange and foreign at first must not remain so. Parents who better understand the reactions of their baby, and the care he/she needs, will be able to adjust to him/her. Through its tonic-postural changes, the baby manifests a need, and the parent sees a signal, requiring an answer. The parent gives meaning to this message which was not specifically addressed to him. Throughout the relationship, a feeling of parental competence arises, and thanks to the adjustments of his responses, the baby assimilates and integrates a repertoire of tonic-emotional expressions, which will serve as a basis for communication. The quality of this communication will rely on the repetition, regularity, and consistency of the responses (responsiveness) of his social partners. Indeed, the baby, whether vulnerable or not, and his parent play a part in this early dialogue.

11.8 Conclusion

A child who experienced neonatal hospitalization, although competent, remains extremely vulnerable long after discharge. The difficulty is thus to perceive his/her competences and to do everything possible to help him/her express and develop them. This involves adults (parents and professionals) observing and listening to the child during all its motor, emotional, and relational expressions. It also requires quality in the care and the practice of all the gestures of everyday life, as well as the desire to provide an adequate environment to the child. In addition, the parents must be encouraged as soon as possible to make quality gestures to help them become self-confident with their baby. The return home also needs to be prepared, so that their baby can develop as harmoniously as possible. The psychomotor support offered during hospitalization must continue during the following months in order to support both the development of motor and relational patterns in the baby and a high-quality parent-infant tonic-emotional attunement. Early psychomotor care is complementary to medical care.

References

1. Wallon H (1942) De l'acte à la pensée. Flammarion, Paris
2. Ajuriaguerra de J, Angelergues R (1962) De la psychomotricité au corps dans la relation avec autrui; à propos de l'œuvre d'Henri Wallon. Evol Psychiatr 27:13–25
3. Als H (1982) Toward a synactive theory of development: Promise for the assessment and support of infant individuality. Infant Ment Health J 3(4):229–243
4. Lickliter R (2000) Atypical perinatal sensory stimulation and early perceptual development: Insights from developmental psychobiology. J Perinatol 20(8):45–54
5. Brunet O, Lézine I, Josse D (2001) Brunet-Lézine révisé: échelle de développement psychomoteur de la première enfance. Editions et Applications Psychologiques, Paris
6. Vaivre-Douret L (1999) Développement fonctionnel moteur de 0 à 48 mois. ECPA, France
7. Guidetti M, Tourrette C (1993) Evaluation de la communication sociale précoce: ECSP. Editions et applications psychologiques, Paris
8. Dubowitz L, Ricciw D, Mercuri E (2005) The Dubowitz neurological examination of the full-term newborn. Ment Retard Dev Disabil Res Rev 11(1):52–60
9. Gosselin J, Amiel-Tison C (2007) Évaluation neurologique de la naissance à 6 ans. Éditions du CHU Sainte-Justine/Masson, Montréal/Paris
10. Brazelton TB, Nugent JK (1995) Neonatal behavioral assessment scale (No. 137). Cambridge University Press
11. Als H, Lester BM, Tronick EZ, Brazelton TB (1982) Toward a research instrument for the assessment of preterm infants' behavior (APIB). In: Theory and research in behavioral pediatrics. Springer, Boston, MA, pp 35–132

12. Einspieler C, Prechtl HFR (2005) Prechtl's assessment of general movements: a diagnostic tool for the functional assessment of the young nervous system. Ment Retard Dev Disabil Res Rev 11(1):61–67
13. Bayley N (2006) Bayley scales of infant and toddler development., 3rd edn. Harcourt Assessment, Psych. Corp, San Antonio
14. Timor-Tritsch I, Zador I, Hertz RH, Rosen MG (1976) Classification of human fetal movement. Am J Obstet Gynecol 126(1):70–77
15. Anzieu D (1985) Le Moi-peau. Dunod, Paris
16. Als H, Duffy FH, McAnulty GB, Rivkin MJ, Vajapeyam S, Mulkern RV, Warfield SK, Huppi PS, Butler SC, Conneman N, Fischer C, Eichenwald EC (2004) Early experience alters brain function and structure. Pediatrics 113(4):846–857
17. Mewes AUJ, Hüppi PS, Als H, Rybicki FJ, Inder TE, McAnulty GB, Mulkern RV, Robertson RL, Rivkin MJ, Warfield SK (2006) Regional brain development in serial magnetic resonance imaging of low-risk preterm infants. Pediatrics 118(1):23–33
18. Amiel-Tison C (2002) Neurologie périnatale. Masson, Paris
19. Feldman R (2005) From biological rhythms to social rhythms: Physiological precursors of mother-infant synchrony. Dev Psychol 42(1):175–188
20. Veldman F (1994) Confirming affectivity, the dawn of human life. The pre-, peri-and postnatal affective-confirming haptonomic accompaniment of parents and their child. Int J Prenatal Perinatal Psychol Med 6(1):11–26
21. Ferrari F, Bertoncelli N, Gallo C, Roversi MF, Guerra MP, Ranzi A, Hadders-Algra M (2007) Posture and movement in healthy preterm infants in supine position in and outside the nest. Arch Dis Child Fetal Neonatal Ed 92(5):386–390
22. Halverson K (2010) The effects of positioning on premature infant development. Pediatr CATs. http://commons.pacificu.edu/otpeds/5
23. Monterosso L, Kristjanson L, Cole J (2002) Neuromotor development and the physiologic effects of positioning in very low birth weight infants. J Obstet Gynecol Neonatal Nurs 31(2):138–146
24. Vaivre-Douret L, Ennouri K, Jrad I, Garrec C, Papiernik E (2004) Effect of positioning on the incidence of abnormalities of muscle tone in low-risk, preterm infants. Eur J Paediatr Neurol 8(1):21–34
25. Grenier A (1988) Prévention des déformations précoces de hanche chez les nouveau-nés à cerveau lésé. Ann Pediatr 35(6):423–427
26. Papousek H, Papousek M (1987) Intuitive parenting: a dialectic counterpart to the infant's integrative competence. In: Osofsky JD (ed) Handbook of infant development, 2nd edn. Wiley, New York, pp 669–720
27. Lester BM, Boukydis CZ, Garcia-Coll CT, Peucker M, McGrath MM, Vohr BR, Oh W (1995) Developmental outcome as a function of the goodness of fit between the infant's cry characteristics and the mother's perception of her infant's cry. Pediatrics 95(4):516–521

Diagnostic Classification: 0-3R. A Tool for Early Interactive Clinical Assessment

12

Matylda Alecian and François Medjkane

12.1 Classification of Mental Disorders in Infant Psychiatry

International diagnostic classifications such as the DSM-5 and the ICD-10 are currently in use both in adult and child psychiatry. They answer the need for a common language, for use between clinicians and researchers worldwide, to improve scientific communication and promote mental health as part of general and public health. Notwithstanding the anthropological criticism and theoretical discussions linked to the concept of objectivity in mental health disorders, we wish to underline how these diagnostic classifications conceived for the description of mental disorders in adults may pose some problems when applied to infancy, toddlerhood, and even childhood and adolescence. Some of the general diagnoses of adults are transposed to childhood problems, such as depression, with adaptation essentially linked to the existence of differences of duration and intensity. Sometimes, the existence of paradoxical symptoms specific to childhood is added to adult descriptors. Mostly, in the DSM, there are but a few specific child diagnoses. Thus, diagnoses based on these tools seem poorly adapted to infant psychiatry and often oversimplistic. Most importantly, international classifications lack developmental and interactive perspective and are therefore insufficiently relevant. The criticisms generally made regarding the adaptation of classifications of adult diagnoses to child diagnoses concern the almost total absence of specific criteria. These criticisms reflect a more general evolution in pediatric psychiatry, which is moving away from the concept of the child as a "miniature" adult, and underline the specific nature of early development at this age in addition to the polymorphic character of its symptomatic

M. Alecian
Maternité, Hôpital Privé de Marne La Vallée, Bry sur Marne (94), Bry-sur-Marne, France

F. Medjkane (✉)
Service de Psychiatrie de l'Enfant et de l'Adolescent, CHU Lille, Universitary Hospital of Lille, Lille, France
e-mail: francois.medjkane@chru-lille.fr

© Springer Nature Switzerland AG 2019

G. Apter et al. (eds.), *Early Interaction and Developmental Psychopathology*,
https://doi.org/10.1007/978-3-030-04769-6_12

expression. It thus appears crucial that a symptomatic interpretation be combined with a developmental one.

Conversely, the nosographic question for infants and children involves a choice between a categorical and a dimensional classification. By definition, infancy, toddlerhood, and childhood represent only a temporal sequence integrated in larger developmental processes. Clinically, it clearly appears more relevant to use a diachronic approach than a synchronic one. For children, each new acquisition changes the modes of expression they use, their modes of thinking, and thus their modes of adaptation to the environment.

The special nature of psychiatric diagnosis for children is now well recognized. Chatoor et al. [1] reported how working groups faced with nosographic classifications of childhood disorders met with numerous hurdles. Chatoor and colleagues distinguished problems relevant to all ages from those that are specific to children aged up to 60 months. The authors point out how difficult it is to assess young children due to their rapid behavioral and cognitive development and also to their emotional regulation abilities. Diagnostic classifications should be able to define pathology as well as determine variations in non-pathological development. On the more specific aspect of early childhood, the authors highlight the validity of the criteria for this age, especially concerning the description of symptoms and their duration. In fact, some symptoms do not seem relevant for this age group or at least will require reformulation. Lastly, they note the need for researchers to create objective evaluation tools to collect symptoms in young children who are not yet able to express their suffering. Such tools are available for ages above 2 years, but there is a significant lack of them for younger ages. All these elements show that a specific classification is needed for 0–3 year olds.

Two texts on diagnostic classification in child psychiatry were available in the last decades. One was proposed by the Group of Advancement of Psychiatry (GAP) in 1983 and constructed with a uniaxial system. The other was the first to be proposed for very young infants. In French, conceived by Kreisler in 1984 [2], it was the first to be founded on a multiaxial model including the observation of social interactions.

The merit of these two attempts is to have prepared the ground for the creation and improvement of evaluation tools for early psychological disorders. These classifications were the first to include attachment disorders and to mention depressive disorders, ie. anaclitic depression (GAP) and essential depression [3]. However, they have limitations. The first was quickly abandoned because of its linear categorizations. The second one is difficult to use due to the lack of a detailed glossary, its specific theoretical framework, and complexity, thus hindering inter rater reliability.

Moreover, these early tools were not constructed with a developmental perspective. Yet, it is commonly accepted that a multidisciplinary and multidimensional approach is best suited to accurately express the infant's developmental and interactional context.

12.2 The 0 to 3R Classification

In 1977,[1] "The National Center for Clinical Infant Programs is founded by internationally renowned leaders in the fields of medicine, mental health, social science research, child development and community leadership interested in advancing the healthy development of infants, toddlers, and families." The Zero to Three Diagnostic Classification (DC: 0-3) was published in 1994. It emerged from an in-depth theoretical and clinical reflection over a 10-year period; and "it presents state-of-the-art approaches to diagnosis and treatment planning for young children with emotional and developmental disorders" [6]. These influential experts coming from various backgrounds (adult, adolescent, and child psychiatrists, psychoanalysts, pediatricians, psychologists, educators, and one philanthropist: Irving Harris) sought to apply the recent discoveries in early development. DC: 0 to 3 has been translated into several languages, among which French, which promotes its circulation and use. The casebook that details the evaluation and treatment procedures for each clinical category described in the DC: 0-3 was published in 1997.

DC: 0-3 is now in its fourth edition. It has been updated through a broad field survey. The "Task Force Revision 0-3" presented the updates and the latest revision of DC: 0-3R, changing it to DC: 0 to 5 at the WAIMH Congress in 2016.[2] Considering the current use of 0 to 3R and the absence of sufficient data on the use of 0 to 5, we will concentrate on the currently most widely used 0-to-3-R classification system.

12.2.1 Design

The classification was developed from a broad theoretical basis, in order to represent, as best it could, the "interactive genesis of infant psychological disorders, between what comes from the baby, and what comes from the environment" [7].

Therefore, the design relies on theories of development and early interaction, relationships and attachment, psychodynamics, how babies organize their experience, their regulatory modalities and individual differences, emotional development, temperament, theories of neurophysiological regulation, and environmental influences.

The revision initiated in 2002 was aimed at making the diagnostic criteria operational [8], that is to say, at expressing disorders in a quantitative way, by using the number of symptoms, their context, and their duration. Therefore, to retain a diagnosis, it is currently required that the child presents at least three symptoms, in at least two different settings and for at least 2 weeks.

The diagnostic classification DC: 0-3R aims to provide a tool for professionals working with very young children. Its purpose is to promote a global evaluation of all clinical situations, without neglecting any essential aspect concerning young

[1] https://www.zerotothree.org/resources/514-zero-to-three-historical-milestones#chapter-263.

[2] www.zerotothree.org.

children whose developmental courses so depend on the environment. Primarily focused on the infant, the classification includes the visible medical expression of the infant's symptoms, the importance of stress-inducing events, as well as an interactive dimension with primary caregivers. The baby has a restricted range of behaviors at its disposal; therefore it is important to also consider contextual and interactive ones, to report negative emotions and the impact this may have.

Due to the importance of clinical experience in infant psychiatry, the classification was designed along a multiaxial categorical model, instead of a linear categorical nosographic tool. The use of the five axes enables the symptomatic expression to be investigated in a dimensional perspective more suitable for understanding a clinical situation as it develops over time and depending on the stage of the unfolding development. For instance, diachronic inspection enables the study of the evolution of symptoms, which is interesting during the peripartum and early childhood when both prevention and prognosis take on such an essential predictive role. Thus, the categories are best seen as descriptive rather than nosographic, so that both developmental trajectories and indicated therapeutic interventions can be assessed.

Moreover, a multiaxial construct makes it possible to take into account a multitude of possible combinations. This offers a better representation of the multiplicity of clinical situations, especially in the first years of life.

12.2.2 Description of the Classification

The five axes that compose the DC: 0-3R were designed as additional tools to existing nosographic classifications such as the DSM or ICD-10 systems. A specific decision-making tree guides the clinician towards diagnostic choices. For example, the impact of external traumatic factors is considered a priority with respect to other diagnoses because of its well-known impact on the parent-child relationship and of its immediate acute consequences. It is also known how difficult it is for an infant to deal with these kinds of events.

The *First Axis* conveys infant primary diagnosis and concerns *clinical disorders*, that is to say, it summarizes the difficulties that dominate the clinical situation. To the categories presented in the DSM-4, the DC: 0-3R adds post-traumatic stress disorders and affect disorders, regulatory disorders, sensory processing disorders, and multisystem developmental disorders (MSDD). For the sake of flexibility and in order to accurately reflect clinical realities, there may be several or no coexisting diagnoses on this axis. Incidentally, comorbidity on this axis has been widely discussed and questioned [7].

The *Second Axis* evaluates the *parent-infant relationship* using the PIR-GAS (Parent-Infant Relationship Global Assessment Scale). It determines the quality of the relationship with a notation ranging from 1 to 100. A score below 40 indicates a pathological relationship. From 41 to 80, the relationship is qualified as "disturbed" or "perturbed," while over 81, it is considered "adapted." The PIR-GAS scale describes the relationship so that the environment in which the child evolves can be understood. However, it does not lead to the identification of a disorder, as explained by Perret in his note on the translation of the revised version [9]. If the relationship is pathological, the Relationship Problems Checklist (RPCL) is used to characterize it more specifically. This checklist includes the following characteristics: "overinvolved," "underinvolved," "anxious/tense," "angry/hostile," and "abusive" (verbally, physically, or sexually). Three aspects of the relationship are relevant for the evaluation of these disorders: its behavioral quality, its affective tonality, and its psychological implication (how the parent reads the behavior of their child).

The *Third Axis* provides an inventory of the *medical and developmental disorders* as rated by the DSM-4 and ICD-10.

The *Fourth Axis* evaluates the impact of *psychosocial stress factors* on the child. Each stress factor is associated with the age of its appearance, its duration, and its repercussion on the child. These psychosocial stress factors may be direct or indirect and extended or not. Their impact will vary according to how the caregiving adult is able to shield and buffer the child. What needs to be determined is the impact of an external event on the child, which depends less on the event itself than on how it is modulated by environmental factors that help the child to cope with it. The number of stress factors is counted, as well as their effects on the child, particularly with regard to the adaptation of the infant toward relationships and communication. For example, severe effects are observed when a child shows detachment behaviors vis-a-vis his parents, such as avoidance of closeness and being unconsolable. Moderate effects refer to perturbations observed in different fields, such as oppositional behavior, sleep disorders, or difficulties in going to pre-school. When the acknowledged stress factors do not interfere with the child's general development and adaptive behavior, the impact is considered slight. The wide range of psychosocial stress factors includes "physical abuse," "sexual abuse," "adoption," "birth of sibling," "violence in the environment," "hospitalization," "trauma to significant other," "parent medical illness," "change of home," and "neglect."

The *level of emotional and social functioning* is reported on the *Fifth Axis* by assessing the quality of play with the main caregivers and the evaluator, on the basis of the observation and collection of data on the child's attitude at home and in other settings, to obtain a summary of its level of functioning. An accurate description of each type of interactive ability or interaction level and of the age of onset is thus provided. This axis also assesses "mutual attention" (at all ages), "mutual engagement" (between 3 and 6 months), "interactive intentionality and reciprocity" (between 6 and 18 months), "communication through affect representation (from 18 months)," "elaboration of representation" (from 30 months), and "differentiation of representations I and II" (from 36 to 42 months, respectively). The question is not only whether the child has reached the appropriate level according to his or her age but also the length of time this capacity can be maintained (e.g., mutual attention should be maintained for at least 5 s at 3–4 months, 30 s at 8–10 months, 2 min at 2 years) and the conditions necessary for its appearance. In other words, what is the child's ability to engage in these processes when he or she is in a state of stress or frustration, or to what extent does he or she need the help of the adult? A summary of the functional levels of emotional and social development is then established.

One of the special features of the classification is the creation of an adapted *decision tree* that includes the infant's narrow range of behaviors. The diagnosis of the *clinical disorder* on *Axis I* should reflect the most salient parts of the child's disorder. To assist the clinician in determining the diagnostic choice, guidelines have been developed based on two rationales. The first [5] concerns the etiological hypotheses of the syndrome, from the syndromes most likely to be linked to environmental influences to those most probably related to the biological vulnerability of the child (regulatory disorders and MSDD) to arrive at those that result from the internalization of a failing relational environment (Affect and Attachment Disorders). Thomas [10] describes a second rationale that includes the previous one but is more specifically focused on therapeutic interventions: mainly environmental interventions (on the practical consequences of trauma), psychotherapeutic interventions (for affective disorders, relating to parent-child relationships), and rehabilitation interventions (for regulation disorders and MSDD, relating to sensory integration). For example, priority will be given to the diagnosis of post-traumatic stress disorder, which requires rapid intervention and is thought to be essentially environment-driven.

12.2.3 Limitations

Since the first publication of the classification, both feedback from users and various studies have emitted a number of criticisms regarding the construction of the tool and the accuracy of some of the criteria used. With a focus on improvement, the authors have today taken these criticisms into account. Some have already led to adjustments of the tool in revised versions. Others still deserve attention in order to optimize the tool for and through clinical practice. In particular, more attention still needs to be paid to diagnostic issues such as the delimitation of disorders and the discrimination of variations in normality. This also covers the problem of the lability of any demarcation lines of disorders in psychopathology, and especially in infancy, linked to both the dynamics of developmental adaptation itself and to scientific advances. The optimization of the criteria to make them as objective as possible is an essential aim which would enable this tool to be used in a research context.

Guedeney [7] and Scholl [11] have presented criticisms of the description of regulatory disorders of *Axis I*. Among these, recapitulation of signs and symptoms is a major issue, since this is done essentially through parent reports. They themselves have different sensitivities and limits to their children's reactions due to their own regulatory characteristics. This makes it complicated to obtain an objective judgment of signs and semiological categorization on their part. Another criticism concerns cultural aspects. They are difficult to integrate into any standardized classification tool, often leading to recurrent and prickly problems of objectification and normativity. The 2005 revision resulted in a review of the diagnostic criteria towards a finer description of regulatory disorders.

The reactive attachment disorder also raises many questions. Its place on *Axis I* is questioned because none of the child's behaviors are used as criteria, with the emphasis being mainly on the environmental description (deficiencies, neglect, maltreatment, etc.) for both diagnostic definition and therapeutic prognosis (an action on the environment would lead to an improvement in the disorders). The authors also discuss more recent work on attachment disorders not included in the classification. This it seems will be dealt with in the new 0–5 revision.

The possibility of using comorbidity on *Axis I* is not exempt from queries. Guedeney et al. [12] collected the questions put forward by several authors. What is the true function of comorbidity? Can it account for the complexity of a clinical situation? Is it used to circumvent the guidelines of the decision tree? Or is it a reflection of a breach in the delimitation of diagnostic categories? In addition, the order of the associated diagnoses is not defined by the classification. Should it be determined according to therapeutic guidelines (which differ according to country and theoretical background) or to the prevalence of disorders in the clinical picture?

On *Axis II*, criticism is focused on the threshold score on the PIR-GAS, the absence of sufficiently objective criteria to determine whether the relationship is normal or pathological, the too global perspective of the relationship, and the fact that the cultural dimension is not taken into account [7]. However, other scales have used scores with subjective cutoffs that actually have clinical validity such as the Spielberger Trait and State Assessments [4].

12.2.4 Why Use the DC: 0-3R?

This classification is the first specific tool developed in the field of early childhood and includes diagnostic proposals and a decision tree.

Its clinical basis enables a precise assessment of the capacities and specific features of the child and of the ways in which it will react to treatment.

In addition, just as in the first version the DC: 0-3R offers an interesting alternative approach to severe developmental disorders that could lead to more specific therapeutic methods. In fact, the DC:0-3 explores the extent to which early detection and intervention preclude later emergence and differentiated structuring of severe developmental disorders. The DC: 0-3R also enables innovative investigation of early affective pathologies.[3]

In his note accompanying the French translation (the DC:0-3 is translated and validated in many languages[4]), Perret [9] discusses the clinical relevance of the classification. While its initial purpose was to determine a diagnosis, it seems that the users of the first version of the tool found it extremely useful in achieving a

[3] See Special Issue of Infant Mental Health Journal (2003;24(4)) for a precise view of all aspects of use of DC: 0–3.

[4] www.zerotothree.org.

comprehensive view of each child's clinical situation. Perret proposes the expression "clinical development process" to address this concept. This has the merit of clearly expressing the idea that a clinical situation needs to be globally apprehended by relying on the five axes that constitute the DC: 0-3R. The clinician thus successively examines the various factors that may contribute to the existence of the disorder in the child. This supports clinical assessment and diagnosis and also helps determine what type of intervention is desirable for the child and his/her family. While the classification makes it possible to identify the child's symptomatology and its potentially explanatory factors, it can also highlight the resources of the child and his/her environment. Identifying these resources helps to find the therapeutic propositions that are adapted to each situation.

Including all the different factors truly represents an added value for clinical practice since this impacts evaluation of the disorder, etiological hypotheses, and therapeutic proposals.

12.3 Use and Implementation in Early Interactive Clinical Assessment

The two clinical vignettes below illustrate how the DC: 0-3R can be used for the assessment of a clinical situation.

12.3.1 Lorenzo: To Sleep or to Interact?

Lorenzo is a child of 12 months who was referred for a sleeping disorder. He is the first son of a young couple, both of whom work. At the age of 6 months, Lorenzo was hospitalized for gastroesophageal reflux (GER). According to his parents, it was from then on that the child presented difficulties falling asleep, suggesting a form of adaptive difficulty linked to this short but anxiously lived separation. The mother describes him as a particularly agitated child. Lorenzo spends half his day with his great-grandmother who has been treated for depression for many years. She is nevertheless described as a "very capable person." Lorenzo's father often stays far from home because of his work. In his absence, Lorenzo co-sleeps in bed with his mother. Lorenzo's mother describes frequent conflicts with the father, that vary according to her state of tiredness.

To summarize the evaluation, it is found that Lorenzo is very active and curious, exploring the environment and engaging with the professionals available to him. He walks into the room and stops to study and manipulate the objects that appear interesting to him. During the interview, he approaches his mother on several occasions in order to seek something from her. His interruptions are met diversely during the interview, sometimes the mother responds adequately thus interrupting what she is doing, sometimes she looks as if she does not acknowledge Lorenzo, and at other times, she shows how frustrating it is to be interrupted while speaking. Her own interactive solicitations of Lorenzo may then seem off-beat. Overall, the impression given to the clinician is one of maternal distress and inconsistency. From Lorenzo's point of view, it seems difficult to predict what the mother's answer will be, and therefore, sometimes Lorenzo reacts by crying or by angrily raising the intensity of his solicitations. From the mother's point of view, Lorenzo is difficult to regulate and needs constant attention with little space for maternal response and improvisation of her own interactive propositions. An interaction with the father is also observed separately. With his father, the interactions are characterized by an excessive sensitivity of the parent to the child's signals. Even though the father expresses a great interest in the well-being and development of the child, paradoxically he is not upheld in playful interactions. The father's affective tone is characterized by anxiety, agitation, and apprehension. Lorenzo, mirroring his father, is then emotionally dysregulated in his interactions.

Lorenzo's motor development seems to be on track: at the age of 6 months, he was able to sit without help, and during the consultation, he could almost walk alone. He knew how to pronounce simple words. He is an affectionate and smiling child. On the Vineland scale, he obtained a score that was appropriate for his chronological age in all domains. There are no other sensory development difficulties. Gastrointestinal disorders have been resolved.

On *Axis I*, the only diagnostic criteria found is that of sleeping disorders. Trauma-related disorder due to the short hospitalization is eliminated due to the lack of post-traumatic symptoms in the child.

On *Axis II*, the relationship with Lorenzo's mother can be defined as having a "tendency toward being disturbed," i.e., a PIR-GAS score of 65 caused by over-involvement. Interaction is characterized from the child's perspective by interference by the mother with the desires and goals of the child, who then shows provocative behavior. The affective tone of the parent, often highly stressed, leads to an interaction that is not consistent and to which the child responds with tears or obstinacy. The mother is then at a loss as to how to react. With the father, the relationship is coded differently, indicated as "troubled" (PIR-GAS 35), tense-anxious. In fact, the interactions between Lorenzo and his father show a small array of possibilities and are never relaxed without help from the environment.

On *Axis IV*, the gastrointestinal disorders were noted which, although resolved, are considered to have produced excessive sensitivity in the child. Other psychosocial stress factors include the hospitalization of Lorenzo at 6 months, the depression of one of the caregivers, the separation from both parents due to their work, and trauma of a member of the family (the grandmother is being treated for a tumor). Nevertheless, the protective capacities of the environment are assessed as high, thus rendering the impact of stressful factors weak. It is deemed that the stress factors cannot be considered as having a negative impact on the child's overall level of adaptation.

On *Axis V*, the level of development and emotional functioning seems appropriate considering Lorenzo's age, even though he still appears vulnerable in some areas. For example, Lorenzo is not yet able to maintain the age-appropriate level of emotional developmental functioning under stressful conditions.

We see here that the multidimensional character of the DC: 0-3R assessment has several advantages in clinical practice. First, the classification makes it possible to take into account several non-exclusive factors. For Lorenzo, for example, the relationship with caregivers, life events, and somatic disorders are all included in the general clinical picture. From an etiological point of view, taking into account the different factors avoids the pitfall of linear causality. This has consequences on the proposed therapeutic approaches. Indeed, such an assessment calls for a combination of varied modes of intervention: therapeutic, educational, and social, for example. It includes support for parents in order for them to better understand their infant's heightened sensitivity, educational, guidance and acknowledgment of specific parental anxiety and depressive issues when they exist.

12.3.2 Yann: How Difficult it Is to Grow when Kickoff Did Not Go Well

Within the framework of the perinatal consultation-liaison system setup at the maternity and neonatal hospital department [13, 14], pediatrician colleagues in the neonatology department referred a 20-day-old infant. Yann is described as a restless child with fluctuating eating disorders. He has been hospitalized since his birth for diagnostic monitoring and early care as a result of an obstructed labor associated with perinatal anoxia. The clinical neuropediatric assessment suspects motor impairment. Extensive diagnostic assessment and etiopathogenic exploration are ongoing.

During the first interview, conducted in the neonatology department, Yann is in his mother's arms, and his father is in the room close by. Yann's father expresses his pain and dismay concerning his son's medical condition, while the mother seems emotionally disconnected from both the interview and her infant. The parents, who are first cousins due to traditional cultural preferences, have been married for a year, and the mother has come to France as part of a family reuninification program. Yann is the couple's first child.

In the first interviews with Yann and his parents, great fluctuation is observed in Yann's behaviors. The overall motor scheme appears to be globally hypotonic, with recurrent sudden and impulsive hypertonic movements. Numerous neurovegetative manifestations in the form of hiccups and startle reactions are observed over short intervals. On the expressive emotional affective level, Yann alternates between moments of crying during hypertonic fine motor movements and other periods of waking apathy and absence of contact. Yann seems oversensitive to sounds and noises as well as to moderate tactile stimulation (caresses), while firmer tactile stimulations appear more comforting. The reaction to the presence of others is variable, and attitudes of interactive withdrawal are observed. His caloric intake is described as erratic, and the speech therapist colleague who offers developmentally oriented oral care highlights difficulties in oropharyngeal coordination during bottle-feeding. Sleep is described as irregular, and observations made during sleep times reveal poor-quality sleep with difficulty in reaching deep sleep.

In terms of interactions, we find significant differences in how Yann is able to react depending on who and how one is paying attention to him. There seems to be more disorganization, autonomous behavior, and less contact when his mother is in charge of nursing care. Relational avoidance and withdrawal are heightened and last for longer periods. Yann seems to organize himself in a more peaceful way in his father's arms, and his attempts at mutual attention meet with more success. Maternal unavailability seems linked to this difference in Yann's reactions to adult interactional involvement. Thus maternal behaviors need to be assessed, and maternal care needs to be supported in order to assess how infant's specific needs could be met. The PIR-GAS score is very low (i.e., 20) for mother-child interaction mainly qualified as underinvolvement, while the PIR-GAS scores high (i.e., 80) for father-infant interaction thus qualified as adapted.

These differences observed in Yann's interaction with his father and mother led to further exploration of parental mental health issues. Yann's mother, very withdrawn and apprehensive of the care team, was able to discuss her own relational issues ever since she had been an adolescent. Indeed, having left school early and being unemployed, the everyday life she describes seems to be hampered by stress, controlled through high levels of ritualized behavior. Psychiatric assessment accepted by the mother then revealed many negative symptoms: affective and relational withdrawal, poverty of discourse marked by a relative lack of logic, as well as volitional difficulties that partly account for apathy as well as social withdrawal. Gradually, supported by her husband, she was also able to describe what seem to have been delusional interpretative persecution experiences during her adolescence. All of these elements pointed toward a diagnosis of schizophrenia with low-key chronic evolution (type F20 according to ICD-10).

Regarding medical diagnosis (Axis III), Yann presented a series of symptoms that may lead to Motor Neurological Disability. This diagnostic hypothesis relies on symptoms such as suction/swallowing disorders, hyperexcitability, irritability with sudden and disorganized movements, startles, and the use of hypertonic attitudes and sleep disorders associated with the context of obstructed labor and perinatal anoxia. The observed elements were also suggestive of a hypersensitivity type I regulatory disorder of a fearful/cautious temperamental type.

Apart from the medical stressors, the use of repeated observations of interaction and evaluation was extremely useful. Assessment and diagnosis of maternal psychiatric illness was thus possible, opening possibilities for maternal care, intensive care, and follow-up programs for both Yann and his parents. The impact of maternal illness in addition to the various other stressors involved was considered as high on the Axis IV scale, adding arguments in favor of intensive and specific mother-baby post-hospitalization treatment.

Early stages of emotional development could not be met in all circumstances even if mutuality between Yann and his father or other caregivers except his mother was obtained in certain conditions (the best ones available, see Chap. 3 part 1).

Thus, the DC: 0–3R, through its comprehensive approach, allowed us to explore other possible factors linked to Yann's negative behaviors. This shift from a perspective centered exclusively on infant symptoms as if independent from the caregivers and the global environment led us to offer, in addition to the proposed neurological and rehabilitative care for Yann, specific psychiatric care for his mother, thus addressing both maternal and infant issues. Neglect or nonrecognition of maternal pathology would have been detrimental to Yann and his family in both the short and the long term.

12.4 To Continue with a Classification Diagnostic Tool for Very Young Children

The diagnostic classification presented here tries to avoid the caveats linked to the task of categorizing disorders in a developing human being. In order to do this, the tool presented here includes a vast array of elements ranging from the infant's symptoms and interactive capacities to its relationships and the environmental impact it is submitted to longitudinally. This requires time and a comprehensive assessment with multidisciplinary resources. Even when these are not totally available, focusing on all aspects of the infant's characteristics and environment provides, we believe, a better dynamic view. The rapidity of development and the necessary interactions between the infant and its environment can help understand both, if the child is at risk, and if the environment is heightening or buffering the child's vulnerabilities. A more dynamic and system-oriented assessment is then possible, leading to a whole new way of analyzing what is going astray as well as to how to try to reorganize the system in a more positive direction.

References

1. Chatoor I, Pine DS, Narrow WE (2007) Diagnosis of psychopathology in infants, toddlers, and preschool children. In: Narrow WE, First MB, Sirovatka PJ, Regier DA (eds) Age and gender considerations in psychiatric diagnosis: a research agenda for DSM-V. American Psychiatric Association, Arlington, VA, p 145150
2. Kreisler L (2004) 112. Sémiologie et catégories cliniques en psychiatrie du très jeune enfant. Problèmes de classification et communication interdisciplinaire. In: Lebovici S, Diatkine R, Soulé M (eds) Nouveau traité de psychiatrie de l'enfant et de l'adolescent, vol 2. Presses Universitaires de France, Paris, pp 1953–1970
3. Lebovici S, Diatkine R, Soulé M (2004) Nouveau traité de psychiatrie de l'enfant et de l'adolescent, vol 2. Presses Universitaires de France, Paris, pp 1953–1970
4. Spielberger CD, Sydeman SJ (1994) State-trait anxiety inventory and state-trait anger expression inventory. Lawrence Erlbaum Associates, Inc, Hillsdale, NJ
5. Thomas JM, Harmon RJ (1998) La classification diagnostique des troubles de la santé mentale et du développement de la première et de la petite enfance un système dynamique pour la connaissance et le traitement des nourrissons, des jeunes enfants et de leurs familles. Devenir 10(1):35–50
6. Berman C, Shaw E, Meisels SJ, Fenichel E (1996) Family-directed child evaluation and assessment under the Individuals with Disabilities Education Act (IDEA). In: Meisels SJ, Fenichel E (eds) New visions for the developmental assessment of infants and young children. Zero to Three, Washington, DC, pp 361–390
7. Guedeney A (1999) La classification diagnostique 0-3 ans. Carnet/Psy 44:28–32

8. Fenichel E, Emde RN, Egger H, Guedeney A, Wise BK, Wright HH (2005) Présentation de la révision de la Classification Diagnostique 0-3 ans (DC: 0-3R). Devenir 17(4):347–360
9. Perret P (2009) L'édition révisée de la Classification diagnostique 0-3 ans et sa traduction française. Devenir (5):7–13
10. Thomas JM, Guskin KA, Klass CS (1997) Early Development Program: Col- laborative structures and processes. Infant Mental Health Journal 18(2):198–208
11. Scholl JM (2007) Classification Diagnostique 0-3 ans Révisée: une nouvelle présentation des Troubles de la Régulation du traitement des stimuli sensoriels. Devenir 19(2):109–130
12. Guedeney N, Mintz AS, Rabouam C, Le Nestour A, Guédeney A, Danon G, Morales-Huet M, Jacquemain F, Roujeau S (2002) À propos des systèmes de classification en psychiatrie du très jeune enfant: utilisation de la classification diagnostique Zero to three. La Psychiatrie de l'Enfant 45(2):483–531
13. Garez V, Devouche E, Bobin-Bègue A, Alecian M, Minjollet P, Vallerent A, Poget M, Oguibenine H, Heroux C, Medjkane F, Apter A (2018) La liaison en "Périnatalogie": Des soins entre réseau, liaison et prise en charge mobile. L'Encéphale 44(3):239–246
14. Vallerent A, Garez V, Minjollet P, Heroux C, Devouche E, Apter G (2016) PPUMMA: Expérience d'une unité mobile de pédopsychiatrie au sein d'un réseau périnatal. Pratiques en Santé Mentale 4:5–9

Growing the Brain: A New Perspective on Child Psychiatry

13

Alexandra Murray Harrison

Over the past several decades, new technologies have supported scientific advances in knowledge regarding the biological etiologies of mental disorders in childhood. Concurrently, developmental research has revealed the essential function of the caregiving relationship in modulating risk factors from both heredity and the environment. As a result, the role of the child psychiatrist is challenged to transform her traditional role as diagnostician and clinician using a standard set of interventions designed to treat specific disorders and adopt a new role. The new role requires her to take a more comprehensive view of childhood symptoms and their etiologies, one that gives the caregiving environment a more central position and one that focuses on restoring healthy function rather than eliminating specific symptoms.

A brief literature review will therefore emphasize (1) the caregiving relationship—the importance from the point of view of healthy development and what happens when things go wrong; (2) the stress regulation system and the therapeutic aim of strengthening it ("growing the brain"); and (3) the de-emphasis of categorical diagnoses, in order to shift the focus of attention away from psychopathology to adaptive function and healthy well-being.

After the literature review, interventions designed to support the caregiving relationship, grow regulatory capacities, and enhance developmental competency and function will be discussed and illustrated with brief clinical examples. The chapter will end with some thoughts about the future of child psychiatry.

A. M. Harrison (✉)
Department of Psychiatry, Harvard Medical School, Boston, MA, USA

The Boston Psychoanalytic Society and Institute, Newton Centre, MA, USA
e-mail: aharrisonmd@comcast.net

© Springer Nature Switzerland AG 2019

G. Apter et al. (eds.), *Early Interaction and Developmental Psychopathology*,
https://doi.org/10.1007/978-3-030-04769-6_13

13.1 The Caregiving Relationship

13.1.1 Factors Promoting Protection in the Caregiving Relationship

Even a rudimentary study of human development impresses the reader with the enormous importance of the early caregiving environment on the developing child [1, 2]. The caregiving environment provides developmental scaffolding and a degree of modulation of both internal and external stressors [3].

Babies are born prepared to be protected, nurtured, and enjoyed by a "good enough" caregiver. The appearance of an infant—with a disproportionately large head; large, expressive eyes; and the ability to cry—easily attracts the attention of an adult, especially a parent. At birth the infant is attracted to mother's smell, including the scent of amniotic fluid; infants are soothed when crying, by their mother's odor, which organizes the infant's behavior for nursing [4].

Corticobulbar pathways are sufficiently developed at birth to allow newborns to signal caregivers with vocalizations and grimaces and to gaze and smile; neural regulation of muscles prepares the newborn for social cueing of caregivers with gestures and facial expressions [5, p. 34]. The infant learns the mother's voice and can learn simple rhymes and narratives in the womb ([6]; see also Part 1 Chap. 3). Melodies that the fetus has heard in utero can be recognized by the infant after birth [7, p. 4]. Infants begin learning speech in utero. In elegant studies, infants' vocalizations have been shown to constitute "protocommunication" that generates vocal responses in the caregiver and creates a parent-infant dialogue that figures prominently in the growing infant-caregiver relationship [8, 9].

Similarly, parents are primed to protect, nurture, and enjoy infants. There appear to be neural circuits connected with parental tasks and behaviors that include thalamus, insula, dorsolateral prefrontal cortex, medial prefrontal cortex, anterior cingulate cortex, and orbitofrontal cortex overlapping with circuits involved in reward and empathic processes [10, p. 5]. When first-time mothers listen to their own but not another baby's cries, increased activity is observed in several brain regions such as the insula, amygdala, cingulate, striatum, midbrain, and orbitofrontal cortex [11, p. 3].

13.1.2 Moderating Effects of Caregiving Relationship

We know that the foundation of health and well-being begins in infancy [3]. We also know that health problems result from a combination of genes and the environment—both the present environment and the past, as the environment interacts with genes to cause epigenetic changes that can affect both physical and mental health. What is becoming increasingly clear is that the caregiving relationship can provide a moderating effect on both genetic vulnerability and destructive features in the environment [3, p. 4–5; 12–14]. When the caregiving relationship fails to protect the infant, this moderating effect does not function, with serious consequences for the developing stress regulation system.

Adverse events in the environment influence brain development at different stages, affecting different functions according to the sensitivity to disruption of the developing nervous system. The brain develops most rapidly early in life, making it particularly vulnerable to environmental challenges in early infancy. Development occurs in a sequential fashion, the lower parts of the brain developing first and the higher and more complex parts of the brain developing last. Simple regulatory functions (respiration, heart rate, blood pressure, temperature) are mediated by lower parts of the brain such as the brain stem and diencephalon. Adverse events occurring early in fetal growth can disrupt these basic regulatory systems. More complex functions (language and symbolic thinking) are mediated by the cerebral cortex, which doesn't fully come online until about 1 year of life. Adverse events occurring at this time can disrupt language and other cognitive function, but earlier interference with regulatory capacity can cause a cascade effect in which higher-level functions are compromised due in part to underlying regulatory issues.

Maltreatment in the caregiving relationship can initiate multiple neurobiological reactions that affect the developing brain. In a recent review, Teicher et al. note that 180 original reports show an association between childhood maltreatment and alterations in brain structure, function, connectivity, or network architecture [15, p. 17]. Domestic violence is another major adverse circumstance even if the child is not the direct victim, since witnessing violence is associated with specific changes in the visual parts of the brain and visual pathways [15, p. 655–656]. Some studies show larger amygdala volumes in individuals experiencing caregiver neglect [15, p. 656]. Teicher et al. hypothesize that the left amygdala may be particularly vulnerable to early abandonment or disrupted attachment, whereas the right amygdala may be more vulnerable to physical, sexual, or emotional abuse [15, p. 656]. The conclusion that psychosocial deprivation accounts for the smaller head circumference and other adverse developmental findings of infants who experienced at least 6 months of institutional care in Romanian orphanages (during the second part of the twentieth century) is documented in numerous papers [2, 15, 16, p. 769].

13.1.3 Regulation

The intricacies of the moderating effect of the caregiver on the infant's stress regulation are demonstrated by observations of face-to-face infant-caregiver interactions, particularly when using the still face paradigm [17]. The caregiver's empathic reactions to the infant's intentional and affective signals are communicated by facial expression, gestures, and vocalizations of the caregiver. When the caregiver is neglectful or empathically absent, such as in the extreme case of the Romanian orphanages but also in highly dysfunctional families, or when the caregiver is depressed, such as in postpartum depression, this crucial moderating effect is compromised or lost [18–20].

A major contribution toward the understanding of self-regulation came from Tronick's work demonstrating that self-regulation is developed through reciprocal interactions between infant and caregiver—"mutual regulation" [21]. Tronick built on the observations of Sander, who identified the establishment of the infant's first accomplishment in self-organization, diurnal rhythm, as emerging from the predictable rhythms of the caregiving routine of feeding, bathing, and diaper changing [22]. Analyzing split screen videotapes of infants and mothers in face-to-face communication, Tronick showed that infant self-regulation occurred simultaneously with an interactive process of match, mismatch, and repair with the caregiver. Tronick elaborated this model in observations of depressed mothers, where he noted that infants had to spend more time in self-regulation because their mothers were preoccupied with their own regulatory needs and unavailable for mutual regulatory responses [21].

Tronick's perturbation of the *Still-Face* in the Face-to-Face situation has become perhaps the most important recent scientific paradigm in the study of early development ([17, pp. 11–12, 323–338]; see Part 1 Chap. 2). In this paradigm, mothers are told to (1) play with their infants as they would at home in the face-to-face situation; (2) at a signal, make a "Still Face," in other words, assume an impassive, unresponsive face, for 2 min; and (3), at a second signal, resume play with their infants. During the still face part of the paradigm, the infants typically attempt to elicit their mothers' attention with gestures and vocalizations. When this fails, they show distress and make attempts at self-regulation.

The Still Face experiment highlights the centrality of the infant-caregiver relationship in the development of self-regulation. In a typical family situation, a responsive caregiver will comfort the baby when the baby is distressed but also leave the baby the space to self-comfort when he initiates a "break" from the interaction. Both infant and caregiver do a dance of up and down—pleasurable excitement and calm—as they "play" together. They can sense what the other is feeling and what the other does or does not want to do, the other's "intentionality," and they respect these communications.

An illustration of an intervention focused on regulation: Whereas the skills of other pediatric specialists—occupational therapists in particular—have an explicit target of regulation, the child psychiatrist can also make important contributions. The first is to make observations about the regulatory competency of the child both from the history and from observation. The second is in parent guidance, helping the parent create expectations for the child and scaffold the child's accomplishments. The third is in the implicit realm and has to do with "matching" the child's vocal and action turns in a way that supports the child's regulatory function.

13.1.4 Categorical Diagnoses

Categorical diagnoses have been a persistent challenge and frustration for this author, a practicing child psychiatrist with more than four decades of clinical experience. That is because one categorical diagnosis or even two never seem to capture the individual child being evaluated. One major problem in using a psychiatric nosology such as DSM V is that of comorbidity. It has been estimated that comorbidity rates in psychiatry are as high as 50% [23, p. 2]. Half of individuals who meet diagnostic criteria for one psychiatric disorder meet diagnostic criteria for a second disorder at the same time, and half of those diagnosed with two disorders meet criteria for a third [23, p. 2]. Although dimensional models such as internalizing (anxious and depressive symptoms) and externalizing (aggressive, delinquent, and hyperactive-impulsive symptoms) are frequently used in studies of childhood psychiatric disorders, clinicians are taught to use the DSM or another categorical system, ICD, and third-party payment systems require categorical diagnoses.

Additional studies suggest that the liability for many disorders is influenced by the same genetic factors, suggesting the value of a "transdiagnostic approach" to psychiatric disorders [23, 24, p. 4]. The longitudinal Dunedin study suggested the existence of a "p factor" that begins with genetic liability, the genes enhancing risk for any and all disorders rather than any single disorder [23, p. 6]. This is also consistent with the thoughts that psychopathology is dimensional [25]. The value of such an approach is validated by the author's clinical experience suggesting that children with many different diagnoses may benefit from the same basic therapeutic approach—a thoughtful and empathic psychodynamic psychotherapy that respects the child's agency, supports the parents, and involves the school.

13.2 Interventions

13.2.1 Caregiving Environment: The Parent Consultation Model and Mini Course in Infant Mental Health

Two examples of how a child psychiatrist has addressed the need to support the caregiving relationship are the Parent Consultation Model and the Infant Parent Mental Health Mini course, named "Protect, Nurture, and Enjoy," for the three tasks of the parent or caregiver.

13.2.2 Parent Consultation Method: Child Psychiatrist as Parents' Consultant

This method of evaluating children with psychiatric symptoms emerged from the author's work in early development with infant research colleagues particularly Elisabeth Fivaz-Depeursinge [26] and Downing [27] and also from her earlier work as a consultant to surgeons. It includes a "parent consultation" in three sessions [28]. The first session is with the parents alone to hear their concerns about their child, to obtain a history of the child and family, and to generate consultation questions for the clinician as the parents' consultant. The second meeting is with the whole family for a play (or talk with older children) session, designed to gather data to answer the parents' questions. These are almost always pleasant meetings, which the consultant directs and does not allow anyone to feel put on the spot. The consultant videotapes these family sessions, since infant research has demonstrated the value of observational data, especially with videotape. In between this meeting and the final meeting, the consultant analyzes the tape to come up with impressions that address the parents' questions. Then, in the final meeting with the parents alone again, the consultant refers to these questions and addresses them one by one, offering her impressions and illustrating what she thinks with short clips of videotape from the family meeting. The final step is helping the parents brainstorm what they want to do. In the author's extensive experience with this method, parents have chosen many options. One option is to go home and try out some of the ideas they have come up with together. Another is to request an extended parent consultation with more observation of the video and more brainstorming about how to change family patterns. Another is to begin a psychotherapy with the consultant or with someone else who takes their insurance or who lives closer to them, for example. The method gives parents a lot of freedom to make choices.

What the author has found over the many years of using this method is that it is rarely necessary to see the identified problem child alone in order to answer the parents' questions and, in those cases in which it is important, that visit can follow naturally from new questions that arise in the third parent meeting. One advantage of this approach is that it is not focused on psychopathology but instead on development—where the child and family are in terms of their desired developmental trajectory and how to help them get closer to where they want to be. Another is that the consultant does not immediately begin to make an individual connection with a child who may not become her patient. A third advantage is that the consultant is free to make many important observations of the child in the context in which he or she lives—the way the child and the family express affect and communicate with language and in non-verbal ways, the way the family manages transitions and sets boundaries and maintains them, etc. These observations are in addition to the typical ones a child psychiatrist makes about the child's behavior and the content of the child's speech or symbolic play.

13.2.3 Example of Parent Consultation Method

Older parents with a 5-year-old daughter, adopted at age 22 months, consulted the child psychiatrist because of the child's temper tantrums. They asked what caused the tantrums and what to do to stop them. With sophisticated professionals, they knew all the ins and outs of the adoption process and had attended multiple adoption seminars. In the family meeting, the child chose the puppet of a turtle to play with, the father chose a black-and-white dog puppet, and the mother chose a brown puppy puppet. In the play, the two dog puppets kept tapping on the turtle's shell, asking it to "come out and play." The girl anxiously kept poking the turtle's head and legs back into the shell, when one or the other popped out. Finally, she had a full-fledged tantrum, screaming and kicking, until her parents carried her out to the car.

When the parents returned for the final meeting, they brought up the tantrum and their sense that their daughter had low frustration tolerance demonstrated by her inability to manipulate the turtle puppet. Viewing the video with the consultant, however, they could not avoid the observation of the turtle's efforts to avoid the controlling intrusions of the two dogs. The consultant noted what she saw as an apparent urgency to make a connection expressed by the two dogs in the play and wondered about separation or loss in the parents' lives. She inquired about what events had occurred in their lives when they were the age of their daughter, 5 years old. The father said, "When I was 5-yo my family moved. We had a dog who kept running away back to the old neighborhood, and we had to give him away to a neighbor in that neighborhood, because he couldn't get used to the new home." The mother looked at her husband in astonishment. "When I was 5, she said, 'we had a dog, and when we moved my parents thought we couldn't keep the dog in the new home, so we gave him to a neighbor in the old neighborhood, but he kept running away from that family to our new home in the next city and barking at the door to be let in. My parents finally agreed to keep him in our new house." Neither parent had been aware of the other parent's story about the family dog that could not adjust to the new home. Although the parents had become familiar with the multiple reactions common to adoptive parents through their seminars and readings, the visual image of them with their daughter suddenly confronted them with the shared unconscious fear that their little daughter would not "bond" to them and become "adjusted to her new home." The consultant pointed out the turtle's self-protective response to the tapping on her shell, and the parents appreciated the turtle's need for a more graded and respectful approach to making a connection. They understood that it was their insecurity about their bond with their daughter that led them to behave in an intrusive way. The answer to their question was that the child was having tantrums partly in response to their over control and that she needed them to become more respectful of her sensitivity to intrusion. In other words, her parents' own emotional needs sometimes led them to overlook their child's regulatory needs.

13.2.4 "Protect, Nurture, and Enjoy": Intensive Infant Parent Mental Health Mini Course (PNE)

In the course of her career, the author's interest in prevention has become a primary concern. Believing that the most cost-effective way to support the infant-caregiver relationship was to train professional and paraprofessional caregivers about infant mental health, the author and a team of infant mental health specialists collaborated with a team from a nursing school to develop a curriculum to teach nursing students in North India.[1] The curriculum includes knowledge about current developmental research and multiple instructional videotapes, as well as clinical demonstrations in

[11]American team members collaborating in giving workshops and designing PNE include Ginger Gregory, Alayne Stieglitz, Elizabeth Levey, Anna Baumgartel, and Abishek Bala; Indian collaborators are Neena Lyall and Himanshu Lyall.

the wards and villages. "Protect, Nurture, and Enjoy" ("PNE") is named for the three main tasks of an infant caregiver.

The clinical demonstration piece of the PNE consists primarily of the Newborn Behavioral Observation ("NBO"), a tool developed by Nugent to support and strengthen the infant-parent relationship.[2] In addition to the NBO, the clinical piece of the PNE includes a discussion of the mother's pregnancy and delivery and an exploration of the support system available to her in her family and community. Finally, the PNE emphasizes the value of music and song, for example, asking new parents to sing to their babies. This addition to the training introduced culture in the context of the tunes, rhythms, and words a particular culture uses to welcome an infant into the world. The addition of songs strengthened the goal of individualizing the PNE to fit the specific group of caregiver participants. Evaluations of the students following the course demonstrated good apprehension of the basic principles and of the information given in the course.

The PNE is now a part of the curriculum of the School of Nursing of the Christian Hospital of Kasganj and has also been given at two institutions serving high-risk populations in Lima, Peru, and Grenada. The course is continually evolving, through updating the study guide and bibliography to make the course current and giving the training in different institutions and different countries and to different caregiver groups. The PNE training also emphasizes the self-care of the caregivers, especially in the case of parents who mistreat or neglect their infants. Reflective supervision groups may be helpful in supporting the caregivers as they face these stressful clinical situations.

13.3 Concluding Remarks

As a result of an explosion of new knowledge in the field of developmental psychology, especially research exploring the caregiving relationship and the stress regulation system, and also as a result of questions about the validity of categorical diagnoses, the role of the child psychiatrist is challenged to transform her role. In this chapter, the author has attempted to describe the pivotal features of developmental theory that have affected her clinical thinking and practice. Consequent to this new knowledge, she has decided that it is essential to take a more comprehensive view of childhood symptoms and their etiologies, rather than performing as an expert diagnostician. In her clinical thinking and practice, she now gives the caregiving environment a more central position, attends carefully to the need to develop regulatory competencies, and focuses on restoring healthy function rather than on eliminating specific symptoms. The chapter offers clinical examples to illustrate the

[2] The Newborn Behavioral Observations (NBO), an adaptation of the assessment tool NBAS, developed by Brazelton and Nugent [29]. The aim of the NBO is to demonstrate to parents the particular competencies and sensitivities of their new infant, in that way promoting a responsive and supportive caregiving relationship.

shift in emphasis and the different clinical interventions resulting from these new perspectives.

It is the author's opinion that the mental health needs of the world's children require the child psychiatrist to take a step back from the role of clinician working one on one with a child and function instead as a teacher and as the leader of a team of other clinicians who will focus on specific areas of function—educational (teachers and special educators); regulatory (occupational therapists); making meaning of self and other—parent consultants; and psychotherapists. Such a role will be perceived as a loss by many who chose child psychiatry because they want to do psychotherapy. However, it is true that in order to fill this more comprehensive role, child psychiatrists must understand the way individuals make sense of their experience and of themselves in relationships. That understanding is central to the role of teacher and consultant in child mental health. In fact, the author believes that it is essential to be well trained in psychotherapy and even to maintain a small practice in order to adequately fulfill these roles. A skilled teacher and consultant uses an awareness of the way human beings make meaning as a fulcrum of this important work.

References

1. Bos K, Zeanah CH, Fox NA, Drury SS, McLaughlin KA, Nelson CA (2011) Psychiatric outcomes in young children with a history of institutionalization. Harv Rev Psychiatry 19(1):15–24
2. Rutter M, Kumsta R, Schlotz W, Sonuga-Barke E (2012) Longitudinal studies using a "natural experiment": design: the case of adoptees from Romanian orphanages. J Am Acad Child Adolesc Psychiatry 51(8):762–769
3. Center on the Developing Child (2011) Building the brain's "air traffic control" system: how early experiences shape the development of executive function: Working paper #11. https://developingchild.harvard.edu/
4. Sullivan R, Perry R, Sloan A, Kleinhaus K, Burtchen N (2011) Infant bonding and attachment to the caregiver: insights from basic and clinical science. Clin Perinatol 38(4):643–655
5. Porges SW (2003) Social engagement and attachment. Ann N Y Acad Sci 1008(1):31–47
6. Partanen E, Kujala T, Näätänen R, Liitola A, Sambeth A, Huotilainen M (2013) Learning-induced neural plasticity of speech processing before birth. Proc Natl Acad Sci 110(37):15145–15150
7. Virtala P, Huotilainen M, Partanen E, Fellman V, Tervaniemi M (2013) Newborn infants' auditory system is sensitive to Western music chord categories. Front Psychol. https://doi.org/10.3389/fpsyg.2013.00492
8. Murray L, Trevarthen C (1986) The infant's role in mother–infant communications. J Child Lang 13(01):15–29
9. Trevarthen C (2012) Communicative musicality: the human impulse to create and share music. In: Hargreaves D, Miell D, MacDonald R (eds) Musical imaginations: multidisciplinary perspectives on creativity, performance, and perception. Oxford University Press, Oxford, pp 259–284
10. Piallini G, De Palo F, Simonelli A (2015) Parental brain: cerebral areas activated by infant cries and faces. A comparison between different populations of parents and not. Front Psychol. https://doi.org/10.3389/fpsyg.2015.01625
11. Lambert KG (2012) The parental brain: transformations and adaptations. Physiol Behav 107(5):792–800

12. Alio AP, Mbah AK, Kornosky JL, Wathington D, Marty PJ, Salihu HM (2011) Assessing the impact of paternal involvement on racial/ethnic disparities in infant mortality rates. J Commun Health 36(1):63–68
13. Montirosso R, Provenzi L, Tavian D, Morandi F, Bonanomi A, Missaglia S, Borgatti R (2015) Social stress regulation in 4-month-old infants: contribution of maternal social engagement and infants' 5-HTTLPR genotype. Early Hum Dev 91(3):173–179
14. Porges SW (2015) Making the world safe for our children: down-regulating defence and up-regulating social engagement to 'optimise' the human experience. Children Australia 40(02):114–123
15. Teicher MH, Samson JA, Anderson CM, Ohashi K (2016) The effects of childhood maltreatment on brain structure, function and connectivity. Nat Rev Neurosci 17(10):652–666
16. Nelson C (2013) Biological embedding of early life adversity. JAMA Pediatr, Published online October 28, E1–E2, jamapediatrics.com.
17. Tronick EZ (2007) The neurobehavioral and social-emotional development of infants and children. Norton, New York, NY
18. Beebe B, Jaffe J, Markese S, Buck K, Chen H, Cohen P, Feldstein S (2010) The origins of 12-month attachment: a microanalysis of 4-month mother–infant interaction. Attach Hum Dev 12(1–2):3–141
19. Perry B (2006) Applying principles of neurodevelopment to clinical work with maltreated and traumatized children: the neurosequential model of therapeutics. In: Webb NB (ed) Working with traumatized youth in child welfare. Guilford Press, New York, pp 27–52
20. Provenzi L, Giusti L, Montirosso R (2016) Do infants exhibit significant corticol reactivity to the face-to-face still-face paradigm? A narrative review and meta-analysis. Develop Rev. Elsevier Inc. www.elsevier.com/locate/dr.
21. Tronick EZ (1989) Emotions and emotional communication in infants. Am Psychol 44(2):112–119
22. Sander L (1977) The regulation of exchange in the infant-caretaker system and some aspects of the context-content relationship. Interact Convers Develop Lang 5(40):579–593
23. Caspi A, Houts RM, Belsky DW, Goldman-Mellor SJ, Harrington H, Israel S, Moffitt TE (2014) The p factor: one general psychopathology factor in the structure of psychiatric disorders? Clin Psychol Sci 2(2):119–137
24. Kendler KS (1996) Major depression and generalized anxiety disorder. Same genes, (partly) different environments—revisited. Br J Psychiatry 168(30):68–75
25. Insel, T. (2013) Transforming diagnosis [Web log post]. http://www.nimh.nih.gov/about/director/2013/transforming-diagnosis.shtml
26. Fivaz-Depeursing E, Corboz-Warnery A (1999) The primary triangle. A developmental systems view of mothers, fathers, and infants. Basic Books, New York
27. Downing G (2004) Emotion, body, and parent-infant interaction. In: Nadel J, Muir D (eds) Emotional development: recent research advances. Oxford University Press, Oxford 429–449.
28. Harrison AM (2005) Herding the animals into the barn: a parent consultation model. Psychoanal Study Child 60(1):128–153
29. Brazelton T (1976) The Neonatal Behavioral Assessment Scale, Clinics of Child Development No. 50. Spastics International Medical Publishing, Philadelphia

Printed by Printforce, the Netherlands